Modern Cardiac Surgery

*Based on the Proceedings of the Eighth Annual
Course on Cardiac Surgery, organised by the
British Postgraduate Medical Federation*

Edited by

D. B. Longmore

*Consultant Clinical Physiologist,
The National Heart Hospital, London*

 **MTP**PRESS LIMITED *International Medical Publishers*

Published by
MTP Press Limited
Falcon House
Lancaster
England

Copyright © 1978 MTP Press Limited
Softcover reprint of the hardcover 1st edition 1978

ISBN-13: 978-94-011-6202-9   e-ISBN-13: 978-94-011-6200-5
DOI: 10.1007/978-94-011-6200-5

Contents

CONTENTS

List of Contributors

SALLY P. ALLWORK
Hammersmith Hospital,
London W12 0HS

R. H. ANDERSON
Royal Liverpool Children's Hospital,
Myrtle Street, Liverpool 7

L. BITENSKY
Division of Cellular Biology,
The Mathilda and Terence Kennedy
Institute of Rheumatology,
Bute Gardens, London W6 7DW

M. V. BRAIMBRIDGE
St Thomas's Hospital,
Lambeth Palace Road,
London SE1 7EH

LORD BROCK
Brompton Hospital,
Fulham Road,
London SW3 6HP

L. H. BURR
Thoracic Unit,
Hospital for Sick Children,
Gt Ormond Street,
London WC1N 3JH

J. P. BYRNE
Thoracic Unit,
Hospital for Sick Children,
Gt Ormond Street,
London WC1N 3JH

S. ĆANKOVIĆ-DARRACOTT
Department of Cardiothoracic Surgery,
St Thomas's Hospital,
Lambeth Palace Road,
London SE1 7EH

J. CHAYEN
Division of Cellular Biology,
The Mathilda and Terence Kennedy
Institute of Rheumatology,
Bute Gardens,
London W6 7DW

W. P. CLELAND
Department of Surgery,
Cardiothoracic Institute,
Brompton Hospital,
Fulham Road,
London SW3 6HP

D. K. C. COOPER
Thoracic Unit,
Hospital for Sick Children,
Gt Ormond Street,
London WC1N 3JH

R. J. DONNELLY
Broadgreen Hospital,
Thomas Drive,
Liverpool 14

D. G. GIBSON
Brompton Hospital,
Fulham Road,
London SW3 6HP

A. GOODWIN
Department of Cardiology,
Newcastle General Hospital,
Newcastle-upon-Tyne

D. I. HAMILTON
Royal Liverpool Children's Hospital,
Myrtle Street, Liverpool 7

SHEILA G. HAWORTH
Hospital for Sick Children,
Gt Ormond Street,
London WC1N 3JH

LIST OF CONTRIBUTORS

D. J. HEARSE
The Myocardial Metabolism Research
Laboratories,
Rayne Institute,
St Thomas's Hospital,
Lambeth Palace Road,
London SE1 1EH

S. C. LENNOX
Brompton Hospital,
Fulham Road,
London SW3 6HP

M. R. de LEVAL
Thoracic Unit,
Hospital for Sick Children,
Gt Ormond Street,
London WC1N 3JH

C. LINCOLN
Brompton Hospital,
Fulham Road,
London SW3 6HP

F. J. MACARTNEY
Institute of Child Health,
Guildford Street
London WC1N 3JH

S. M. MANOHITHARAJAH
Leeds Regional Thoracic Surgical Centre,
Killingbeck Hospital,
Leeds 14

D. G. MELROSE
Royal Postgraduate Medical School,
Hammersmith Hospital,
Du Cane Road,
London W12 0HS

WINIFRED G. NAYLER
Cardiothoracic Institute,
2 Beaumont St,
London W1N 2DX

CELIA M. OAKLEY
Royal Postgraduate Medical School,
Hammersmith Hospital,
Du Cane Road,
London W12 0HS

H. OELERT
Klinik für Thorax,
Herzurd Geffässchirurgie,
D-3000 Hanover, West Germany

M. PANETH
Brompton Hospital,
Fulham Road,
London SW3 6HP

G. PETERSEN
Rigshospitalet,
Copenhagen, Denmark

M. QUERO
C. S. La Paz,
Madrid, Spain

D. S. REID
Freman Hospital,
High Heaton,
Newcastle-upon-Tyne NE7 7DN

J. K. ROSS
Western Hospital,
Oakley Road, Mill Brook,
Southampton SO9 4WQ

I. H. RYGG
Rigshospitalet,
Copenhagen, Denmark

F. E. de SALAMANCA
Ciudad Sonatorio Carlos Haya,
Malaga, Spain

C. G. SBOKOS
2nd Department of Surgery,
Athens University School of Medicine,
King Paul's Hospital,
Athens 609, Greece

Å. SENNING
Surgical Clinic A,
University Hospital of Zurich,
CH-8091, Zurich, Switzerland

N. E. SHUMWAY
Department of Cardiovascular Surgery,
Stanford University,
Stanford, California 94305, USA

A. M. SLADE
Cardiothoracic Institute
2 Beaumont St,
London W1N 2DX

AUDREY SMITH
Royal Liverpool Children's Hospital,
Myrtle Street, Liverpool 7

J. STARK
Thoracic Unit,
Hospital for Sick Children,
Gt. Ormond Street,
London WC1N 3JH

E. B. STINSON
Department of Cardiovascular Surgery,
Stanford University
Stanford, California 94305, USA

R. J. SZARNICKI
Thoracic Unit,
Hospital for Sick Children,
Gt Ormond Street,
London WC1N 3JH

D. E. M. TAYLOR
Department of Applied Physiology and
Surgical Sciences,
Royal College of Surgeons,
London

J. F. N. TAYLOR
Thoracic Unit,
Hospital for Sick Children,
Gt Ormond Street,
London WC1N 3JH

T. A. TRAILL
Brompton Hospital,
Fulham Road,
London SW3 6HP

M. TYNAN
Evelina Children's Department,
Guy's Hospital,
London SE1

M. UGARTE
Clinica Puerta de Hierro,
Madrid, Spain

W. H. WAIN
Brompton Hospital,
Fulham Road,
London SW3 6HP

D. A. WATSON
Leeds Regional Thoracic Surgical Centre,
Killingbeck Hospital,
Leeds 14

J. L. WILKINSON
Royal Liverpool Children's Hospital,
Myrtle Street, Liverpool 7

M. YACOUB
The National Heart Hospital,
Westmoreland Street,
London W1M 8BA

Foreword

Modern Cardiac Surgery is based on, but does not consist completely of, papers submitted at the annual course of cardiac surgery run by the combined Institutes and Post-Graduate Hospitals involved in cardiac surgery in London (1977). The subjects which have been chosen and included fulfil one of two criteria; either they are subjects which were not included in the previous book, *The Current Status of Cardiac Surgery*, or they cover subjects which needed to be updated.

Because this is a teaching course and not a symposium, the emphasis has been on being informative rather than on presenting masses of results. The book has been prepared partly from manuscripts submitted by the authors and partly from annotated tapes of the proceedings of the meeting. Throughout the editing and production of this book careful consideration has been given to the requirements of the readership.

The book is aimed at all students of cardiac surgery and cardiology at all levels, and as much information as possible has been packed into it. Nevertheless, the editor wishes to thank the authors for the efforts they have made to be concise and clear in their presentation and for their tremendous co-operation in alterations which have been incorporated to make it a more readable treatise. This means that this is a book which is of value to nurses interested in cardiology in intensive care, to physiotherapists and students wishing to look up particular topics before their final examinations.

The work includes a variety of authors, representing several continents and many important cardiac surgical centres, who together represent experience from many thousands of patients, and a wide range of cardiac surgical procedures ranging from the simplest through to cardiac transplantation. Since the book is based on a teaching programme, where results are presented they represent the bare facts without the optimism which is sometimes shown at surgical meetings.

The courses which have formed the basis for *The Current Status of Cardiac Surgery* and *Modern Cardiac Surgery* really exist because of the efforts and vision of Mr William Paton Cleland, and the course which formed the basis for this book was the last one organized under his chairmanship. He retires from the National Health Service this year. He qualified MB, BS (second place on the honours list), from Adelaide University in 1934 at the age of 21. His father, Sir John Cleland, was Professor of Pathology at the University of

Adelaide and was a most distinguished scientist. Bill Cleland and all his four sisters have had distinguished academic careers. After a severe attack of pneumonia he became a chest physician in 1936 and became a member of the Royal College of Physicians at that time. During World War 2 he became a thoracic surgeon under Sir Clement Price Thomas, and then became a fellow of the Royal College of Surgeons after the war. During his appointment at the Hammersmith Hospital he was associated with the group who pioneered the heart/lung machine and cardiac surgery in Europe. It is because of this broad base that courses organized by Bill Cleland have been so comprehensive and that it has been possible to publish two books covering whole subjects in considerable detail from the basis of just two courses and a modest number of extra contributions.

The Editor wishes to thank all his colleagues who have contributed to this book, particularly for their forbearance in being asked to make many additions and alterations to their original contribution. He also wishes to thank Merilyn Smith and Marie Alcorn for handling all the correspondence and manuscript-checking in their spare time. He also wishes to thank the publishers for their help and advice.

D. B. Longmore

Section I
Invited lectures

Transplantation of the heart

E. B. STINSON AND N. E. SHUMWAY

The clinical programme in heart transplantation at Stanford was launched in concept almost 20 years ago when Drs Shumway and Lower first achieved successful orthotopic heart transplantation in a canine model in 1958. After this milestone there ensued nearly a decade of orderly laboratory experience during which several important objectives that should precede the initiation of a clinical programme were accomplished. These included refinement of the operative technique to the point of routine technical success, characterization

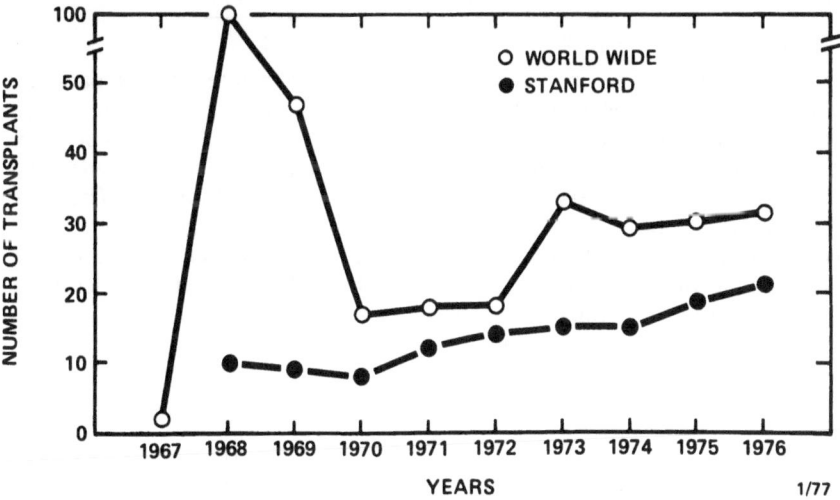

Figure 1 Number of transplant procedures performed worldwide and at Stanford University during calendar years 1967–76. The Stanford experience is included in the worldwide figures

of acute cardiac allograft rejection in terms of morphology and pathophysiology and, most importantly, achievement of long-term survival with appropriate immunosuppression.

The first human cardiac transplantation procedure was performed not at Stanford, however, but in Cape Town, South Africa in December 1967. Figure 1 illustrates that initial efforts at human cardiac allografting were followed by a virtual epidemic of such procedures around the world and, indeed, during the ensuing 12 months 101 cardiac transplant operations were performed. As can be inferred from the graph in Figure 1, however, there followed a precipitous decline in the rate of clinical cardiac transplantation as involved investigators became more aware of the complex problems and challenges that this project incorporated. Our own programme was initiated in January 1968 and for the next 3 years remained at a low, but steady level of activity. Over the past few years, however, our programme has grown to the point of an average two transplant procedures per month.

Table 1 summarizes current worldwide statistics in clinical heart transplantation. A total of 333 transplant procedures have been performed in 325 recipients by 65 teams scattered in 22 countries throughout the world. At the time of this analysis the longest current survivor is still living more than 8 years after biological heart replacement.

Table 1   Cardiac transplantation worldwide experience

Transplant teams	65
Transplants	333
Recipients	325
Alive	68
Longest current survival	8.4 years

Our own series now includes 129 transplant procedures in 124 patients. Table 2 illustrates the primary disease aetiology in patients submitted to cardiac transplantation. The most common has been advanced coronary artery disease associated with global left ventricular dysfunction unamenable to standard aortocoronary bypass and reconstructive techniques. The next most common aetiological category includes patients with idiopathic cardiomyopathy. In general, the latter patients have been younger, and they have come to constitute in recent years nearly half of all patients undergoing transplantation. The youngest patient in our series is 14 years old and suffered from this type of cardiac disease.

Table 2   Stanford cardiac transplantation—recipient diagnosis

Coronary artery disease	74
Idiopathic cardiomyopathy	46
Post-traumatic aneurysm	1
Valve disease with cardiomyopathy	3
	124 patients

At the present time Stanford serves as a unique referral centre for cardiac transplantation in the United States. By virtue of renewed interest in clinical cardiac transplantation by other centres, as well as the explantation of former trainees in the Stanford programme, however, it can be expected that several additional regional programmes will develop within the next 5 years. At present, approximately 200 patients per year are referred for consideration for cardiac transplantation, but because of the stringency of recipient selection criteria only approximately 15% of this total number are officially selected for transplantation; 80% of these patients eventually undergo transplantation, while the remainder die before a suitable donor becomes available.

Criteria for the selection of appropriate cardiac recipients are relatively straightforward. Patients must present with advanced cardiac disability with an estimated survival limited to weeks or months. Data to support our ability to establish prognosis in such patients are provided by the extremely limited survival experience of officially selected patients for whom a suitably matched donor does not become available for several weeks; average survival of such non-transplanted, but selected recipients is 55 days. We have limited transplantation to patients under the age of 55 years because of a higher incidence of severe complications in older age groups, a finding analogous to general experience in renal transplantation. Excessively elevated pulmonary vascular resistance above 8–10 Wood units is a contraindication because of the limited ability of the normal donor right ventricle to acutely elevate its external workload in the face of excessive pulmonary hypertension. Other systemic disease that would separately limit survival constitutes, of course, another contraindication. We have also found that recent, unresolved pulmonary infarction frustrates a successful outcome after transplantation in a high percentage of patients (approximately 32% of those with infarction) because of the vulnerability of such lesions to development of severe infection after the institution of immunosuppression.

The operative technique for clinical heart transplantation needs little review. The key to technical success, as developed in 1958 in the canine model, is excision of the recipient heart at the mid-atrial level, rather than through each of the individual left- and right-sided venous connections. Mirror-image tailoring of the donor heart facilitates performance of the requisite anastomoses which can be performed within a 35–45 min ischaemic interval. By virtue of retention of the posterior and lateral portions of the recipient's atria the recipient's sinoatrial node remains *in situ* after transplantation. Collateral blood supply from the mediastinal vessels that enter through the areas of pericardial reflection posteriorly supports viability of the residual recipient atria, and these remnants therefore remain electrically and mechanically active. Because of preservation of autonomic nervous innervation these atrial remnants in the recipient respond in an appropriate fashion to activation of efferent reflex stimuli. In contrast, the donor heart is completely severed from all neural connection and the donor sinoatrial node, transplanted intact with the donor heart, is insulated from direct neural influence. The result is juxtaposition in the circulation of two sinoatrial nodes in series, one of which remains innervated and one of which is denervated.

5

This anatomical relationship sets up the conditions for interesting electro-physiological phenomena, inasmuch as unidirectional neural modulation of the rate of the recipient sinoatrial node by the pumping action of the dissociated rhythm of the donor heart may occur. An example of the separate, dissociated rhythms of donor and recipient pacemakers is shown in Figure 2. In no patient, studied up through 7 years of transplantation, has efferent autonomic reinnervation of the cardiac graft been documented. This finding is in contrast to the canine model in which vagal and sympathetic reinnervation has been shown to occur. The persistence of the denervated state of cardiac grafts in humans does provide unique investigative opportunities for separating direct versus neurally mediated actions of many interventions, including drugs such as digitalis, quinidine, and beta-blocking agents, as well as various physiological manoeuvres.

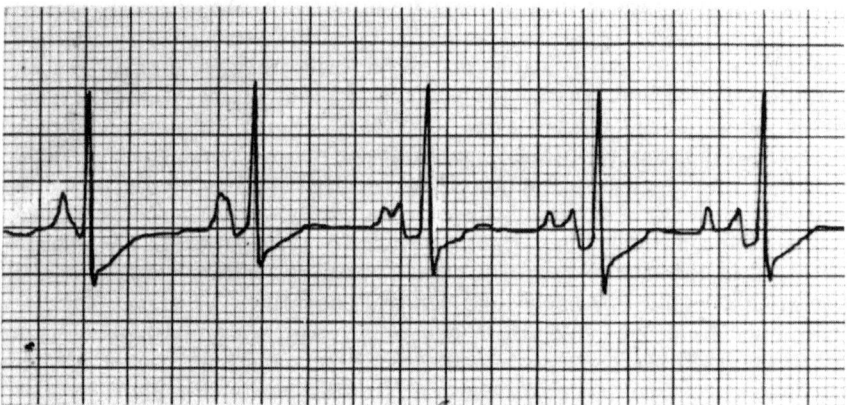

Figure 2 An example of double P waves, originating from recipient and donor sinoatrial nodes. The recipient atrial rate is dissociated from the rhythm of the donor heart

Just as in renal transplantation pharmacological suppression of host immune responses is necessary after cardiac transplantation. We have utilized a 'triple' immunosuppressive regimen. It incorporates prednisone, azathioprine (an antimetabolic agent) and antihuman antithymocyte globulin, a heterologous antiserum raised in rabbits immunized with human thymocytes. Administration of the latter biological is individualized on the basis of circulating levels of rabbit globulin, as measured by radioimmune assay. These measurements permit calculation of rabbit globulin kinetics in individual cardiac recipients and thus modulation of dosage necessary to achieve therapeutic levels, as defined by depression of the thymus-dependent sub-population of peripheral lymphocytes (T-lymphocytes) to a range of 10% of normal or less during the first several postoperative weeks. Episodes of threatened cardiac graft rejection which occur in nearly all cases during the first 8 weeks after transplantation are treated by augmentation of doses of antithymocyte globulin alone or by this manoeuvre combined with high dose pulses (1 g/day) of methylprednisolone administered intravenously.

It is obvious that the key to successful negotiation of the early post-transplant period is early, sensitive diagnosis of impending graft rejection episodes. Over the past several years we have surveyed many potentially useful indices for rejection diagnosis, including examination of serum enzyme levels, various radiographic techniques, and echocardiography. Those indices that we have found to be the most reliable, sensitive, and specific for the diagnosis of cardiac rejection include simply auscultation for detection of abnormal diastolic heart sounds (a clue to changes in ventricular compliance that accompany the rejection process), the standard electrocardiogram (diagnostic features include a generalized decrease in QRS voltage and atrial arrhythmias), and in recent years percutaneous transvenous endomyocardial biopsy. It is self-evident that the importance of early diagnosis of rejection lies in the institution of effective immunosuppressive manoeuvres before the development of irreversible morphological changes in the cardiac graft. At present, the 'gold standard' for rejection diagnosis is endomyocardial biopsy.

The biopsy instrument used at Stanford is a highly modified version of previously developed cardiac bioptomes, designed for improvement in flexibility, control of intracardiac manipulation, and ease of cleaning and sterilization. The Stanford biopsy forceps was thoroughly validated by Dr Philip Caves in 1971 as a highly sensitive and specific diagnostic tool for rejection diagnosis before its introduction into the clinical programme in 1972. The technique for endomyocardial biopsy is simple. Utilization of the Seldinger technique for percutaneous introduction of the biopsy forceps into the right internal jugular vein under local anaesthesia permits repetitive and safe biopsy of the donor right ventricular endomyocardium without undue inconvenience to the patient. Indeed, this technique provides a unique tool in the field of human organ transplantation because of the ability to examine graft histology on a serial basis. After insertion into the right internal jugular vein the biopsy forceps is guided under fluoroscopic control through the tricuspid valve and into the region of the right ventricular apex. The open jaws of the forceps are then pressed against the endomyocardium and a 2–3 mm specimen then removed. Such specimens are sufficient for not only routine light microscopy, but also for ultrastructural and special immunological studies. Figure 3 shows an over-penetrated chest radiograph during a biopsy procedure and illustrates the open jaws of the instrument in the apical portion of the right ventricle.

The present protocol for postoperative cardiac graft biopsy calls for routine biopsy at 5–7-day intervals during the first 8 weeks after transplantation or immediately upon suspicion of rejection as evidenced by clinical or electrocardiographic findings, after treatment of threatened rejection episodes for purposes of monitoring histological response to therapy, and at annual evaluation of long-term survivors. Some patients whose early postoperative courses have been complicated by recurrent rejection episodes have undergone more than 20 endomyocardial biopsy procedures during the first several weeks after operation, and altogether more than 1200 endomyocardial biopsies have been performed within the context of the transplantation programme without serious morbidity or mortality. Minor complications have included atrial arrhythmias and pneumothorax (0.3%).

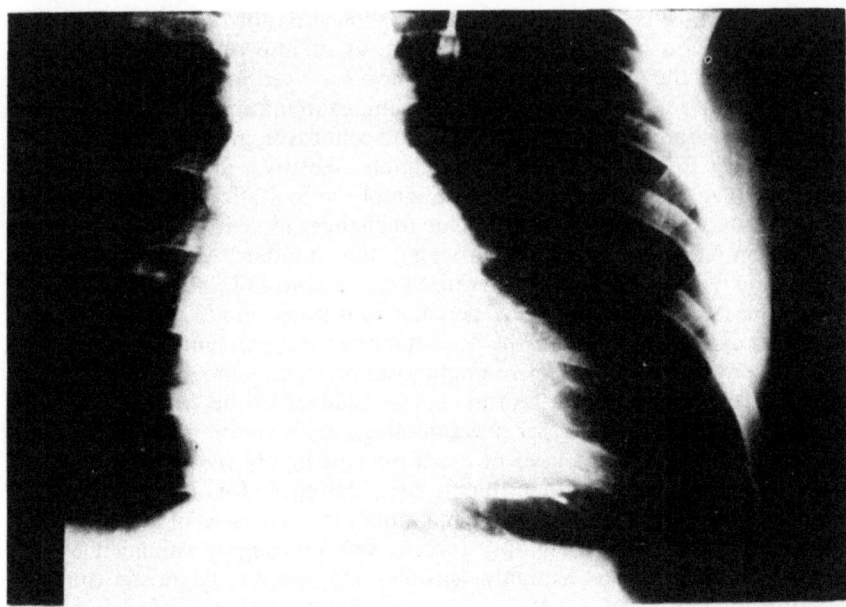

Figure 3 Over-penetrated chest radiograph showing a transvenous cardiac biopsy forceps with jaws open in the region of the apex of the right ventricle. The biopsy instrument has been passed percutaneously into the right internal jugular vein and guided under fluoroscopic control through the right atrium and tricuspid valve

Figure 4 illustrates classical histological features of acute cardiac rejection as observed in a biopsy specimen. Principal pathological changes include interstitial oedema and infiltration with mononuclear cells, similar to the morphological expression of rejection of other types of solid organ grafts. These pathological changes also involve the endocardium which is characteristically greatly thickened by oedema and cellular infiltration. The metabolic activity of infiltrating cells is assayed by special histochemical stains such as methyl green pyronine. All of these changes are fully reversible following effective augmentation of immunosuppression; severe rejection episodes, however, may be marked by residual irreversible features such as myocyte degeneration (myocytolysis) and replacement fibrosis. In virtually all cases the diagnostic histological features of acute cardiac rejection are distributed diffusely throughout the heart; therefore, right-sided endomyocardial biopsy is a highly specific and sensitive diagnostic tool. A special advantage of the ability to assess objectively graft histology on a serial basis after cardiac transplantation consists of the ability to rule out rejection in patients with extracardiac complications (such as pneumonia) and thus avoid needless and potentially dangerous augmentation of immunosuppression.

As mentioned earlier, doses of immunosuppressive agents are increased transiently upon diagnosis of an acute rejection process by endomyocardial biopsy. Classically, antirejection therapy incorporates high-dose pulses of a corticosteroid agent such as methylprednisolone, but because of the cumu-

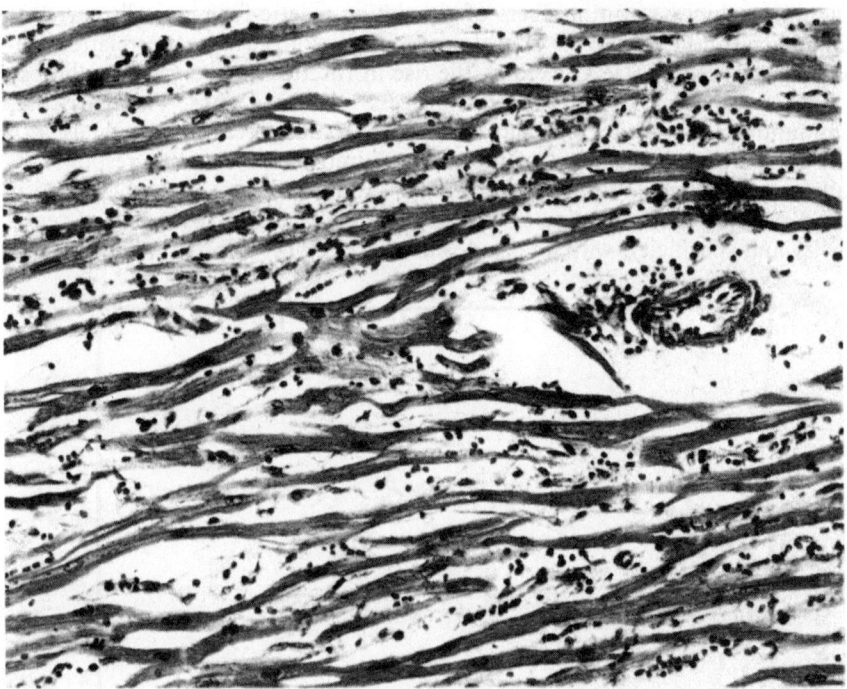

Figure 4 Photomicrograph showing interstitial oedema separating the myocytes and an interstitial and perivascular mononuclear inflammatory infiltrate, characteristic of acute cardiac rejection (haematoxylin and eosin, × 170)

lative infectious and metabolic toxicity of corticosteroids we have recently explored the usefulness of antithymocyte globulin treatment alone. The ability to measure serially circulating levels of rabbit globulin and calculate kinetics of disposition allows individual modulation of this type of immunosuppressive strategy. Figure 5 illustrates serum levels of rabbit globulin and circulating numbers of peripheral lymphocytes capable of spontaneous formation of rosettes with sheep red blood cells (operationally defined as T-lymphocytes, the lymphocyte subpopulation considered primarily responsible for allograft rejection) in a patient who sustained two early postoperative rejection episodes treated solely with antithymocyte globulin. A mirror-image inverse relationship between levels of rabbit globulin and numbers of T-lymphocytes is evident, confirming the efficacy of antithymocyte globulin for control of T-lymphocyte values, at least during the initial weeks after transplantation. It is also evident from Figure 5 that the onset of biopsy-confirmed rejection episodes was heralded by premonitory increases in circulating T-lymphocyte levels, and for this reason the serial measurement of T-lymphocytes constitutes a method for immunological monitoring.

Immunological monitoring by this technique is a recent development in our programme. During the first 6 weeks after transplantation statistically significant increases in numbers of circulating rosette-forming cells correlate highly with the onset of biopsy-proved rejection, with a correlation co-efficient exceeding 0.9. Generally, the rise in rosette fraction precedes biopsy confirmation of an acute rejection process by 3 to 4 days. This particular immunological monitoring assay, therefore, would appear to provide us with an indication of activation of the efferent limb of the immune response. It allows more directed timing of graft biopsy and facilitates very early diagnosis of impending graft rejection episodes. Because of its very high rates of sensitivity and specificity, with a false-positive rate of only approximately 5%, we

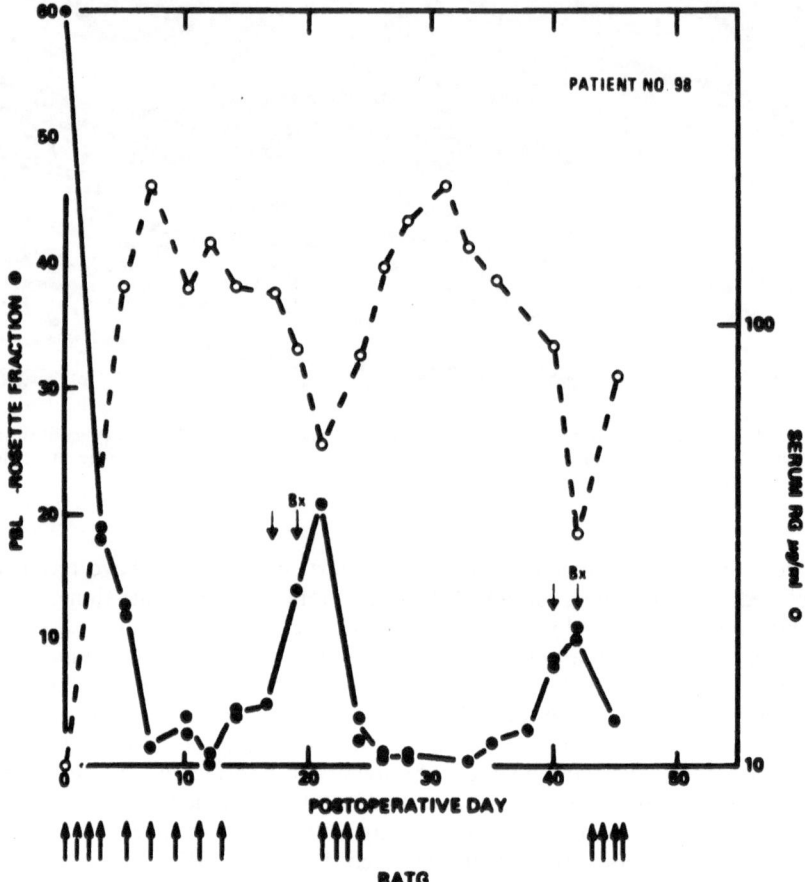

Figure 5 Serum levels of rabbit globulin (RG) and peripheral rosette-forming cells (T-lymphocytes) in a patient who experienced two acute rejection episodes early post-operatively, both treated with antithymocyte globulin alone. PBL = peripheral blood lymphocyte, and RATG = rabbit antithymocyte globulin, administration of which is indicated by vertical arrows. Courses of antithymocyte globulin, both the routine early postoperative course and later administration for acute rejection, were associated with reciprocal depression of peripheral T-lymphocyte levels. Rejection episodes were confirmed by biopsy (Bx)

have recently begun to initiate treatment with antithymocyte globulin during the early postoperative period solely upon the basis of changes in circulating T-lymphocyte levels. This type of strategy for immunosuppressive management during the initial postoperative period has resulted in better control of early rejection with lower overall doses of prednisone, the agent we consider responsible for the greatest morbidity early after transplantation.

Approximately 95% of acute rejection episodes can be successfully reversed by means of the diagnostic indices that I have summarized and by appropriate augmentation of immunosuppression. Overall, 85% of patients are discharged from hospital after transplantation at the present time. Follow ing discharge recipients continue to sustain hazards such as graft rejection or infection, but these occur with a greatly decreased frequency as compared to the early postoperative period. An additional complication that emerged during our early experience with cardiac transplantation, however, was a phenomenon that we have termed accelerated graft atherosclerosis. Our hypothetical formulation for the pathogenesis of this lesion in the graft coronary arteries is indicated in Figure 6. The pathological findings are consistent with the concept that immune injury to the coronary artery intima exposes a thrombogenic surface, leading to the aggregation and activation of platelets with release of mitogenic factors that promote proliferation of myointimal cells that have migrated through the internal elastic lamina. The initial result is a thickened intimal layer due to cellular proliferation and increased amounts of ground substance. Subsequent infiltration or *in situ* production of lipids leads to an atheromatous lesion that is virtually indistinguishable on a morphological basis from that of native, spontaneously occurring atherosclerosis.

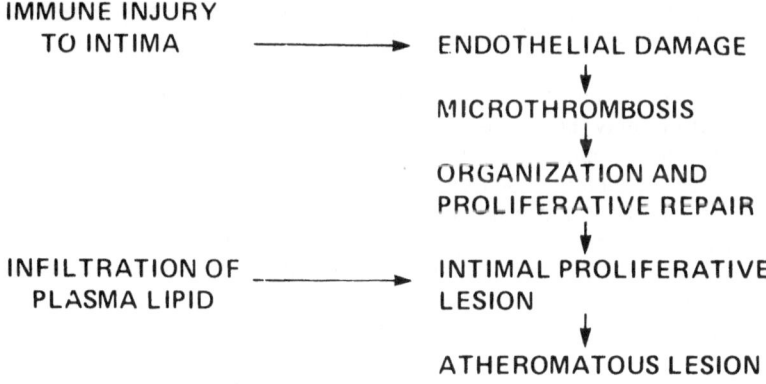

Figure 6 Hypothetical formulation of the pathogenesis of donor coronary artery atherosclerosis (see text for details)

During the first several months after transplantation the appearance of such lesions is predominantly proliferative, as shown in Figure 7. The cross-section of the atrioventricular nodal artery shown in Figure 7 was recovered from the graft of a patient who sustained repeated acute rejection episodes during the first several months after transplantation and succumbed of a Stokes–Adams attack. In this case conduction system abnormalities were due apparently to severe obliterative disease of arterial supply to the atrioventricular node.

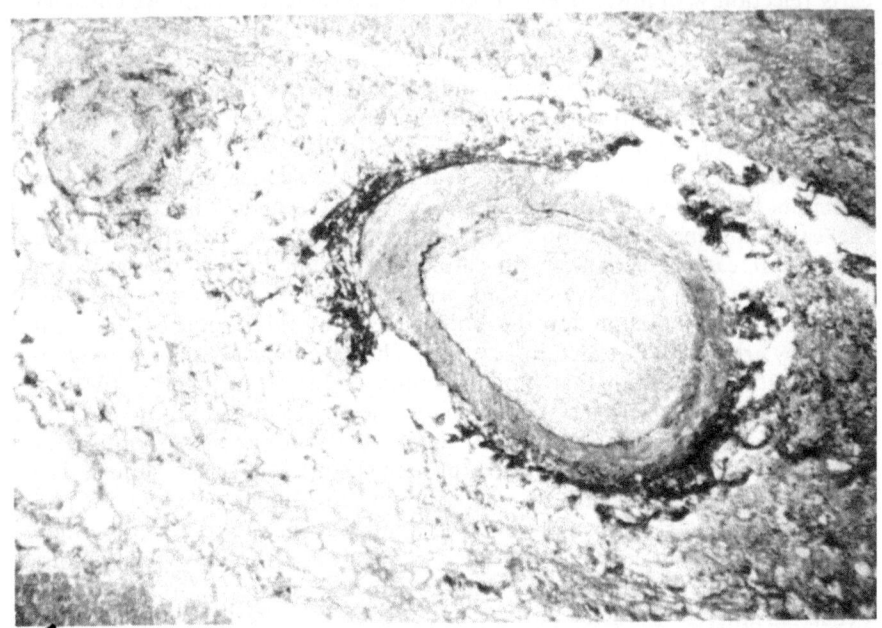

Figure 7 Photomicrograph of nearly occluded atrioventricular nodal artery, due to proliferation of myointimal cells, in a patient who sustained repeated acute rejection episodes during the first several months after transplantation.

After approximately 1 year following transplantation, lipid and eventually mineralization may be incorporated into the hyperplastic intimal lesion, leading to the development of a complicated atheromatous plaque. The consequences of such include ischaemic left ventricular dysfunction, ventricular arrhythmias, and myocardial infarction which is painless due to persistence of the denervated state. The coronary arteriogram presented in Figure 8 was obtained in a patient 3 years after transplantation, and shows a high-grade lesion of the left anterior descending coronary artery and complete occlusion of the circumflex system. Such lesions would appear to be amenable to coronary artery bypass grafting, but, in fact, the accelerated graft atherosclerosis process is diffuse and involves the entire length of epicardial coronary arteries and proximal portions of penetrating branches.

In 1970 accelerated graft atherosclerosis appeared to constitute a barrier to long-term survival after heart transplantation. One may recall that Dr Barnard's first long-term recipient died of this complication 19 months after operation. At that time we therefore formulated a prophylactic regimen directed against some of the intermediate steps in the pathogenesis summarized earlier. The components of this prophylactic regimen included indefinite

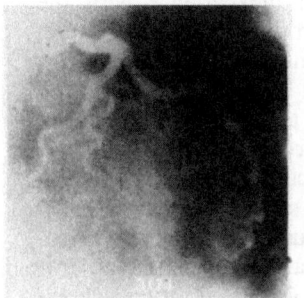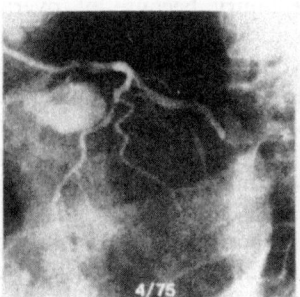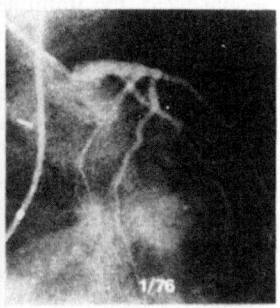

Figure 8 Serial selective left coronary arteriograms in a patient who developed donor coronary atherosclerosis. The left panel (3/74) shows normal anatomy. The centre panel (4/75) shows a high-grade lesion of the left anterior descending coronary artery and complete occlusion of the left circumflex coronary artery, demonstrated 3 years after transplantation. Elective retransplantation was performed, and several months later repeat left coronary arteriography of this patient's second transplanted heart was obtained (right panel 1/76)

administration of an oral anticoagulant, warfarin sodium, along with a platelet antagonist, dipyridamole, in addition to more strict attention to reduced intake of saturated dietary fats and maintenance of ideal body weight. We subsequently analysed our experience with two consective sets of patients. The first group included nine 3-month survivors who underwent transplantation before January 1970 and who had not been treated with such a regimen. The second group included the subsequent 44 patients who survived the first 3 months after transplantation and who had been treated with the prophylactic regimen, beginning 1 week after transplantation. The definition of graft atherosclerosis utilized for this retrospective analysis of a non-concurrent series consisted of 20% or greater luminal narrowing of any major epicardial coronary artery, as defined by arteriography or post-mortem examination. The time of appearance of such a lesion was defined as midway between the last time the coronary arteries in a particular graft were known to be normal and the first time that evidence of occlusive coronary disease in the graft was detected. There were no significant differences between the two groups in regard to many preoperative factors that one might consider influential in the development of coronary lesions, including sex, age of the cardiac donor, sex of the cardiac donor, underlying aetiological diagnosis (coronary artery disease versus cardiomyopathy), hypertension, obesity, serum lipids, and number of HLA-antigen mismatches. Postoperative factors that did not distinguish between the two groups included the frequency of rejection, the total rejection score, late postoperative rejection frequency, maintenance doses of prednisone and azathioprine, late postoperative histories of smoking, hypertension, and obesity, and serum cholesterol levels up through 4 years postoperative. Some significant differences between the two groups did exist, but were probably not influential. Group 1, the untreated group, sustained in general an earlier onset of rejection, but in terms of overall rejection history this group did not experience more severe rejection. Indeed, it might be argued that, in fact, patients in Group 1 might, by virtue of a selection process have included patients whose grafts were less jeopardized by immune injury because of overall inexperience with the management of rejection at that time. The patients in the treated group were, on the average, 5 years younger than those in the untreated group, but this difference was of borderline statistical significance. Overall, there were no significant differences in factors that would appear to definitively modulate the progression of graft atherosclerosis in the two groups.

Actuarial curves illustrating the time-related incidence of graft atherosclerosis in the treated and untreated groups are shown in Figure 9. By 3 years postoperatively 100% of patients in Group 1 developed atherosclerotic lesions, an observation confirming our earlier concern with this complication as a barrier to long-term survival. In Group 2 patients, however, the incidence of graft atherosclerosis at the same interval was 18%. The probability that this difference in incidence between the two groups was due to chance alone is less than one in one million. This retrospective analysis of our experience in human heart transplantation constitutes one of the best indications, that in a human model of coronary atherosclerosis pharmacological intervention may in fact exert an important role. Obviously, our patients constitute a highly selective and relatively small group, but other populations at high risk for accelerated coronary atherosclerosis exist, and institution of a controlled pharmacological trial in such subjects would be warranted. These include patients on long-term haemodialysis, patients with homozygous familial type 2 hypercholesterolaemia, or patients with homocystinaemia.

This experience with a prophylactic regimen directed toward prevention of

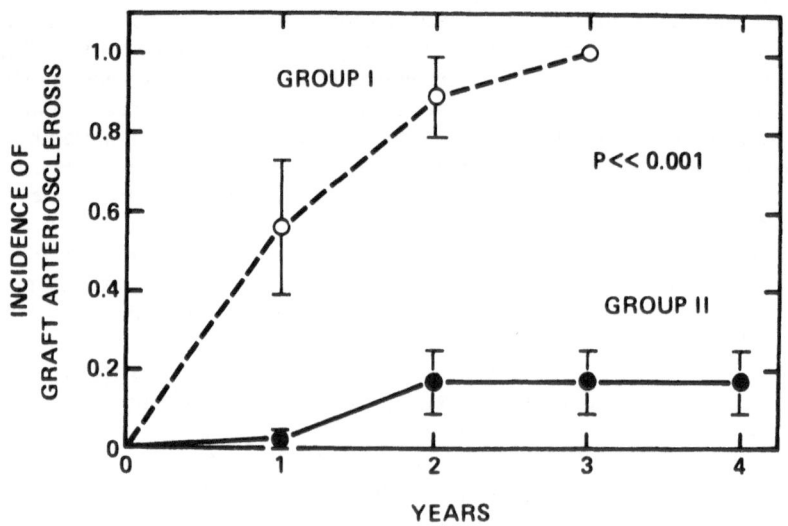

Figure 9 Actuarial curves of the incidence of graft arteriosclerosis in two transplant patient groups, illustrating the effects of a prophylactic regimen directed against the development of donor coronary arteriosclerosis (see text for details)

cardiac graft atherosclerosis has proved encouraging since it has demonstrated that this particular pathological entity, despite incomplete understanding of all of the processes involved, no longer restricts longevity after cardiac transplantation. For example, the selective left coronary arteriogram shown in Figure 10, illustrating normal coronary anatomy, was obtained recently in a patient 7 years after transplantation.

Another dimension of cardiac transplantation that we have successfully explored during our recent experience is cardiac retransplantation in selected cases. One indication for graft replacement, clearly, is accelerated atherosclerosis in that minority of patients who continue to sustain this complication late postoperatively. As mentioned earlier, the manifestations of occlusive coronary disease in the graft include ischaemic ventricular dysfunction with congestive heart failure, painless myocardial infarction, and ventricular arrhythmias that may lead to sudden death. All of these complications have been encountered in our experience. For this reason our current policy is to consider graft replacement in any patient whose serial postoperative coronary arteriograms show significant, progressive arterial lesions. Two patients have undergone retransplantation because of graft atherosclerosis in our series. One presented in moribund condition after myocardial infarction and

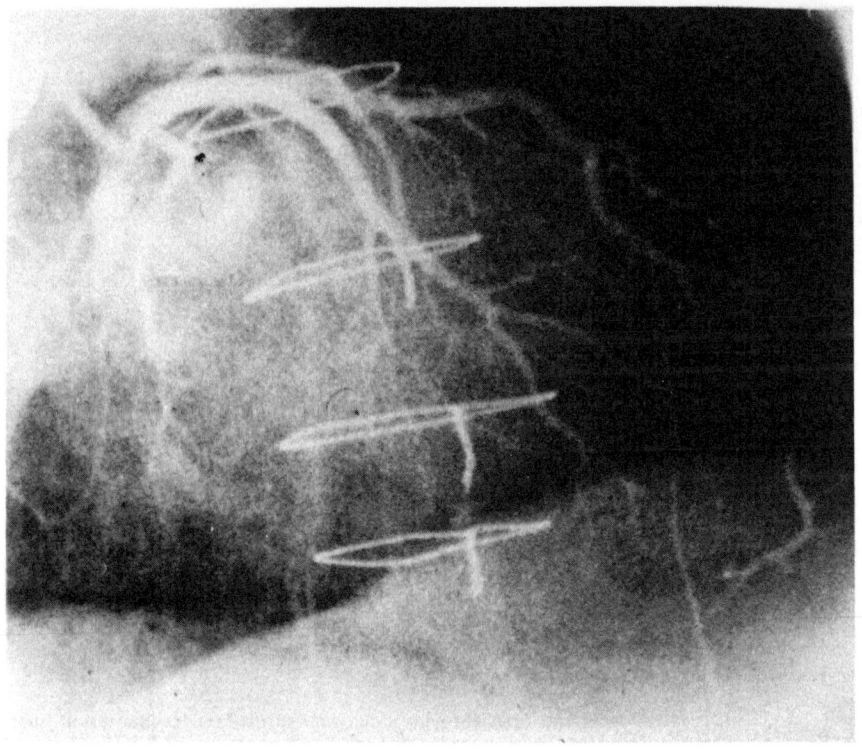

Figure 10 Selective left coronary injection in a cardiac transplant patient 7 years postoperatively. Normal coronary anatomy is illustrated

retransplantation was unsuccessful because of disseminated infection with *Candida*, present at the time of reoperation. The second patient underwent retransplantation slightly more than 2 years after his original operation because of the development of graft coronary disease. Reoperation was successful and follow-up coronary arteriography after receipt of this patient's third heart showed a normal coronary system.

The other identified requirement for consideration of cardiac retransplantation is intractable, recurrent acute rejection early postoperatively. Three patients have undergone reoperation for this reason, two successfully. Figure 11 illustrates postoperative events in the case of a 15-year-old boy who underwent transplantation because of advanced heart failure due to idiopathic cardiomyopathy. His early postoperative course was complicated by persistent acute rejection, treated on five occasions with high dose augmentation of immunosuppression. On the basis of repeated graft biopsy it became apparent that reversal of the rejection process could not be achieved and retransplantation was performed on the 57th postoperative day. After replacement of the first graft no further acute rejection was detected and this patient has continued to do well more than 3 years after transplantation. This experience with cardiac retransplantation has documented both the feasibility

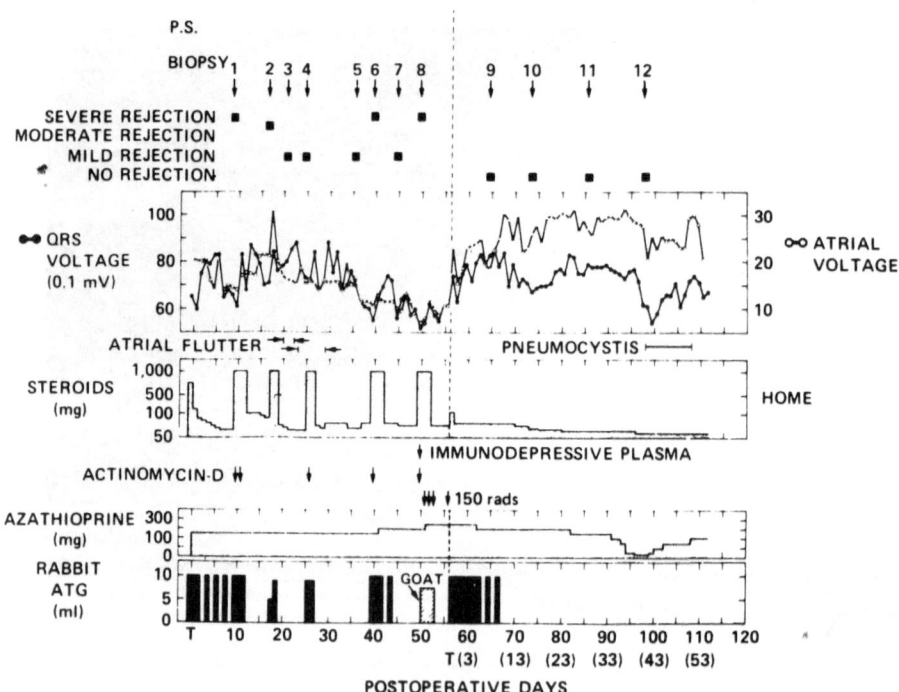

Figure 11 Postoperative events in a patient who underwent cardiac retransplantation on the 57th postoperative day. Repetitive episodes of acute graft rejection after initial heart transplantation were confirmed by serial endomyocardial biopsy. After retransplantation no further episodes of acute rejection occurred

and value of this manoeuvre. It should be considered as realistic strategy in any patient with irreversible graft failure who is free from active infection.

Equally important as survival rates after transplantation of the heart is the quality of life sustained by patients undergoing this procedure. We have attempted to define rehabilitation as simply the restoration of physical and psychosocial capacity to a point that provides a patient with a voluntary option to return to employment or to an activity of choice. As of the present time 49 patients in our total series of 124 patients have survived for at least 1 year after heart transplantation. According to the definition of rehabilitation stated above 90% of these patients have been rehabilitated. Studies of the functional capacity of the long-term recipients by both non-invasive techniques as well as cardiac catheterization and angiography have documented nearly normal function of the transplanted heart despite persistence of autonomic denervation.

Long-term survival rates, calculated by the actuarial method, for the entire series are illustrated in Figure 12. It is obvious that many mistakes were incorporated into our learning curve during the early years of our programme; nevertheless, the overall survival rate of 1 year after transplantation is 53% and the attrition rate thereafter is approximately linear, reaching a survival rate of 26% 5 years after operation. Also illustrated in Figure 12 is the survival experience of patients who were selected for transplantation but who died before a suitable donor became available. Clearly, these patients do not constitute a true control group for patients undergoing transplantation, but they do serve to emphasize the severity of cardiac disease present in

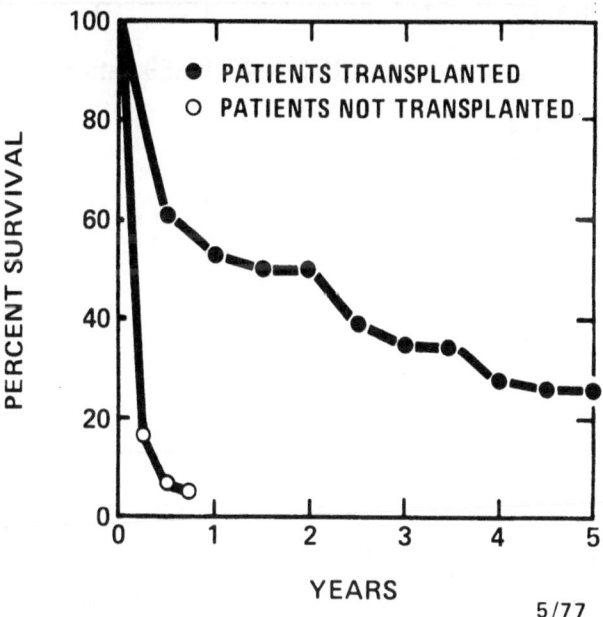

Figure 12 Actuarial postoperative survival rates for the entire cardiac transplantation series

patients whom we select for transplantation; average survival in these 39 patients not undergoing transplantation after acceptance was 55 days.

It is more pertinent to evaluation of the current status of cardiac transplantation to illustrate the survival experience of patients undergoing operation since late 1973, when rabbit antithymocyte globulin as an immunosuppressive agent and endomyocardial biopsy as a diagnostic tool were routinely incorporated into the programme. The 59 patients thus included provide a maximum follow-up interval of approximately $3\frac{1}{2}$ years. The survival rates of this more recent subgroup of patients at 1, 2 and 3 years postoperatively are 69%, 62%, and 59%, respectively. These survival rates are significantly superior to those observed in patients undergoing transplantation prior to 1973 and they illustrate the current expectations for survival after heart transplantation at our centre (Figure 13).

I would conclude this review of cardiac transplantation by submitting that this procedure, despite its somewhat halcyon history, does constitute a genuine therapeutic alternative for highly selected and carefully managed patients. The survival rates that have been illustrated are comparable or superior to those generally reported for renal transplantation for unrelated donors. It is evident that there is a renaissance of interest in cardiac transplantation throughout the world at the present time and we would support the reinitiation of programmes in qualified centres. We believe, however, that it is appropriate that this complex procedure continues to be restricted to institutions with continuing serious interest in this field and a responsive, appropriate laboratory background.

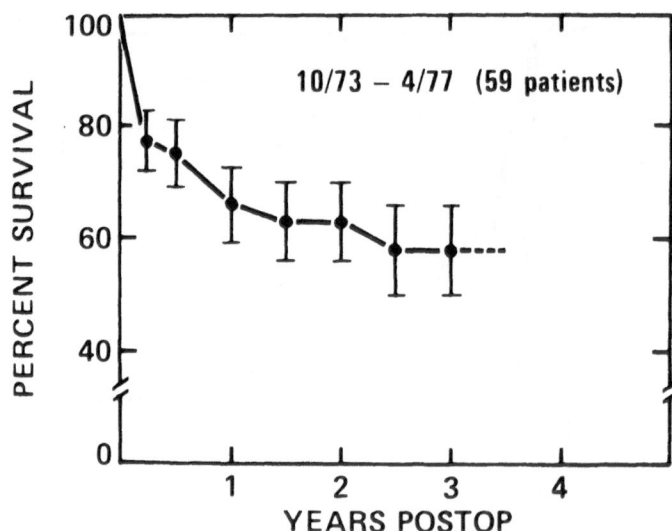

Figure 13 Actuarial survival experience of patients undergoing cardiac transplantation since October 1973, when rabbit antithymocyte globulin as an immunosuppressive agent and endomyocardial biopsy as a diagnostic tool were routinely incorporated into postoperative management. These survival statistics (69%, 62%, and 59% survival rates at 1, 2, and 3 years postoperatively) illustrated current expectations for survival after heart transplantation

18

Aortic valve replacement with autologous fascia lata

Å. SENNING

INTRODUCTION

In the search for biological autologous material to replace heart valves, fascia lata was tried experimentally. The collagenous structure of the fascia lata is theoretically ideal for valvular grafting since it is easily incorporated by surrounding tissue without the risk of immunological reaction. From experience in general surgery it was known that fascia lata used in autologous transplantation continues to survive, and maintains its structure for many years. Valves could be constructed allowing a central flow without turbulence and minimal pressure gradient across the valve; also, the risk of thromboembolism appeared minimal. A series of fascia lata replacements of the aortic cusp was started in 1962 and altogether 207 patients have been operated on between then and 1971.

TECHNIQUE

The operative technique has been reported previously (Senning, 1966). The heart was exposed either through a median sternotomy or through a right-sided thoracotomy in the fourth intercostal space with transection of the sternum (for associated mitral and tricuspid valvular disease). Cardiopulmonary bypass was instituted by cannulating the right and left atrium and returning the oxygenated blood via an aortic or iliac cannula. Haemodilution technique was employed using dextrose–saline prime. The oxygenator was of a rotation cylinder type (Crafoord, Norberg and Senning, 1957). Perfusion was started with a left heart bypass and the blood was cooled rapidly until hypothermic fibrillation occurred. At this point total heart–lung bypass was started and the aorta was cross-clamped and opened through a longitudinal

S-shaped incision. The body temperature was then stabilized at 28–31 °C. Coronary perfusion was used until 1967; afterwards all aortic valvular replacements were done without coronary perfusion, by keeping the heart submerged in ice-cold saline.

A strip of fascia lata was taken from the patient's thigh, meticulously cleaned and tailored to size. A single row of continuous 3/O mersilene was used for suturing the fascia lata strip into the aortic root. The commissures were attached to the wall of the aorta with separate, Teflon-felt anchored sutures. During the perfusion the operative area was frequently bathed with ice-cold kanamycin solution (2 g/l). After the completion of the operation the blood was rewarmed, the heart electrically defibrillated and the total heart–lung bypass discontinued. The heart was supported through a left heart bypass for a variable period of time until the haemodynamic situation became stabilized. All patients with fascia lata replacement received antibiotics after the operation. Ten million units of penicillin and 6 g of methicillin were given daily for 4–6 days, followed by chloromycetin 2 g/day for the next 7 days. Apart from the first 40 patients no anticoagulants were used, except in cases of concomitant mitral prosthetic replacement; nor was any long-term antibiotic prophylaxis given.

Postoperative cardiological evaluation was performed at the out-patient clinic at 3, 6 and 12 months after the operation; afterwards the patients were seen once yearly.

Resection of fascia lata from the patients' thighs did cause haemorrhages with haematomas in a few cases. Even meticulous haemostasis is not effective during extracorporeal circulation when heparin is used. Therefore the thigh wound was closed first after the heparin had been neutralized. The follow-up showed that around one-third of the young males had visible muscle herniations through the defect of the fascia. These muscle herniations had neither functional nor cosmetic importance. Dubied and co-workers (1973) reported two young males with a deterioration in the isometric muscle strength in hyperflexion and knee extension. None of our patients has complained of difficulties when walking. Dubied and co-workers (1973) carried out an analysis on gait and this showed that an extensive fascia lata resection produced no serious functional disorders.

PATHOLOGY

Normal fascia lata consists of at least three layers of relatively acellular tense collagen. The collagen fibres in each layer run parallel but at an angle to one another. In the deep layer which forms the important element of the valvular graft the fibrils run parallel to the main axes; in the thin layer they are oriented perpendicular to it. Small blood vessels are seen between the collagen layers and have elastic fibrils related to them. After preparation for valve surgery one surface of the fascia is smooth and shiny, and practically free from surrounding tissue. This side has been used as the aortic side of the cusp in our material. The other side of the fascia is somewhat rough and may have tags of areolar tissue even if it is extremely carefully cleaned. Sometimes it contains small blood vessels.

When placed in the valvular position, changes occur on and in the fascia lata tissue. Within a very short time, perhaps minutes or seconds as shown by scanning electron microscopy (SEM), a thin layer of proteinaceous and fibrinogenous deposits cover the fascia tissue. The next change seems to be swelling of the fascia due to oedema. In the early months the number of original cell-nucleides in the fascia diminish but they later increase by invasion of what are mainly fibroblasts.

The changes which then take place in the fascia vary not only from individual to individual but also from cusp to cusp in the same valve graft and there seem to be indirect correlations between the fascia lata transplant duration and extent of lesion, e.g. the first patient operated in 1962 still seems to have an acceptable function of his aortic valve graft. On the other hand there are grafts which have had to be replaced within the first year.

Histological examination of grafts excised between 1 and 12 years has shown some characteristic changes. At the time of transplantation the fascia lata of the constructed valve is no thicker than 0.6–0.9 mm. Even if the fascia has thickened by deposition and reparative events during the first years, the normal texture of the fascia was often easily recognizable through the white gelatinous coating. In most transplants the form of the valvular pocket was preserved although the valves exhibited various degrees of thickening and retraction. The free edge of the valve was sometimes normal but more often indented and thickened. The commissures were present, free of adhesions or dehiscences of the sutures. During the first years of the transplantation the graft contained only small focal calcifications. With time, the calcifications became more and more pronounced, especially at the base of the cusp. Light microscopy shows the valvular surface scattered with deposits of varying thickness. The deposits are dense, either homogenous or pitted with small lacunae containing cellular fragments.

Pictures of a cusp with a smooth surface taken by the SEM show a fibrin and hyaline substance on the surface in deep lacunae. In these lacunae there are often fibrin thrombi with numerous platelets.

One year postoperatively the valve is still thin and beautiful and in the middle part is less than 1 mm and at the base about 2 mm thick. It seems though that the valve has been elongated along the axis perpendicular to the free edge. The deposits on the surface of the fascial cusps increase in thickness especially towards the basis of the cusp. They became organized from a connective tissue layer, that coats both surfaces of the cusps, especially the ventricular side of the cusp and also infiltrate the fascial tissue.

After 5 years some cusps are about 2–3 mm thick. The thickness varies from cusp to cusp and also within the cusp. The deposit layer is clearly thicker on the ventricular side of the cusp. In some cases the difference is remarkable. On the one side the deposit layer can be 0.5 mm and on the other side (the ventricular side) around 2 mm thick.

Electron microscopy shows that some of the collagen fibrils of the fascia lata tissue are already degenerating. The fascia is covered with a thin homogeneous protein layer of hyaline nature. The superficial layer is pitted sporadically by irregularly edged lacunae containing numerous cellular fragments, thrombocytes and fibrin. Most importantly, although an occasional

21

isolated cell of endothelial type can be found, a real endothelium is never present on the surface of the fascia grafts. As the deposition layers increase, areas of necrosis appear which occasionally even fibrolyse the entire thickness of the graft. With time there is a scanty invasion of vessels from the base. The fibres of the fascia seem stretched and broader and they start to separate from each other. This is especially the case in the bottom of the cusps. The fibres start to disintegrate and rupture along the free edge of the cusps.

With increasing thickness of the deposits the areas of necrosis are more numerous and enlarged. In some areas calcifications are observed, in other areas a reparative cellular proliferation is present composed of numerous fibroblastic cells. However, instead of forming fibres in a parallel arrangement they exhibit a totally random pattern. This reparative fibrotic tissue increases with time and the cusps become thick and rigid and the free edge becomes retracted. The thick and rigid, partly retracted free edge of the valve can not close effectively during diastole. The bottom of the cusp can still be thin and flexible and even a little aneurysmatic. In some cases the aneurysmatic dilatation of the bottom of the cusp is more pronounced, although the free edge is still pliable enough to give a good closure during diastole. When this aneurysmatic dilatation becomes severe the valve will be insufficient, because the aneurysmatic dilatation of the bottom of the cusp may stretch the valve, hindering closure.

Generally the fascia lata cusps function well for 4–5 years. With increasing thickness, dilatation of the cusps and calcification, the cusps become insufficient 4–5 years after implantation and several have become stenotic after 8–9 years. These changes to the fascia have determined the clinical course of the patient after surgery.

RESULTS

X-ray follow-up after 1 year shows a decreased heart size. Five years after the operation the heart is the same size as postoperatively and thereafter gradually increases in size. Severe valvular insufficiency then develops requiring reoperation.

ECG studies show that the Sokolow index is practically normal after 2–6 months postoperative but 2–3 years after surgery the index tends towards the pathological condition, especially in patients with combined aortic disease. Patients with pure aortic insufficiency, however, are still practically normal after $3\frac{1}{2}$ years. As is more usual the dysfunction of the valve starts about 4–5 years after surgery, complications being mainly early insufficiency.

There have been 79 reoperations in 207 patients. In 15 cases the reoperations were necessary because of early malfunction. The fascia lata cusps seem to be very sensitive to endocarditis and 11 patients were reoperated because of damaged cusps. Fifty-three reoperations were necessary because of late deterioration.

In some cases sutures have torn holes in the fascia. In one case not only the free edge fringed but also there was a central hole in the cusp causing a severe aortic insufficiency and a severe haemolysis. These early malfunctions which occurred were first noticed in the latter part of the series. One explanation could be that in the earlier part I cut the fascia myself, and I looked for a good part of the fascia. Later in the series this task was given to different surgeons assisting the operation.

The fascia cusp is very sensitive to bacterial endocarditis. During the first postoperative year there were ten cases of endocarditis, eight of these died, only two survived. Sixteen patients have developed a late endocarditis which occurred between 2 and 10 years post-operatively. Seven of those patients have been reoperated on and the valve replaced with an artificial valve prosthesis. The cumulative rate of endocarditis after 9 years is 23%. One explanation which could be given is, that the architecture of the valve is not only different from a normal valve, but also the surface of the valve is uneven and therefore bacteria adhere more readily to the surface of these valves. In one case cocci could be seen on the surface of the valve, although the patient was without signs of endocarditis. In another patient, although he had a well functioning valve there were several small emboli. The valve, when opened showed on the ventricular side small granulations and the histology shows the typical picture of an endocarditis.

In 161 patients, an isolated aortic valve replacement was performed. There were 14 hospital deaths. These patients have been closely followed. Four patients have been unfortunately lost to follow-up and in eight there has been an incomplete follow-up. We have a complete follow-up on 135 patients with an average of at least 8 years.

Hospital mortality

I think today that most of the deaths were caused from insufficient myocardial protection. In contrast, results from a recent series indicate a mortality of around 1.5%.

From the 135 patients with a complete follow-up a total of 85% of the patients are alive 5 years later, 70% of which have a fascia valve. The 15% difference consists of those patients who have been reoperated and had their valve replaced with a prosthetic valve, mainly a Björk-Shiley prosthesis. After 10 years only 40% have a functioning fascia lata valve. Thanks to reoperation, altogether 69% of the patients followed for 10 years are still living. If compared with other series of homologous valves it is obvious that the autologous fascia lata replacement does not have any advantage over other biological valves.

Chronic haemolysis which leads to an anaemia in some instances is a feature of some of the artificial valve prostheses. There has been no significant haemolysis induced by fascia lata grafts in the valvular position when regurgitation is absent. There was only one instance of haemolytic anaemia and this occurred in a patient who suffered from a severe aortic incompetence caused by a bacterial endocarditis and this valve had to be replaced. In agreement with our findings, Dubied and Culhed have found a high degree of haemolysis and also anaemia in three patients who had to undergo reoperation because of dysfunction of the stenosed fascia lata graft.

Lactate dehydrogenase (LDH) values were slightly elevated to an average of 256 IU/l (195 IU/l is the upper normal limit). In the Dubied and Culhed series the LDH-values were also slightly elevated and they found that slight regurgitation did not cause a significantly higher haemolysis than did a stented competent valve, and neither the size of the supporting ring of the prosthesis nor the presence of a pressure gradient across the fascia lata graft appeared to affect the degree of the haemolysis. In our series haptoglobin binding values were slightly below normal, the average value being 35.4 mg/100 ml (the lower limit of normal being 40 mg/100 ml). In the Dubied and Culhed series the haptoglobin binding values were around 50% of the original value but non less than 15 mg/100 ml. In this series there has been not one single embolus in spite of the fact that most patients were never anticoagulated. With regard to bacterial endocarditis, a few small septic emboli have occurred.

The greatest benefit in this and other series, in contrast to the experience in London published by Joseph and co-workers, must be the total absence of thromboembolic episodes in spite of withholding anticoagulants. This has made it possible for several young women to have children without any complications before the valve has had to be replaced.

Encouraging reports have been published with fascia lata replacement of the aortic valves, e.g. from Trimble and co-workers with 31 survivors of the 36 operated patients at least 3 years post-operatively and Rodewald too gave a report about good results. I have a feeling that their fascia lata valves, even if stented, will ultimately suffer the same fate as the unstented valves.

DISCUSSION

The great problem with fascia lata cusps is that no 'self-rinsing' occurs as no blood-repellent endothelial layer is formed. Therefore a continuous deposition onto the surface takes place. Apparently this deposit is of thrombotic origin, as platelets and old fibrin were found in the most superficial layers. The successive layers are organized by proliferating fibroblasts. The increasing proliferation of collagen tissue on both sides of the valves not only makes the cusps increasingly thicker but also disturbs the nutrition of the fascia in spite of the scanty ingrowths of small vessels from the base, with necrosis as a consequence. Reparative processes by fibroblastic cells with fibrils, cicatrization and calcification together make the cusps more and more stiff and the free edges become retracted.

It appears that in some cases the fascia is traumatized and overstretched perpendicular to the free edge resulting in the formation of aneurysms at the bottom of the cusp, which changes the geometry of the valve so that it prevents the free edge of the cusp from closing.

The often non-ideal architecture and the lack of a self-rinsing endothelial layer seem to be factors which make the valves more sensitive to bacterial invasion and endocarditis. The high incidence of bacterial endocarditis seems to be a great problem in all series with stented or non-stented fascia lata cusps. The early laceration and dysfunction of cusps in the aortic position is likely to be caused by the fact that non-ideal parts of the fascia have been used.

The great advantage of the fascia lata valves is the good flow characteristic with minimal haemolysis.

Section II
The mitral valve

1
Echocardiography

T. A. TRAILL

Echocardiography is now widely used for the investigation of patients with mitral valve disease. The rapid opening and closing movement of the valve are characteristic so that it is usually easy to identify.

Figure 1 shows a normal echocardiogram, recorded with a simultaneous

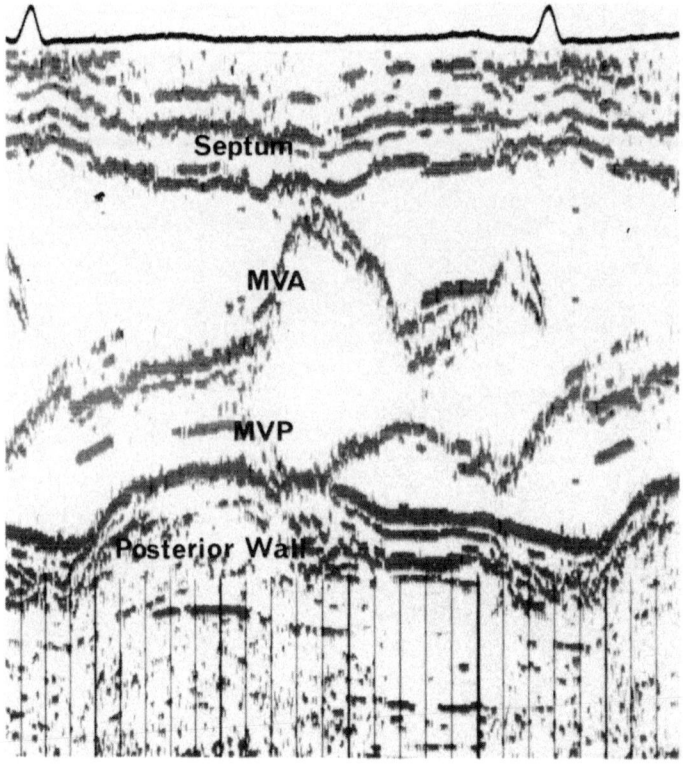

Figure 1 Normal echocardiogram showing both leaflets of the mitral valve (MVA and MVP). Anterior to the valve lies the interventricular septum and posterior to it is seen the endocardium of the posterior left ventricular wall

27

ECG. The tracing represents echoes reflected from different depths within the patient, anterior being at the top and posterior at the bottom of the record. The structure in the centre, labelled MVA, is the anterior cusp of the mitral valve. It opens rapidly at the onset of diastole and then moves posteriorly again to a half-closed position which it reaches by the end of the rapid filling period. At the fast recording speed it is clear that its early diastolic closure is not along a straight line but is better described by a curve. In late diastole there is a second opening movement at the time of atrial systole. The posterior cusp, labelled MVP, shows a similar pattern of diastolic movement but in mirror image and with a smaller amplitude. In systole the cusps are together. Anterior to the mitral valve at this level lies the interventricular septum, labelled Septum, and posterior to it the posterior or free wall of the left ventricle. Note that the endocardial surfaces are clearly apparent as continuous echoes.

Figure 2 shows the mitral echogram from a patient with mitral stenosis. At the top is the ECG and below it a phonocardiogram showing the opening

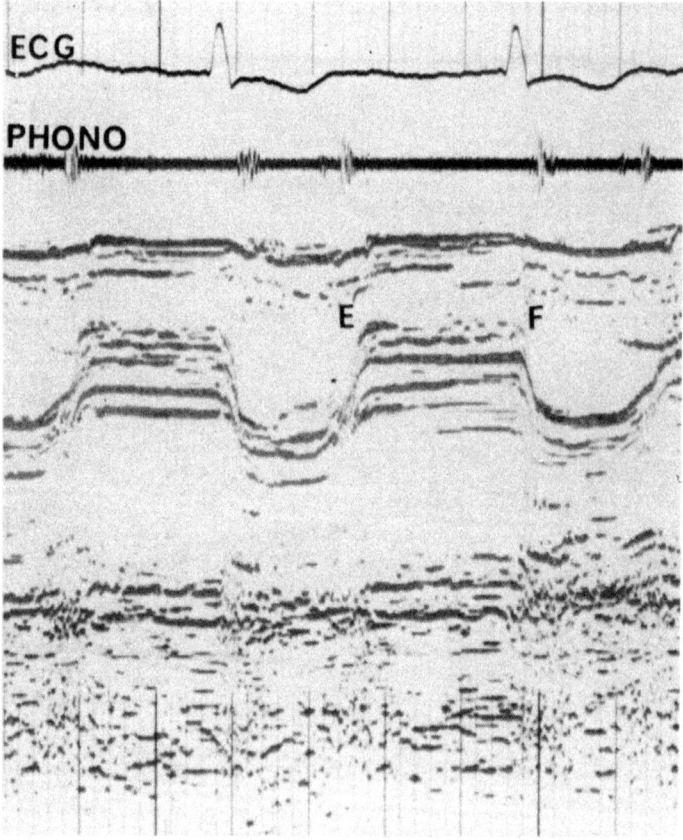

Figure 2   Mitral stenosis, showing thickening of the valve cusps, forward movement of the posterior cusp and a reduced diastolic closure rate (EF slope)

snap. In contrast to the normal patient the cusps are thickened and the excursion of the anterior cusp is reduced. The latter is not always the case, and the reduction of amplitude of movement reflects the degree of chordal shortening. The pattern of movement is quite different from normal for there is no rapid early diastolic closing movement, but instead the valve remains in its open position throughout diastole. It has frequently been suggested that measurement of this so-called EF slope is an indication of severity of mitral valve stenosis, but in practice the numerical correlation between this and other measures of severity has been poor, and the sign is itself non-specific, for a reduced diastolic closure rate is seen frequently in patients with left ventricular hypertrophy and reduced cavity size, and also, for example, in the presence of right ventricular preponderance due to pulmonary hypertension. As causes of slow diastolic closure, these are easily distinguished from mitral stenosis by the pattern of movement of the posterior cusp, for in the normal patient it moves as the mirror image of the anterior cusp, whereas in mitral stenosis it is clear that the posterior cusp, because of commissural fusion, is pulled forwards in diastole by the anterior cusp. Such anterior diastolic movement of the posterior cusp is specific for mitral stenosis.

In mitral regurgitation systolic separation of the cusps is uncommon, so that the mitral echogram may give no clue to the presence or severity of the disease. However, there are exceptions and Figure 3 illustrates one of them. Although the diastolic movements of the valve are normal, it is obvious that

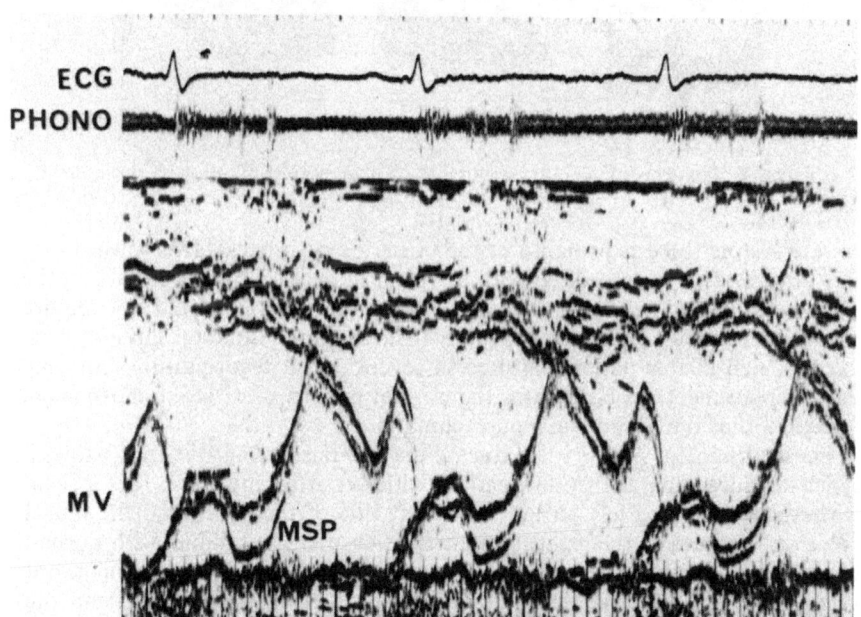

Figure 3 Non-rheumatic mitral regurgitation—mid-systolic prolapse. Part of the mitral valve leaflet is seen to prolapse backwards in late systole. A simultaneous phonocardiogram shows the loud systolic click

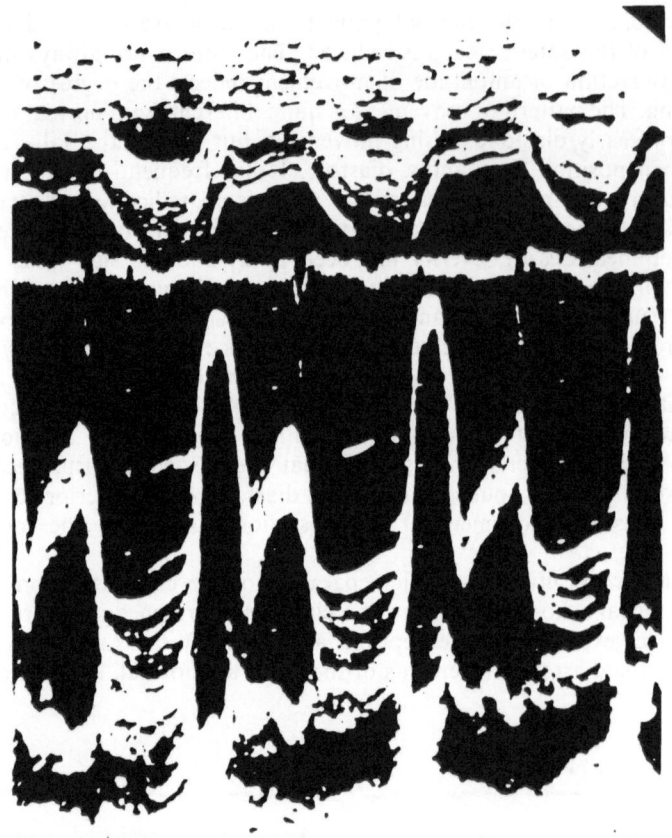

Figure 4 Non-rheumatic mitral regurgitation, pan-systolic mitral valve prolapse

in late systole there is prolapse of the posterior cusp backwards towards the left atrium. This is associated with a typical mid-systolic click shown on the phonocardiogram at the top. This is a benign lesion and would not require surgical treatment. By contrast Figure 4 shows pan-systolic prolapse of both cusps which in this patient resulted in severe mitral regurgitation requiring valve replacement. In both cases the normal pattern of diastolic movements indicated that the lesion was non-rheumatic.

Physical signs of mitral valve disease may be misleading. Figure 5 shows a typical echocardiogram from a patient with left atrial myxoma. It is a scan, with aortic root and left atrium at the left side of the figure and the mitral valve and septum at the right. The anterior cusp is identifiable, with normal opening and closing movements and immediately behind it, within the mitral valve orifice in diastole, there is a dense mass of echoes arising from the myxoma. In systole they swing back into the atrium. Similar clusters of echoes, usually smaller and less dense may arise from mitral valve vegetations, or the flail ends of ruptured chordae. Cor triatriatum should be suspected

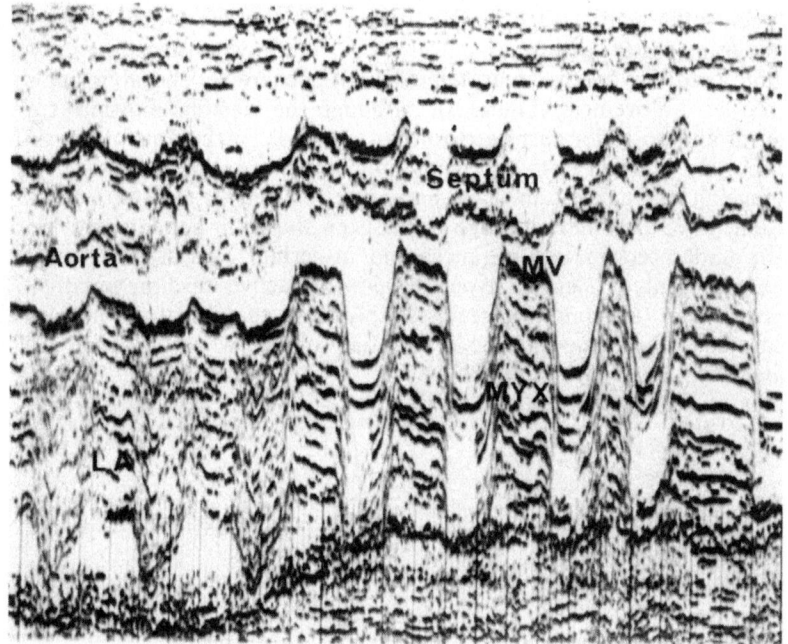

Figure 5 Left atrial myxoma. At the left of the 'sweep' is seen the aorta and posterior to it the left atrium. To the right is seen the anterior mitral valve cusp lying posterior to the septum. Behind the valve cusp in diastole and almost filling the left atrium is seen a dense mass of echoes reflected by the tumour

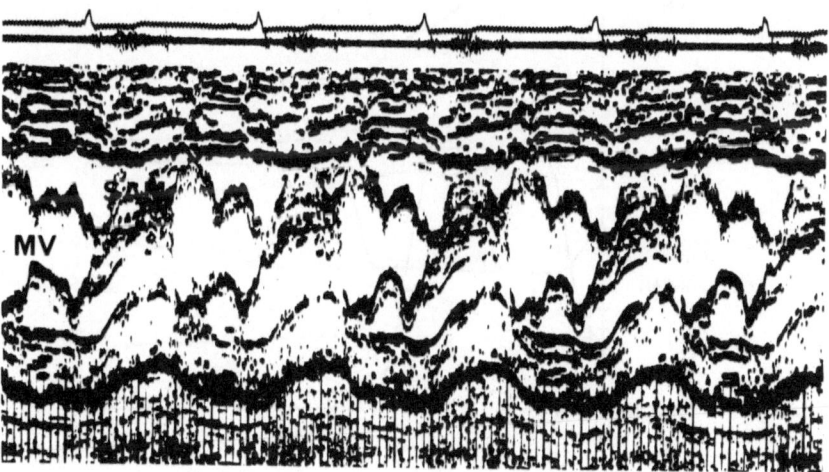

Figure 6 Hypertrophic cardiomyopathy. Although the diastolic movements of the mitral valve are normal, during systole a mass of echoes moves forwards to touch the septum. This systolic anterior movement (SAM) is related to the murmur and possibly to the genesis of outflow obstruction

when, despite having detected by catheter that there is a diastolic gradient between pulmonary wedge or left atrium and the left ventricle, the echocardiogram shows a normal mitral valve. Outflow obstruction in hypertrophic cardiomyopathy is associated with a characteristic abnormality of mitral valve movement (Figure 6). Although the diastolic movement of the anterior and posterior cusps are normal, in systole at the time of the systolic murmur the anterior cusp and its attachments move rapidly forwards, often impingeing on the septum. This finding is referred to as 'systolic anterior movement' (SAM) and although it has been shown in patients with normal hearts under certain circumstances and in certain congenital lesions, it is most commonly a sign of hypertrophic obstructive cardiomyopathy. The mechanism in this condition seems simply to be that all of the mitral valve apparatus is pushed up into the base of the ventricle when the apical cavity is obliterated.

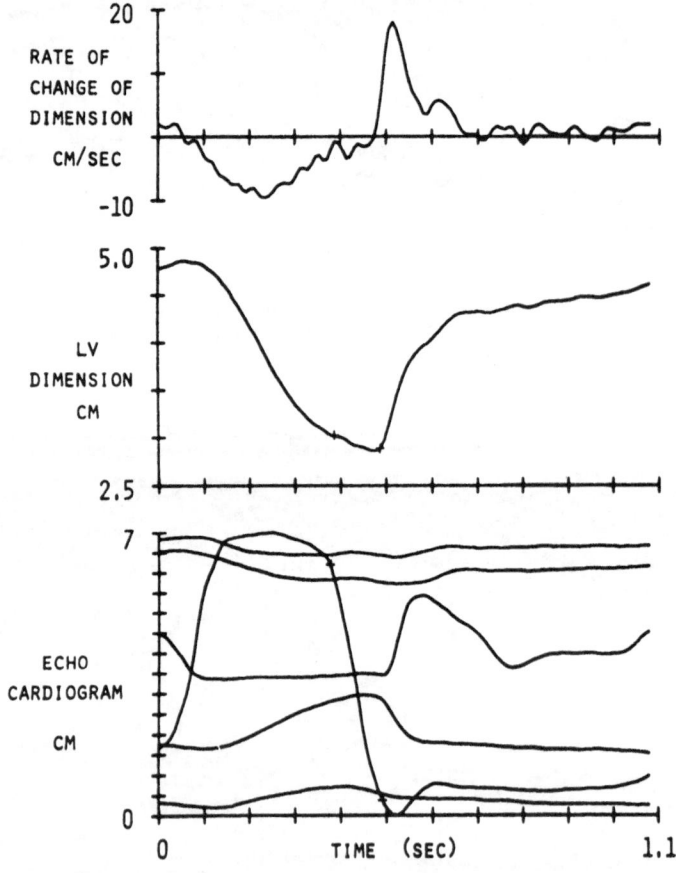

Figure 7 Normal subject; computer plot-out from digitized echocardiogram. The bottom panel shows (reproduced) the original data with (superimposed) the apex cardiogram and crosses representing the time of aortic valve closure and mitral opening. The middle record is the continuous plot of left ventricular dimension and at the top is plotted its first derivative

Not only is echocardiography of considerable value for diagnosis of anatomical abnormalities in patients presenting with mitral valve disease, but we also consider it to be the method of choice for quantifying the physiological disturbance produced. For this however we examine not the valve, but the left ventricular cavity, in particular the rate and pattern of filling. Figure 7 shows a computer plot-out derived from a normal echocardiogram. The bottom panel simply shows tracings of the mitral valve, septum and posterior wall from the original echogram which have been digitized by hand and then replotted by the computer. By subtracting the ordinates of their positions the instantaneous transverse cavity dimension is obtained, which is plotted on the middle panel. It is reduced during systole which ends with the first cross corresponding to the time of aortic valve closure. After this there is a further small inward movement before mitral valve opening, marked by the second cross, which is when filling begins. The normal pattern of filling, typified here, has two phases. There is an initial rapid filling period, followed by relatively slow outward wall movement during diastasis. This can perhaps be more easily appreciated from the top graph which shows the first differential with time of the continuous dimension. From minimum dimension the rate of increase rises rapidly to a peak at about 18 cm/s (the normal range is between 12 and 21 cm/s) and it then declines to an obvious discontinuity, which marks the end of rapid filling at between 100 and 200 ms.

In mitral regurgitation the filling pattern shows an even more clear cut discontinuity between rapid filling and diastasis, and typically the rate of early filling is strikingly increased. Thus in this patient (Figure 8) the peak

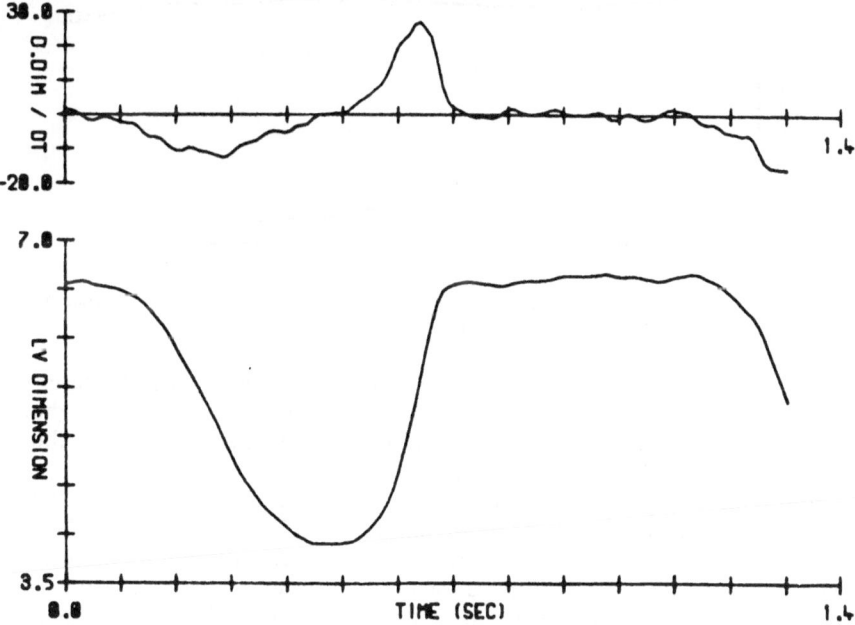

Figure 8 Continuous plots of left ventricular dimension and its first derivative in a patient with severe mitral regurgitation

33

rate of outward wall movement is 30 cm/s, which is well outside the normal range. The end diastolic dimension is increased, and the end systolic dimension is normal, so that overall wall excursion is increased and the lesion is therefore likely to be 'organic' as opposed to 'functional' associated with left ventricular disease.

In mitral stenosis the pattern of filling is entirely different (Figure 9).

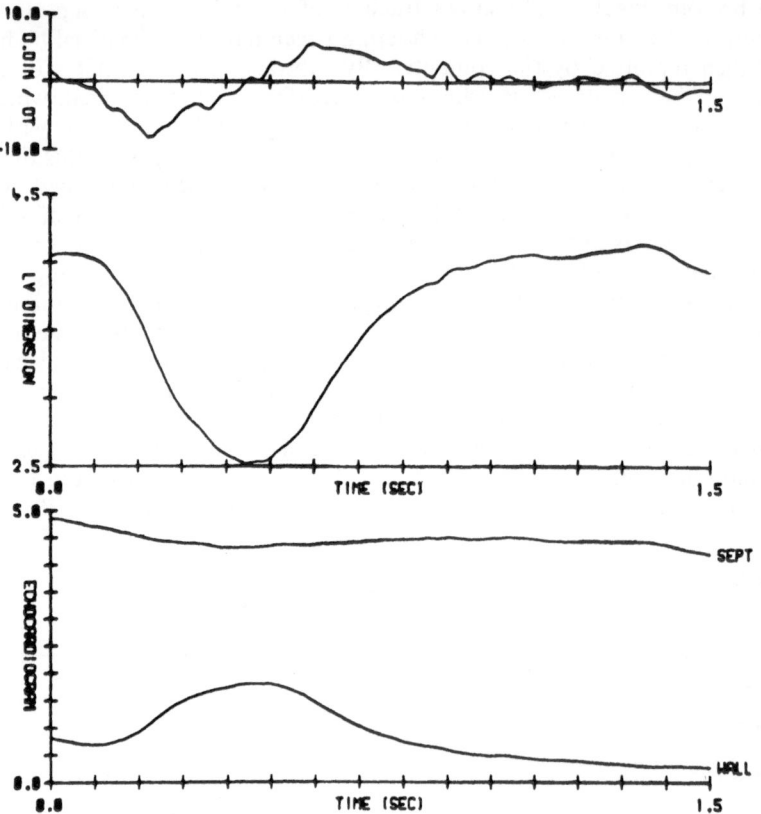

Figure 9 Plots of echocardiogram, left ventricular dimension and rate of change of dimension in a patient with mitral stenosis

In particular, there is now no longer a discontinuity between two phases of filling, and the dimension increases at a more or less steady rate throughout diastole. The peak rate of increase is reduced, in this instance to about 6 cm/s, and the filling period prolonged to more than 400 ms.

Lest it be thought that this sort of information is available only to those with access to a computer and digitizing table, an illustrative case is shown. Figure 10 shows echocardiograms taken from a woman in her forties with a typical history and signs of mitral stenosis. The left-hand panel shows an obvious rheumatic mitral valve with cusp thickening, slow early diastolic closure and anterior diastolic movement of the posterior cusp. The right-hand panel shows an echo taken slightly lower down in the ventricle to show the septum and posterior wall. It can be seen in the long diastole in the middle how the pattern of wall movement is typical of the slow and protracted filling in this condition, and although a computer is not required, Figure 11 demonstrates that the filling curve is indeed just like the example in Figure 10. This patient is of particular interest, because at catheterization, although the cardiac index was only slightly reduced, the measured 'gradient' across the valve, between pulmonary wedge and left ventricular pressures, was only 3 mmHg. Furthermore a left ventriculogram showed reduced wall excursion in all regions and hence a reduced ejection fraction. On their own, therefore, the catheter results might have been taken as showing mild mitral valve disease with cardiomyopathy. However, cardiomyopathy would not account for the filling pattern and she was submitted for operation with an excellent surgical result. At recatheterization left ventricular wall movement was improved and ejection fraction increased. Thus, the presence of mitral stenosis can mimic left ventricular disease and makes catheter assessment of left ventricular performance unreliable.

In summary, we consider that echocardiography is frequently helpful for describing the structural abnormalities in patients with mitral valve lesions, and that study of the left ventricular filling pattern reflected by the change in a single transverse dimension provides a useful means to assess their functional effect and severity. It is now the exception rather than the rule at the Brompton Hospital to perform cardiac catheterization on patients with mitral valve disease.

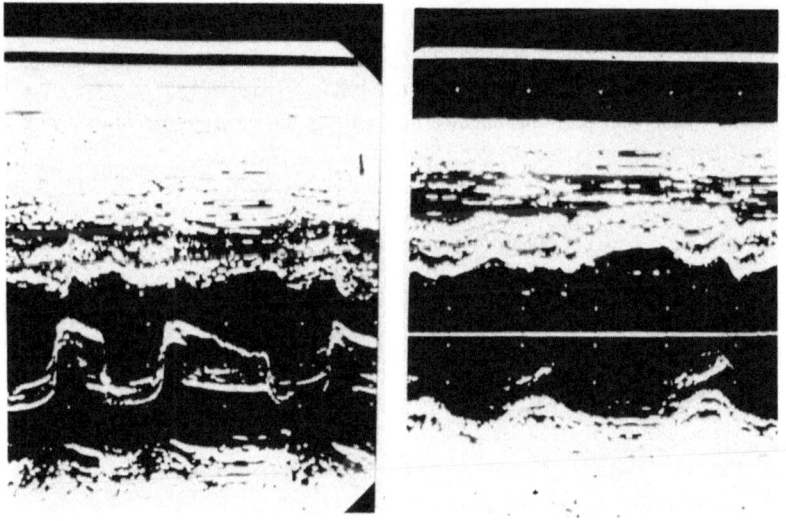

Figure 10 Echocardiograms from a patient with mitral stenosis. The left-hand panel shows cusp thickening, a slow diastolic closure rate and forward movement of the posterior cusp. The right-hand panel shows the left ventricular cavity, demarcated by the endocardial surfaces of the posterior wall and interventricular septum

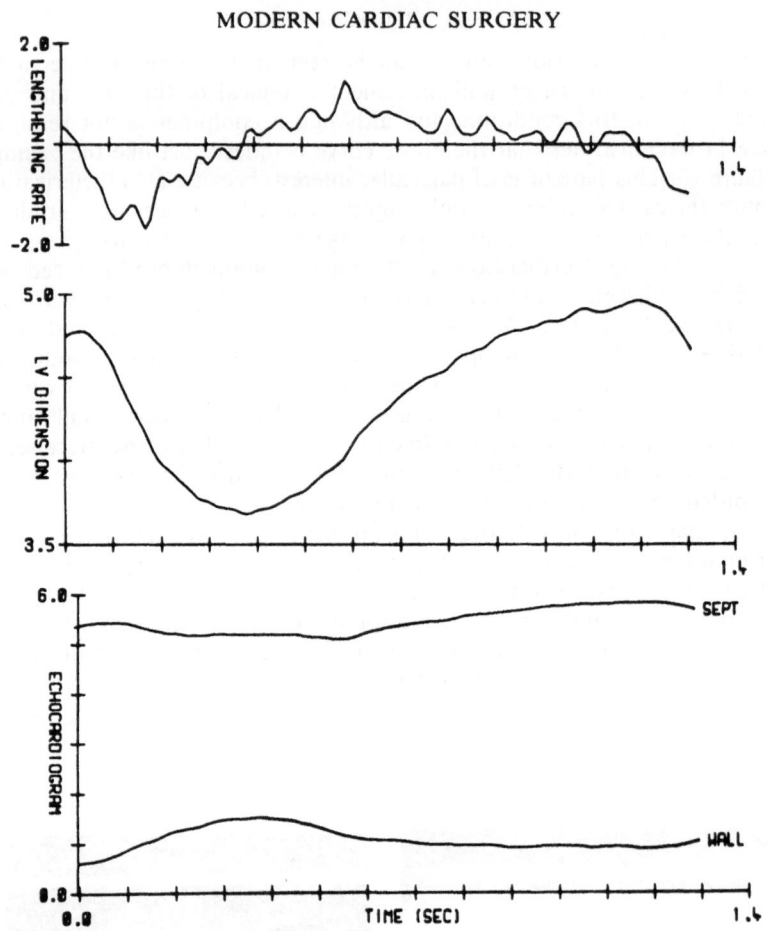

Figure 11 Computer plot-out obtained by digitizing the echocardiogram in Figure 10

2

Mitral valve disease: the case for cardiac catheterization

CELIA M. OAKLEY

Advancement in surgical techniques, with the alternatives of open or closed valvotomy, repair or prosthetic replacement of the mitral valve, has made necessary the acquisition of more detailed information about the valve and left ventricle than sufficed when the surgical choice was mitral valvotomy or nothing.

BACKGROUND

When a decision had to be made regarding closed mitral valvotomy all that was needed was the knowledge that the valve orifice was sufficiently reduced and that there was no substantial mitral regurgitation. Clinical auscultation became so accurate for this limited purpose that Edler's[1] development of echocardiography in 1954 was received without enthusiasm and remained in obscurity until the late 1960s. Occasionally cardiac catheterization was carried out to estimate severity when this was in doubt, with retrograde left ventricular angiography to assess the importance of any accompanying mitral regurgitation.

In the 1960s mitral valve replacements became available and increasingly used. It became necessary to recognize which valves were ideally suited for valvotomy because only those gave good and lasting results from the closed technique. So-called 'mitral restenosis' is more often a reflection of the inadequacy of the initial valvotomy than an actual restenosis. A 'placebo' operation on an unsuitable valve was no longer acceptable and mitral valve replacement was the alternative. Auscultation became further refined; for example Nixon[2] demonstrated that a loud first and opening snap meant flexibility of the anterior leaflet.

The new demand for detailed anatomical information led to a growing popularity for echocardiography in order to show mitral valve mobility, the severity of mitral stenosis and the efficiency of left ventricular contraction. Unfortunately it gradually became apparent that the severity of mitral stenosis was not well depicted by echo, and that measurement of the lesser dimension of the left ventricle gave very little information about left ventricular contractile efficiency, especially when the patients also had atrial fibrillation. The echo volumes matched poorly with the left ventricular angiographic volumes. Even the seeming thickness and mobility of the mitral leaflets could be misleading since the echoes from the anterior leaflet are so much better seen than those from the posterior leaflet and it is the shrunken tethered posterior leaflet which so often precludes a good mitral valvotomy or makes necessary mitral valve replacement. Unfortunately mitral valve replacement is not the panacea which had been anticipated, and attention once again turned to mitral valve repair.

PRESENT NEEDS

Coming up to date two additional facets of the patient with mitral valve disease now concern us: one is the integrity of the left ventricle and the second is the suitability of the mitral valve for open plastic reconstruction. It is on these that the current case for cardiac catheterization hinges.

The left ventricle in mitral valve disease

Left ventricular failure has become known as the most important cause of an unsatisfactory result following mitral valve replacement. It comes close to thromboembolism as the major cause of late death after mitral valve replacement. It has accounted for an unknown number of operative deaths (unknown because of our previous failure to appreciate the frequency of left ventricular malfunction in patients being considered for mitral valve surgery). It is next to impossible to determine left ventricular efficiency clinically in a patient with mitral valve disease. Occasionally there are major signs such as clinical left ventricular enlargement in a patient with other features of pure mitral stenosis or ECG indicators such as a conduction defect, left ventricular disorder or changes of past infarction. More often there are no such clues. Ultrasound has been shown to be of very limited value because left ventricular shape can be greatly distorted in the presence of mitral valve deformity and atrial fibrillation further makes interpretation difficult.

A major reason for cardiac catheterization nowadays is to assess left ventricular function in patients with mitral valve disease. The finding of poor left ventricular function does not necessarily prohibit surgery but it allows one to judge the greater operative risk and lesser surgical benefit that the patient must face. Poor left ventricular function in a patient with mitral stenosis is particularly ominous since increasing the preload by removing the obstruction seems to engender deterioration in function. Conversely, poor left ventricular function in a patient with severe mitral regurgitation may not preclude surgery provided the mitral regurgitation itself is at least moderately severe. This is because the ailing left ventricle may have fixed systolic and diastolic dimensions; to correct reflux and divert that fixed stroke volume forwards would improve stroke output and lower the raised left atrial pressure. Even patients with primary cardiomyopathy and secondary mitral regurgitation may benefit. Either primary dilated cardiomyopathy, restrictive cardiomyopathy or hypertrophic cardiomyopathy may masquerade as primary mitral valve disease. Rarely, mitral valve surgery may be needed. In dilated cardiomyopathy the benefit can be surprising. In restrictive cardiomyopathy (endomyocardial fibrosis) mitral regurgitation results from involvement of the posterior mitral leaflet and chordae in the scarring process with tethering of the leaflet (Figure 1). Stripping of the endocardium plus mitral repair or replacement may be carried out with benefit. In hypertrophic cardiomyopathy (Figure 2) organic changes in the mitral anterior leaflet may result from turbulence in the left ventricular outflow tract leading to an acquired non-rheumatic mitral stenosis. Mitral replacement is then needed, removal of hypertrophic papillary muscles improves ventricular capacity and removal of the anterior leaflet relieves outflow obstruction.

The finding of segmental dysfunction in a patient with mitral valve disease may reflect coronary artery disease; it is now the usual practice to carry out coronary angiography in any patient with mitral valve disease whose ECG suggests a myocardial fault, and in selected patients with mitral valve disease

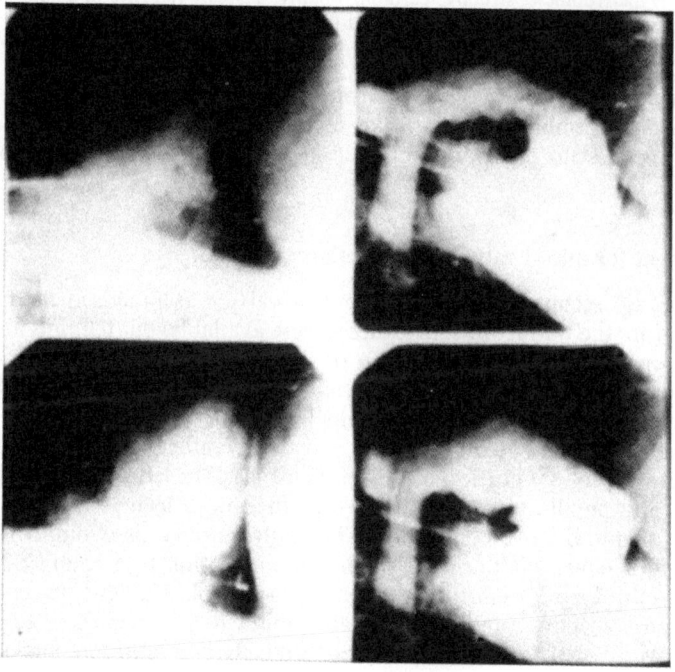

Figure 1 Restrictive cardiomyopathy. Left ventricular angiograms at the top, and right ventricular angiograms underneath. Diastole on the left and systole on the right. The typical apical blunting of the left ventricle is shown with obliteration of the right ventricular cavity and marked mitral and tricuspid reflux

39

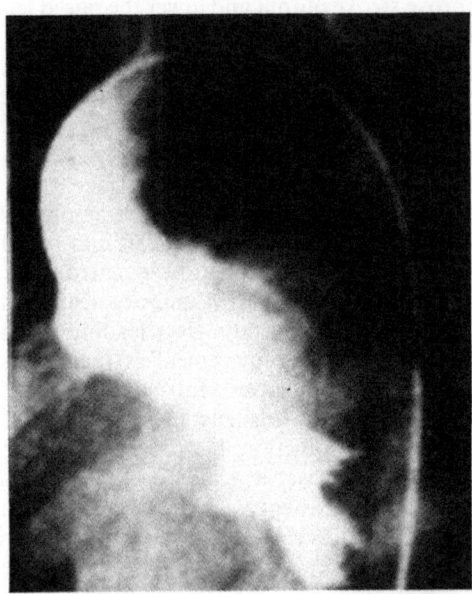

Figure 2 Hypertrophic obstructive cardiomyopathy. The left ventricle in axially tilted left anterior oblique view showing the deformed mitral valve

over the age of 50 who may have coronary atheromatous obstructive disease. Past coronary embolism may leave segmental ventricular dysfunction but usually there is no persisting obstruction to be found in a major coronary artery.

Assessment for mitral valve reconstruction and repair

Open plastic reconstruction of the mitral valve was practised in the early 1960s before the mitral valve prostheses were available, but fell into abeyance as everyone rode on the bandwagon of the new prostheses. The crash came with the recognition that the prosthetic devices are still carrying a relatively high instance of thromboembolism which cannot be abolished by the use of anticoagulants. They also carry a second disadvantage: the imposition of a splint into the inflow portion of the left ventricle. The left ventricular muscle, annulus and papillary muscles, as well as the mitral leaflets themselves, are needed for mitral valve competence. The mitral orifice is ovoid, it is innervated and it constricts during systole. The imposition of a round rigid ring into the mitral orifice effectively puts a considerable segment of ventricular muscle out of action, and it is probably this which precipitates actual left ventricular failure in patients who preoperatively had been just managing in the face of already compromised left ventricular function.

The possibility of conserving the valve again became attractive so the cardiologist began to try and separate the patient with a reparable valve from the patient whose valve needed replacement. The rather unsatisfactory results of mitral valve replacement deterred the cardiologist from referring the patient to the surgeon early. Autonomous deterioration in valve function over the years applies as much to the abnormal mitral valve as it does to the aortic valve and it is not the result of continuing rheumatism. Valvular inefficiency leads to turbulence and endothelial damage; poor mobility leads to progressive immobility. The mitral valve is not in a static state and the possibilities for its successful reconstruction may well be brighter at an earlier stage in the decline of the valve than they will be years later. Patients who are put forward for valve repair should probably be sent up many years earlier than would be proper if they were going to have a mitral valve replacement. This faces the physician with the absolute need to pick the patient and the timing correctly so that the mitral valve repair can be optimal.

How then are we to differentiate a mitral valve which is suitable for repair from one which needs to be replaced?

Neither the clinical findings, fluoroscopy, phonocardiography, impulse cardiography, systolic time intervals nor echo pictures nor any combination of these are reliable, although of course they provide pointers. Suitable patients are usually younger but not always. In non-rheumatic mitral valve disease plastic techniques may provide a watertight and durable repair of mitral

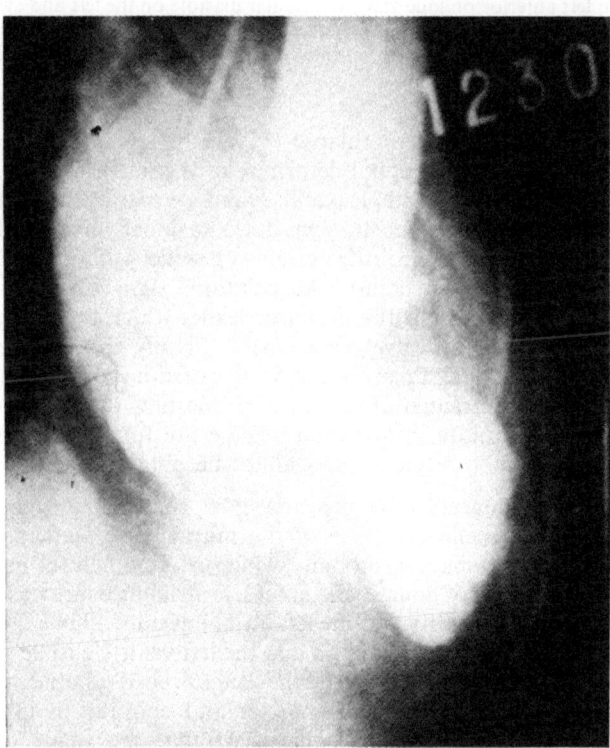

Figure 3 Gross posterior mitral leaflet prolapse with mitral reflux

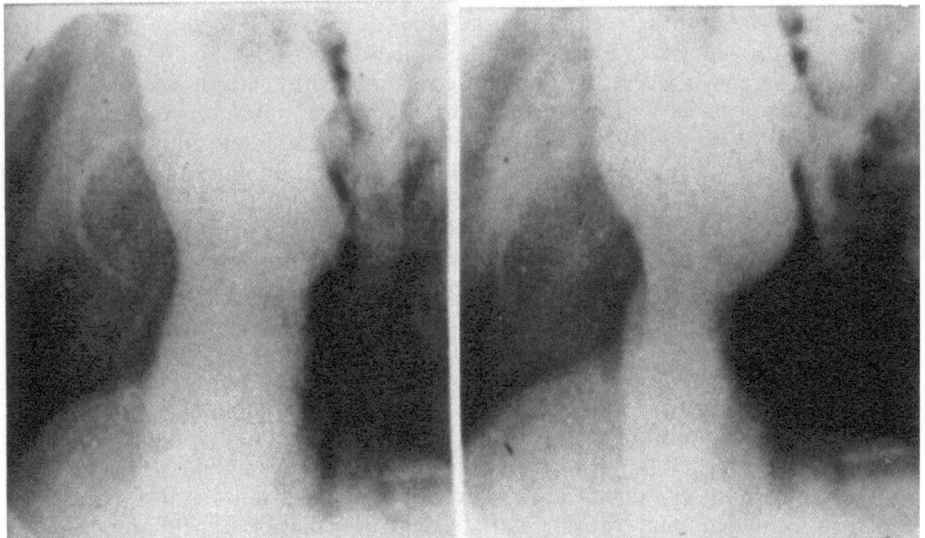

Figure 4 Severe mitral reflux caused by mitral chordal rupture. Retrograde left ventricular angiography in left anterior oblique view, ventricular diastole on the left and systole on the right. This is not a good view for assessing either the mitral valve or the left ventricle, but it may show up anterior leaflet prolapse; in this case the severity of the reflux obscures the detail of the valve

regurgitation caused by leaflet prolapse (Figures 3 and 4) Left ventricular angiography may reveal congenital deformity of the mitral valve such as the insertion of all chordae into a single papillary muscle (parachute mitral valve). A calcified valve is a bad prognostic sign, but occasionally heavy calcification may be confined to a portion of the annulus or leaflet without involving the major part of the valve structure. Auscultatory signs of anterior leaflet mobility tell us nothing about the posterior leaflet which through shrinkage may determine a need for valve replacement. Finally the echo, the bright hope of a few years ago, fails on the vital questions of the subvalvular apparatus and left ventricular function. The question then is can invasive investigation provide more information? There are four areas wherein the information obtained by angiography cannot be obtained by other means:

(1) Left atrial angiography by the transeptal route in a right anterior projection gives an excellent picture of the mitral valve leaflets providing evidence of their thickness and mobility which is most helpful in assessing reparability. In addition of course the direct left atrial pressure measurement is of value in assessing severity and the left atrial injection allows the presence of left atrial thrombus to be recognized and the left ventricle to be visualized.

(2) Left ventricular angiography is the single most reliable method of assessing the state of the papillary muscles and chordae in mitral valve disease. It has been observed for some years that the shape of the left ventricle often appears very abnormal in rheumatic mitral valve disease. This

is easily mistaken for segmental dyskinesia when the abnormality is really a filling defect caused by thickened papillary muscles and chordae tethering a mitral leaflet. When both papillary muscles are recognized the appearance may be mistaken for left ventricular hypertrophy because of the seeming increase in size of the papillary muscles. The recognition therefore of a misshapen left ventricle provides good evidence of a valve which may prove impossible to repair. Conversely the finding of a smoothly ellipsoidal left ventricle provides good support for a plan to repair the valve.

(3) Retrograde left ventricular angiography is the best method we have of determining left ventricular myocardial integrity. Calculation of the ejection fraction is easy, reasonably accurate and reproducible and in atrial fibrillation the ejection fraction, though variable, should not fall below 60% for any beat. Segmental dyskinesia provides a clue to localized ischaemic damage either from obstructive coronary atheroma or past coronary embolism.

(4) Coronary angiography is now established as a necessary procedure in many patients over the age of 50 undergoing valve replacement, particularly if they have overt risk factors, and this means that many of our patients will need an invasive investigation anyway. It is not uncommon to find obstructive atheroma with mitral valve disease, particularly as more of our patients are older and as coronary artery disease occurs earlier in the female population.

We have been comparing the left ventricular and angiographic experience with the surgeon's description and with the appearances of the excised mitral valve in our patients, and have found excellent correlation so far between severe mitral valve disorganization and angiographic deformity of the left ventricular outline.

In conclusion then it seems that cardiac catheterization is required in the assessment of patients with mitral valve disease in order to determine the prospects for valve conservation, to assess left ventricular function and to detect accompanying coronary artery disease.

References

1. Edler, I. and Hertz, C. H. (1954). Use of ultrasonic reflectoscope for continuous recording of movement of the heart wall. *K. Fysiogr. Saellsk. Lund, Foerh.*, **24,** 40
2. Nixon, P. G. F., Wooler, G. H. and Radigan, L. R. (1960). The opening snap in mitral incompetence. *Br. Heart J.*, **22,** 398

3

Closed mitral valvotomy

W. P. CLELAND

There have been considerable changes in the indications for closed as opposed to open mitral valvotomy in the past 8 or 10 years, due partly to the increasing safety of cardiopulmonary bypass but also to the development of echo-cardiography which enables the clinician to select suitable cases for the closed procedure.

The operation is essentially that which reached its perfection in the 1950s. The valve is split with an expanding dilator (Tubbs), inserted through the apex of the left ventricle and controlled with the right index finger inserted into the atrium through the appendage or atrial wall.

At the present time the conditions for accepting a patient for a closed valvotomy are based essentially on the pathology of the valve and the presence or absence of mitral regurgitation. The assessment can be made by clinical or radiological means but especially by echocardiography. There is little place for cardiac catheterization or angiography in the assessment of the condition of the valve. The following suggest a pliable valve suitable for valvotomy:

1. the presence of a loud accentuated first sound at the apex;
2. the absence of calcification on chest X-ray;
3. non-thickened valve demonstrated on echocardiography;
4. the absence of a systolic murmur or other evidence of mitral regurgitation.

With these criteria I have accepted for closed valvotomy approximately 60 patients from January 1972 to March 1976. These patients have been followed up from 12 months to 4 years.

The advantages of a closed valvotomy as opposed to an open valvotomy can be summarized as follows:

1. the operation is a simple and fairly quick procedure and does not require the elaborate preparation or involvement of staff that cardiopulmonary bypass demands;

2. blood transfusion requirements are considerably less than for open valvotomy;
3. a good valvotomy that eliminates the gradient is obtained in 80% of patients;
4. with the use of preoperative anticoagulants the embolic rate is virtually nil.

The main disadvantages of the closed procedure are the risks of dislodging calcific or thrombotic emboli, the risk of tearing the valve and producing mitral regurgitation, and the difficulty in producing a complete valvotomy with separation of both commissures. These points are dealt with in the review of my patients.

Hospital complications

In the 60 patients there was only one early death and this from a Gram-negative septicaemia. Two patients had postcardiotomy syndrome requiring treatment. Only one patient developed a pleural collection of fluid sufficient to warrant aspiration.

Later complications

There were three late deaths, one from a cerebral embolism $2\frac{1}{2}$ years after operation, one from congestive heart failure and a chest infection in a very poorly split valve, and the third after open heart surgery for replacement of the tricuspid valve.

Quality of valvotomy

In all patients at least one commissure was fully split, but in only one patient in three were both commissures split. Experience has shown that repeated efforts to split a second commissure after the first has been opened often result in tearing of the valve and the production of regurgitation. Experience has also shown that a good split of one commissure usually results in the elimination of the gradient. However, it would seem probable that the incidence of restenosis would be higher in those patients who have only had one commissure divided.

Regurgitation

Three patients were found to have some mitral reflux at the time of operation, but in none of these was the regurgitation increased after valvotomy. Regurgitation was additionally produced in seven patients (11%) but was never more than slight in degree. In three patients followed up all evidence of regurgitation had disappeared, but in the four others a systolic murmur persisted.

CLINICAL RESULTS

Of 41 patients assessed clinically there were good or excellent results in 35 of them, or 83%. Only one patient to date has required valve replacement.

HAEMODYNAMIC RESULTS

Of 31 patients assessed either by echocardiography or catheterization and angiography, 24 have signs of mild or minimal mitral stenosis with or without slight regurgitation and can be regarded as entirely satisfactory. In seven patients (23%) there was more severe stenosis and/or regurgitation and it would seem likely that valve replacement would be required at some future date.

IN SUMMARY

Closed mitral valvotomy gives excellent clinical and haemodynamic results in over 80% of patients selected on the basis of a thin and pliable valve. The operation can be carried out expeditiously with minimal requirements of blood and without the necessity for cardiopulmonary bypass.

4

Open mitral valvotomy

S. C. LENNOX

There is still considerable controversy as to whether mitral stenosis should be treated by an open or closed operation. The results of closed mitral valvotomy are well known. However, at a time when more sophisticated techniques of repair are available it must be remembered that valvotomy is only suitable for those patients with pure mitral stenosis, and therefore the results of the operation are dependent upon accurate selection. This is of course less critical when an open operation is performed. The appropriate operation, whether it be valvotomy, repair or replacement, can be decided at the time of operation. Many people regard this as the weakness of advising patients to have an open operation since they feel that the tendency will be to replace the valve rather than to perform a conservative operation. The purpose of this paper is to attempt to assess the place of open valvotomy. Since 1968 I have only performed open operations for mitral valve disease. At the onset I decided that all patients referred for valvotomy would have a conservative operation, irrespective of the state of the valve found at operation.

Between July 1968 and July 1975, 111 patients underwent operation (Table 1). Of these 100 had a valvotomy alone, while 11 patients had a mitral valvotomy plus aortic valve replacement. There was one early death in this series and one late death, both in patients who had a lone mitral valvotomy.

In this series there was the usual female bias, with 76 females compared to 24 males and their ages ranged from 14 to 64 years, the majority being

Table 1 Open mitral valvotomy (July 1968–July 1975)

Number of patients	111
Mitral valvotomy alone	100
Mitral valvotomy plus AVR	11
Early mortality	1
Late mortality	1

AVR = aortic valve replacement

between 30 and 60 years old (Table 2.); 17 patients had had a previous operation, 11 had one closed valvotomy, five two valvotomies, and one had had an aortic valve replacement and mitral valvotomy (Table 3). In 12 patients there was a large amount of clot present in the left atrium and this had to be removed. Four patients required control of a small amount of regurgitation following the valvotomy by annuloplasty, and a further patient required a tricuspid annuloplasty; 31 patients had significantly calcified valves.

Table 2 Open mitral valvo-tomy (July 1968–July 1975)

Female	76
Male	24
Ages	
14–20	4
21–30	9
31–40	27
41–50	30
51–60	22
61–64	6

Table 3 Open mitral valvotomy (July 1968–July 1975)

Previous Operations	
One closed valvotomy	11
Two closed valvotomies	5
AVR plus valvotomy	1
Additional Procedures	
Removal of clot	12
Mitral annuloplasty	4
Tricuspid annuloplasty	1
Calcified Valves	
Number of patients	31

AVR = aortic valve replacement

These patients have been followed up from 21 to 105 months with an average follow-up of 59.25 months. During this time two patients have died (one early death), six patients have required mitral valve replacement, one patient is only moderately well, while the remaining 89 are in good health. Two patients had neurological lesions following operation, one has made a complete recovery, while the other has still some residual defect. There have been three embolic episodes, all during the first year following operation, but none of these has left neurological problems. Many patients with atrial fibrillation have been electively anticoagulated and this has probably altered the embolic rate. Two patients had a postpericardiotomy syndrome, while one patient had a major wound dehiscence (Table 4).

On examination 64 patients have murmurs (Table 5). In 33 there is only a systolic murmur present. However, these patients have got a small heart and no haemodynamic evidence of significant mitral regurgitation. More

50

Table 4   Open mitral valvotomy (July 1968–July 1975)

Mortality	
Early	1
Late	1
Morbidity	
Neurological	
Early	2
Late (2–12 months)	3
Post-pericardiotomy syndrome	2
Wound dehiscence	1

Table 5   Open mitral valvotomy (July 1968–July 1975)

Post-operative murmurs	64
Systolic murmur only	33
No murmurs	34

recently these patients would have had some form of repair to correct the small amount of regurgitation. Six patients have required mitral valve replacement. Five of these had severely calcified valves and these were replaced from 16 days to 15 months after operation. One patient had mixed mitral valve disease and had his valve replaced at 12 months. None of these patients had done well after operation and in retrospect should have had replacement at the first procedure (Table 6).

Table 6   Mitral valve replacement

16 days	Calcified valve
7 months	Calcified valve
15 months	Calcified valve
14 months	Calcified valve plus failed annuloplasty
5 months	Disorganized valve
12 months	Mixed valve disease

The advantages of open mitral valvotomy include the following:

1. the clot can be removed at the time of operation;
2. the valve can be examined visually and therefore the optimum procedure can be performed;
3. full valvotomy can be achieved;
4. if regurgitation is produced this can be controlled by repair;
5. if the valve is unsuitable it can be replaced;
6. this procedure can be demonstrated to others and therefore is helpful in training junior staff;
7. at the same time other valve lesions can be dealt with.

In comparing the results with those in closed valvotomy our experience shows that there is no increase in mortality or morbidity, and indeed these two parameters are less than the average attributed to the closed operation.

Considering the economics of the operation, undoubtedly it costs more to perform an open operation and one requires the added equipment and manpower associated with open heart surgery. However, this added cost has to be equated with the possibilities of achieving a better operation. This, I believe, can now be obtained.

5

Reconstruction of the mitral valve

M. PANETH

Before attempting to repair a malfunctioning mitral valve, a clear concept of its anatomical components must be borne in mind (Table 1). Each of these components may make a separate contribution to malfunction, and before a repair is attempted such contributions must be accurately assessed.

Table 1 Anatomical components of mitral valve apparatus

1. Annulus	4. Chordae tendinae
2. Leaflets	5. Papillary muscles
3. Commissures	6. Left ventricular wall

From January 1975 to June 1976, 209 procedures on the mitral valves were carried out either in isolation or with other intracardiac procedures, such as aortic and tricuspid valve repair or replacement (Table 2). In more than 50% of these cases a conservative procedure was carried out.

Table 2 Analysis of mitral surgery (January 1975–June 1976)

Conservative mitral operations		129
Mitral plication suture repairs	100	
Open mitral commisurotomy	17	
Closed mitral valvotomy	7	
Other repairs	5	
Mitral valve replacements (Björk–Shiley)		80

Analysing the first 100 consecutive repair procedures using the mitral plication suture, one can see that in 72 regurgitation was the predominant lesion, and in 15% the valve was calcified (Table 3).

Each sub-unit of the mitral valve complex received individual treatment. Thus, abnormal commissures were incised to within 2 mm of the ring,

Table 3 **Mitral plication suture repairs: patient data**

100 patients–58 women, 42 men		
Mean age–42.2 years (range 10–78)		
Predominant lesion–stenosis		28 patients
–regurgitation		72 patients
Atrial filbrillation		51 patients
Mitral valve calcium		15 patients
Detected preoperatively	7	
Found at operation	8	

calcification was removed restoring leaflet mobility, valve clefts or perforations were sutured or patched, and adherent chordae were separated; this separation included the corresponding papillary muscle which would be split longitudinally so as to increase the size of the subvalvular opening and permit free chordal action.

In any repair procedure the size of the anterior leaflet of the mitral valve and its relationship to the size of the mitral annulus will be the decisive factor. The posterior leaflet usually only acts as a baffle which the anterior leaflets float up against, thus closing the mitral orifice since, following rheumatic fever, thickening and rigidity of the posterior leaflet is almost a constant finding. Provided the anterior leaflet area is big enough to close a normal-sized orifice, and provided it can be mobilized sufficiently to float freely into the open and closed position, then a repair procedure has a high degree of success. The final step in the repair is the placement of the mitral plication suture (Figure 1) which stabilizes the annulus and will control regurgitation which occurs most frequently at the commissures. It consists of

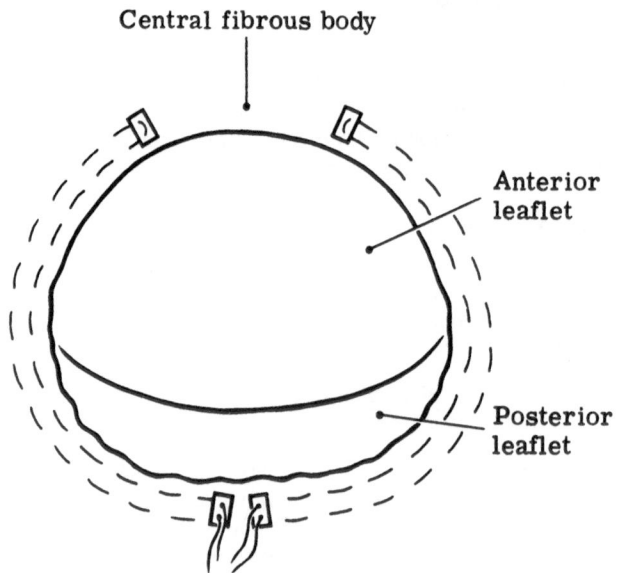

Figure 1 Placement of the mitral plication suture

a double suture of 2-O Ethiflex, guarded by teflon pledgets, sutured circumferentially around the annulus in 2–3 mm interlocking horizontal steps. It is best to start this suture, appropriate for each commissure, anteriorly at the margins of the central fibrous body and to proceed towards the posterior half of the mitral ring, centering each circumferential suture on its corresponding commissure. By tightening each suture in turn, regurgitation at its commissure can be controlled, and provided that (i) the area of the anterior leaflet is normal, and (ii) each suture is only tightened sufficiently just to control regurgitation, stenosis will not be produced. Although it at first would seem to be attractive to use only one continuous suture since the two posterior pledgets are close together in the double suture techniques, nevertheless it is important to realize that each suture controls its commissure independently and may require different tension and tightening from its fellow controlling the opposite commissure.

With experience the surgeon can very soon estimate that the repair is going to be effective, while the plication sutures are being placed, and to test the repair the left ventricle is filled by temporarily rendering the aortic valve regurgitant.

An analysis of the repairs is given in Table 4 with the deaths in parentheses. By immediate failure is meant that either the regurgitation could not be controlled, or to control it resulted in an unacceptable degree of stenosis. In these patients a prosthesis was inserted at the time.

Table 4   Analysis of repairs

	Number	Immediate Failures	Late Failures
Isolated mitral repair	52 (3)	8 (1)	5
Double valve repair			
MV and TCV	15	1	0
MV and AV	2	0	0
Mitral repair and AVR	29 (1)	1	0
+ TCV repair 8		0	2
+ TCV replacement 1		0	0
Mitral repair + CABG	1	0	0
Mitral repair + congenital	1 (1)	0	0
TOTAL	100 (5)	10 (1)	7

MV = mitral valve; TCV = tricuspid valve; AV = aortic valve; CABG = coronary artery bypass graft

Late failures were treated by mitral valve replacement at a subsequent operation, but in only two patients was the failure found to be due to the plication suture cutting out. In the others mitral valve replacement became necessary because the degree of mitral regurgitation or stenosis had been underestimated at the first reparative procedure.

POSTOPERATIVE ASSESSMENT

We believe that the best non-invasive assessment of mitral valve function is obtained by analysing left ventricular filling rate. Using real-time M-mode echocardiograms, linear traces of left ventricular dimension and rate of change of cavity size were derived. The 'peak rate of dimension change' (PRDC) was developed which indicates the instantaneous distance relationship between the anterior and posterior walls of the left ventricle with time and then reflects peak volume of blood flow through the mitral valve (Table 5).

Table 5   Comparison: repairs and replacement valves

	PRDC	Filling pattern
Normal mitral valve	10–20	Normal
Mitral plication suture repaired valve	8–23	Normal
Björk–Shiley valve	8–10	Abnormal
Hancock porcine valve	8	Abnormal
Starr–Edwards	6	Abnormal

PRDC = 'peak rate of dimension change' in cm/s

This new measurement can indicate whether the valve orifice is normal (10–20 cm/s), stenotic (10 cm/s), or regurgitant (20 cm/s). Not all patients have been studied by this technique but 23 out of 31 patients had normal PRDC values; four were in the mildly stenotic range and four more were mildly regurgitant (Table 6).

Table 6   Postoperative echocardiogram

PRDC*	Number	Late failures
10 cm/s (stenotic)	4	1
10–20 cm/s (normal)	23	1
20 cm/s (regurgitant)	4	1

PRDC = 'peak rate of dimension change', the peak rate of change of left ventricular transverse diameter by echocardiography.
Unit of measurement: centimetres per second (cm/s)
Normal range: 10–20 cm/s

The technique and results represent the first 18 months of an aggressively conservative approach to the mitral valve. All patients were unselected and all were considered initially to be reparable irrespective of the presence of calcium, multiple valve lesions, previous surgery or advanced disease. During the first 12 months of this 18-month period, 67 out of 137 patients were repaired and this rate (49%) is higher than that reported by others.

During the last 6 months a further 56 repairs have been performed with two deaths and two failures resulting in a 4.5% mortality for this procedure overall, whether performed in isolation or combined with tricuspid repair and/or aortic valve replacement.

The technique is simple and reliable and maintains annulus flexibility. Though the follow-up period is short, there is so far no reason to believe that deterioration in function will occur later.

SUMMARY AND CONCLUSIONS

(1) Mitral valve repair with the technique described can be carried out with a high degree (90%) of success.

(2) The failure rate and mortality (4.5%) are decreasing with experience.

(3) Systematic assessment and treatment of each anatomical component of the mitral valve complex is essential.

(4) The technique is simple, effective and cheap.

(5) Echocardiographic measurement of peak ventricular filling rate is a better index of the function of the mitral valve than the diastolic closure rate, since the latter may simply indicate a stiff valve which by itself need not interfere with left ventricular filling. Using this index the satisfactory repairs are superior to any commonly used mitral prosthesis.

6

Fluid dynamics of prosthetic heart valves

D. E. M. TAYLOR

The initial intention in the development of prosthetic heart valves was to provide a substitute for the normal and it was hoped that when a prosthetic valve, whether of biological or of non-biological origin, was inserted it would behave in a manner analogous to the normal valve. Increasing experience, however, is showing that the behaviour of prosthetic valves approximates to that of the diseased valve which it is replacing rather than to the normal valve[1-3], the difference between the two being merely one of degree. Thus, all prosthetic valves at present in use are associated with a degree of stenosis and also with a degree of regurgitation, closure being determined by flow reversal rather than by other fluid dynamic forces. To understand the reasons for this type of behaviour and, therefore, to be in a position to lay down criteria for improved valves, one has to consider the behaviour of the normal, the diseased and the prosthetic valve from two points of view. Firstly, the types of flow pattern which occur in the vicinity of valves and secondly, the way in which the energy loss (that is the fall in pressure head across the valve) is determined. The latter has three components: a frictional component accounted for by the viscosity of blood and being related directly to the cardiac output; an inertive loss due to the energy required for acceleration and deceleration of blood not fully recovered, which is related to the heart rate; and a turbulent loss which is related to the square of the cardiac output [4,5].

FLOW PATTERN

Far from being the complete mixing system with established turbulence as was formerly thought, it is now known that the flow patterns within the heart and around the cardiac valves are a stable system. This has been shown both in model studies[6,7] and in *in vivo*[8,9]. In the case of the aortic valve, the valve goes to a position such that the free cusp margins have a wider diameter than the valve orifice and a vortex system forms behind the cusps within the sinuses of Valsalva, this being a major factor causing closure of the heart valve[6]. For the mitral valve a stable vortex system is also formed. Here the jet of blood entering through the mitral valve diverges in the region of the cardiac apex to form vortices behind the cusps, that in the outflow track region tending to be larger than that formed behind the posterior cusp (Figure 1).

In both situations there is only transient turbulence and valve closure is determined largely by fluid dynamic factors with a zero regurgitant fraction[7,9].

When one considers the diseased valve, the flow patterns are totally different, particularly where there is marked stenosis. A rapid jet passes through the valve and in the region beyond the cusp margin degenerates into turbulent flow (Figure 2). Little or no stable vortiseal patterns form and valve

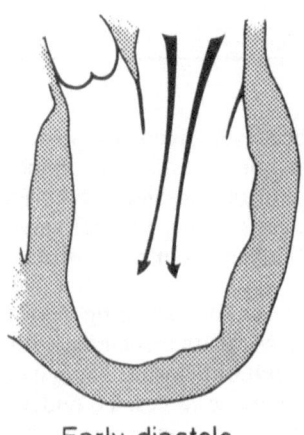

Early diastole

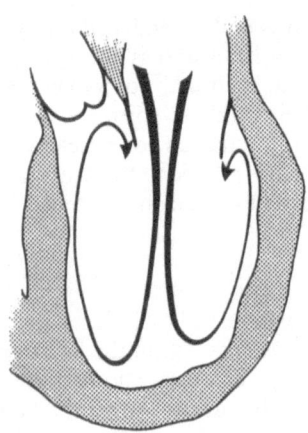

Mid diastole

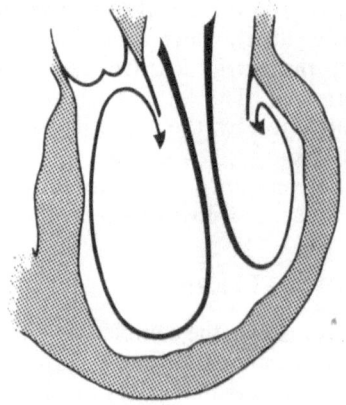

Late diastole

Figure 1 Flow patterns around a normal mitral valve during diastolic filling. Note the formation of stable vortex systems on the ventricular aspects of the cusps

closure, if it is possible, is determined by a reversal of flow and is, therefore, accompanied by a regurgitant fraction[2].

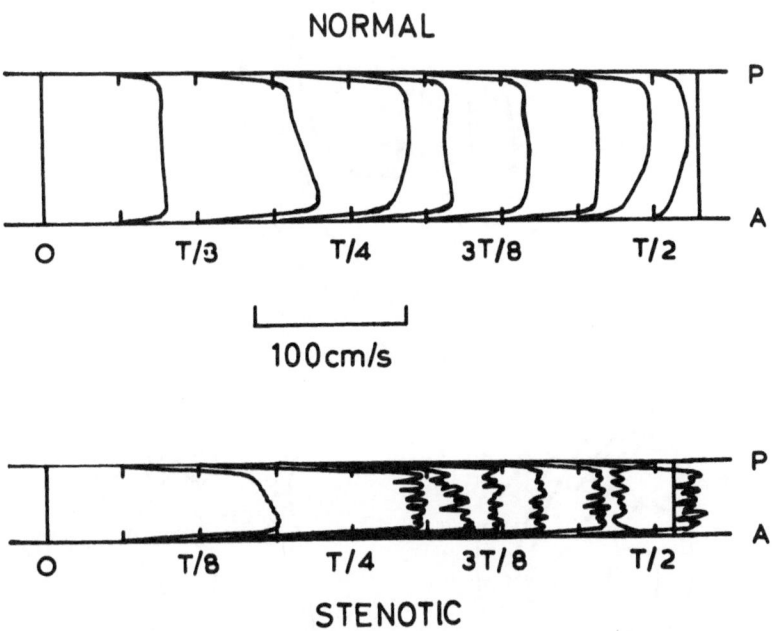

Figure 2 Velocity profile through a normal and a stenotic mitral valve. The profile is smooth for the normal valve, indicating a stable flow system without turbulence, but for the stenotic valve there are much higher velocities and marked turbulence. Note also that there is a period of backflow before closure with the stenotic valve

The prosthetic valves which have been studied, both *in vitro*[1,3] and *in vivo*[2], may show the formation of vortices, but while these are stable in valves such as the Björk–Shiley (Figure 3) they are not stable and tend to break up into turbulence in central occluder valves such as the Starr-Edward or Beall[1-3]. In addition the forces which develop on the occluder will not tend to close the valve as forward flow ceases, so that closure must always be accompanied by reversal of flow and therefore a regurgitant fraction, which can be from 3 to 30%, tending to be greatest at low heart rates associated with additional leakage throughout the closed phase[3]. In addition, the forces produced by the flow patterns around the occluder tend to give partial closure after the early stage of filling, so that although on immediate opening the valve will have primary and secondary flow orifices of the dimensions one would deduce from a physical examination of the valve, in the fully opened position that once flow has become established the occluder tends to return towards the partly closed position, resulting in a reduction in the size of the secondary orifice (Figure 4)[2]. This effect accentuates the relative stenosis necessitated by the primary orifice being smaller than the annulus of the excised valve[1].

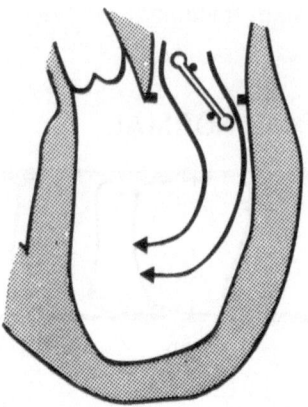

Early diastole

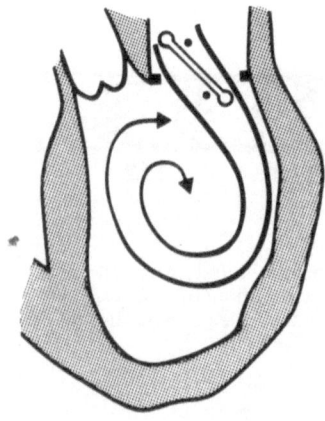

Mid diastole

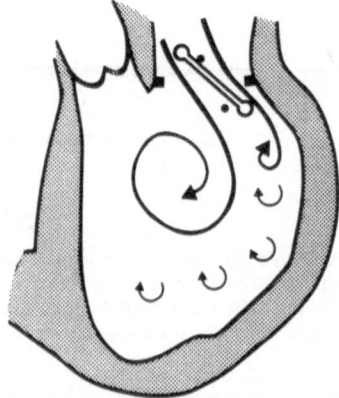

Late diastole

Figure 3 Flow patterns around a Björk–Shiley valve in the mitral position during diastolic filling. Although flow initially is stable with the formation of a single vortex, in late diastole the occluder partially closes and while a central vortex is still present flow adjacent to the wall becomes turbulent

ENERGY LOSS PATTERNS

As has been stated previously there are three main sources of energy loss in a valve. In a very simple mathematical form it may be stated as:

$$\varDelta E = AV + BV^2 + C\dot{V}$$

where $\varDelta E$ = energy loss
V = velocity
$\dot{V}$ = acceleration (rate of change of velocity).

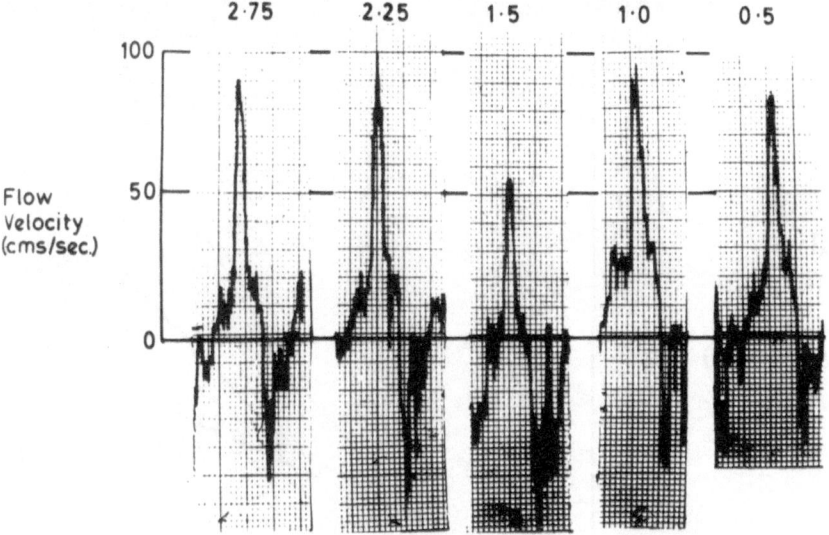

Figure 4 Velocity tracings across the aorta 2 cm distal to a Starr–Edward Ball valve in the aortic portion. The tracings are irregular, indicating turbulence, and there is an annular jet at the tertiary orifice with a zone of marked flow disturbance in the centre of the stream. Note the backflow phase before valve closure

At a simple orifice almost the entire loss is accounted for by the turbulent fraction, the pressure drop being related to the square of the velocity. This forms the basis of the various area formula, such as that of Gorlin and Gorlin[10]. The energy loss across the healthy valve falls between the square law predicted for a turbulent loss and the linear relationship predicted for flow along a tube (Figure 5)[5,11].

Applying AC electrical theory, the fluid resistance will be equivalent to electrical resistance and the turbulent and inertive losses will correspond to the reactance of an electrical circuit. Carrying out this type of AC analysis on pressure drops it has been shown[12] that although the resistive loss follows a predicted relationship the reactive loss shows only a slight change over a wide range of pulse rates and cardiac outputs. In electrical terms this is equivalent to impedance matching and has been reported previously in the vascular system with respect to the aorta[13].

In simple terms what this means is that the normal valve, and the portions of the circulation adjacent to it, behave so that they adapt over a wide range of pulse rate and cardiac output to optimize the loss of pressure head. Therefore, a great range of cardiac output is obtainable without imposing an unnecessarily large change in the pressure head required to get blood through the valve region. Such impedance matching does not occur at the stenotic valve[14], where both resistive and reactive forces behave in the manner one would predict of a fixed circuit analogue showing no adaptation.

The prosthetic valves, in terms of the constituents of pressure loss, behave in a manner very similar to that of the stenotic valve[2,3] and, therefore,

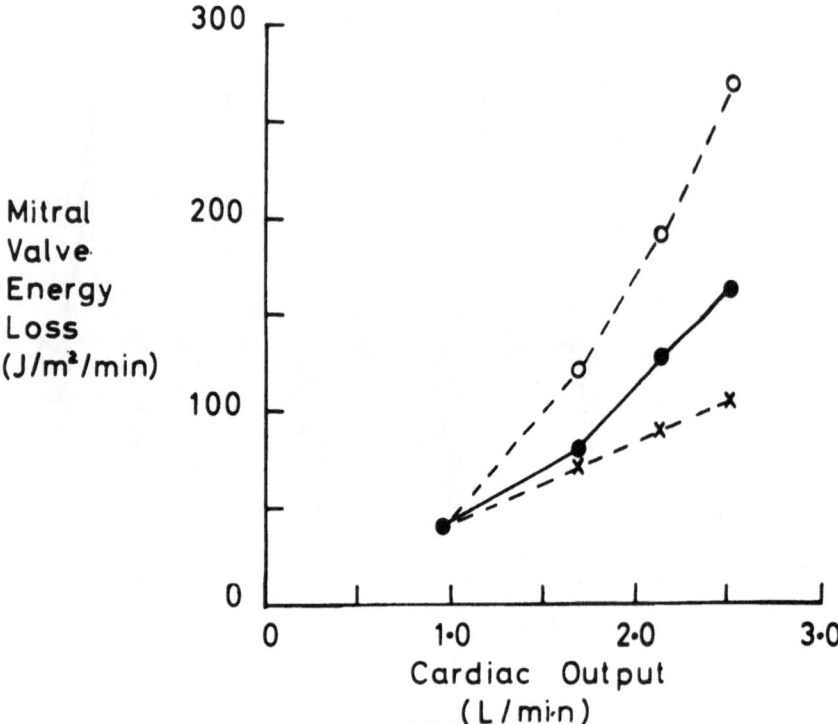

Figure 5 Loss of energy across a normal mitral valve compared to that for stream line flow in a tube (lower) and flow through an orifice (upper). Most prosthetic valves and all stenotic valves behave in the manner predicted for the orifice model

although a valve may show a satisfactory pressure drop at a low cardiac output, its performance is less than satisfactory when one considers the high cardiac output of exercise or the increased pulse rate produced by emotional stress.

SUMMARY AND CONCLUSION

Studies over recent years have shown that prosthetic valves generally show flow patterns and energy loss patterns analogous to those seen with the diseased valve, rather than those encountered in the normal. There are qualitative differences between different types of valve, so that a valve which is satisfactory at a low heart rate, may be less satisfactory at a high heart rate[3,5].

At the present state of cardiac surgery, other causes of morbidity with prosthetic valve, such as thromboembolism, are of far more significance than haemodynamic factors. Should the present major causes of morbidity be successfully countered, one must take serious account of the current haemodynamic failings of prosthetic valves and an endeavour should be made to produce a valve which will show a behaviour pattern similar to that of the normal valve. The latter is one which is capable of adaptation so as to minimize energy losses over a wide range of pulse rates and cardiac outputs, and one which shows the formation of stable flow patterns around the valve and in the circulation in the immediate vicinity.

Acknowledgment

This work was carried out under grants from the British Heart Foundation, the Scottish Home and Health Department and the Freemason's Anniversary Trust.

References

1. Bellhouse, B. J. and Bellhouse, F. H. (1976). Fluid mechanic performance of five prosthetic mitral valves. In D. Kalmanson (ed.). *The Mitral Valve*, p. 247. (Acton, Mass.: Publishing Sciences Group)
2. Taylor, D. E. M. and Whamond, Joan S. (1976). Velocity profiles and impedance of prosthetic mitral valves. In D. Kalmanson (ed.). *The Mitral Valve*, p. 261. (Acton Mass.: Publishing Sciences Group)
3. Wright, J. T. M. (1976). Flow dynamics in prosthetic valves—an assessment of hydrodynamic performance. In D. Kalmanson (ed.). *The Mitral Valve*, p. 271. (Acton, Mass.: Publishing Sciences Group)
4. Yellin, E. L., Laniado, S., Peskin, C. and Frater, R. (1976). Analysis and interpretation of the normal mitral valve flow curve. In D. Kalmanson (ed.). *The Mitral Valve*, p. 163. (Acton, Mass.: Publishing Sciences Group)
5. Taylor, D. E. M. and Whamond, Joan S. (1977). The assessment of haemodynamic function of diseased and prosthetic heart valves in patients. *J. Med. Eng. Technol.* **1**, 81
6. Bellhouse, B. J. and Talbot, L. (1969). The fluid mechanics of the aortic valve. *J. Fluid Mech.*, **35**, 721
7. Bellhouse, B. J. (1972). Fluid mechanics of a model mitral valve and left ventricle. *Cardiovasc. Res.*, **VI**, 199
8. Hider, C. F., Taylor, D. E. M. and Wade, J. D. (1966). Action of the mitral and aortic valves *in vivo* studied by encloscopic ciné photography. *Q. J. Exp. Physiol.*, **51**, 372
9. Taylor, D. E. M. and Wade, J. D. (1973). Pattern of blood flow within the heart: a stable system. *Cardiovasc. Res.*, **VII**, 14
10. Gorlin, R. and Gorlin, S. G. (1951). Hydraulic formula for calculation of the area of the stenotic mitral valve, other cardiac valves, and central circulatory shunts. *Am. Heart J.*, **41**, 1
11. Taylor, D. E. M. (1972). Mitral valve geometry and flow dynamics at varying heart rates in the dog. *J. Physiol.*, **227**, 37
12. Carnie, Norah, Mukhtar, A. I., Pollock, C. G., Taylor, D. E. M. and Whamond, Joan S, (1973). Impedance spectra change across the aortic valve at different heart rates in the sheep. *J. Physiol.*, **238**, 48
13. Abel, F. L. (1971). Fourier analysis of left ventricular performance. *Circ. Res.*, **28**, 119
14. Eastell, R., Taylor, D. E. M. and Whamond, Joan S. (1975). Impedance change to differing heart rate and cardiac output across the acutely stenosed aortic valve. *J. Physiol.*, **248**, 33

7

Aortic homograft valves for mitral valve replacement

M. YACOUB

The early and long-term survival, as well as the quality of life after mitral valve replacement can be influenced by the type of valve substitute used. The 'ideal' valve substitute has not, as yet, been found; therefore it is felt that it is essential to continue to evaluate, critically, the results achieved by using different valve substitutes.

The purpose of this chapter is to analyse the results of the use of fresh antibiotic-sterilized aortic homografts inserted without the use of metal stents, as previously described[1].

PATIENTS AND METHODS

Between August 1969 and October 1976, 493 patients underwent aortic homograft replacement of the mitral valve at Harefield Hospital. Of these 329 had isolated mitral valve replacement (Figure 1), 164 had either additional valve replacement or other procedures. The details of these procedures are listed in Figure 1. The percentage of patients undergoing mitral valve replacement, when compared with the total number of patients having open operations on the mitral valve over the years, is shown in Figure 2. In 1970 approximately 75% of patients had replacement; in contrast, in 1976, only 15% required replacement. This is probably due to the fact that with further experience in valve-conserving operations it is possible to conserve most valves. Of 377 patients undergoing mitral valve replacement without replacement of the aortic valve, 329 underwent isolated replacement, while the rest underwent additional procedures. Details of these are shown in Figure 3. The age and sex distribution of the total number of patients (493) is shown in Table 1. All patients were severely symptomatic. Advanced age, severe pulmonary hypertension, or the presence of additional valve or coronary artery disease, were not considered as a contra-indication to operation. The aetiology of the mitral valve lesion in the 377 patients undergoing single valve replacement is shown in Table 2. The methods of sterilization, storage and insertion have been previously described[1-3].

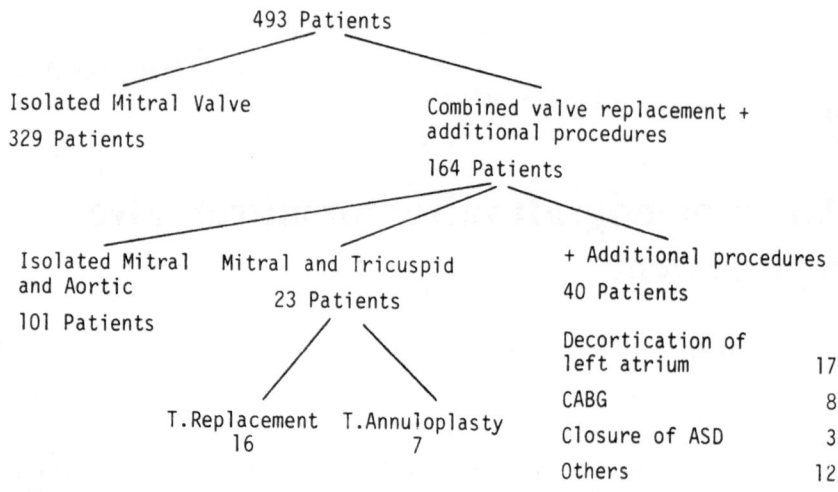

Figure 1 Aortic homograft replacement of mitral valve (Harefield Hospital August 1969–October 1976)

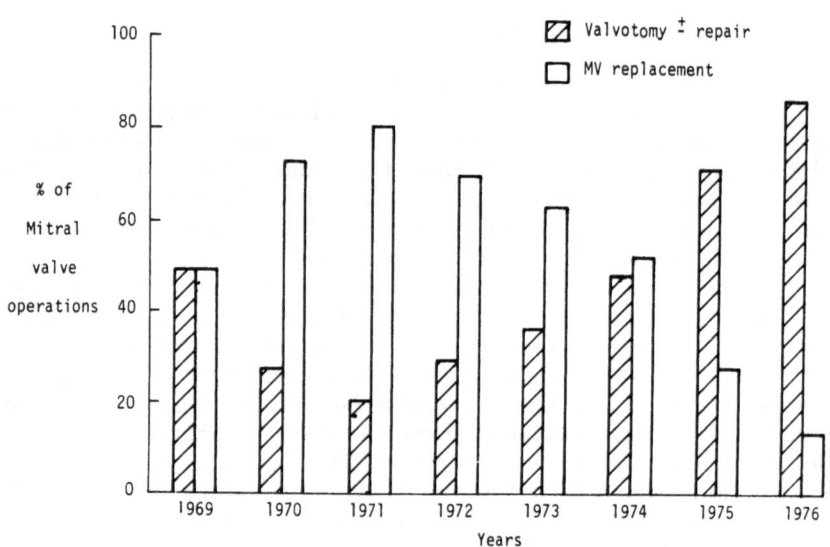

Figure 2 Yearly comparison of numbers of mitral valve repairs and replacements (Harefield Hospital)

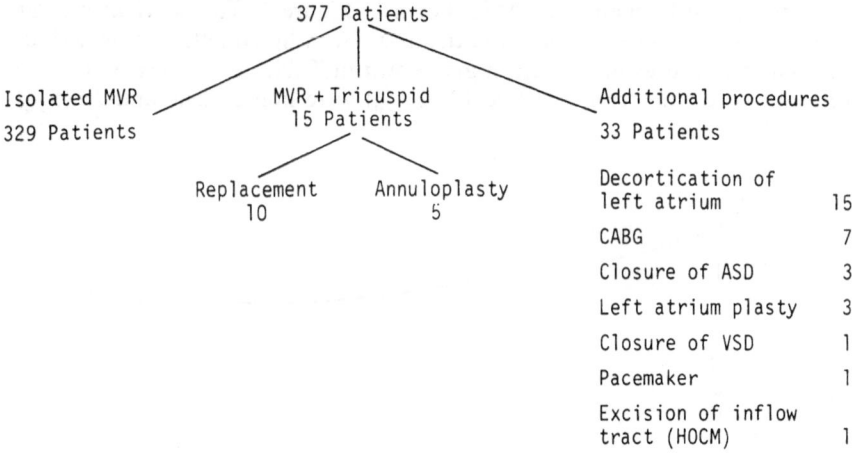

Figure 3 Aortic homograft replacement of mitral valve (Harefield Hospital August 1969–August 1976)

Table 1 Aortic homograft replacement of the mitral valve (Harefield Hospital August 1969–January 1977) 377 patients–mean follow up 48 months, hospital and late mortality

Operation	No.	Early		Late		Total	
		No.	Percentage	No.	Percentage	No.	Percentage
MVR + additional procedure	377	37	9.8	61	16.0	98	25.8
Isolated MVR	329	27	8.2	50	15.1	77	23.3

MVR = mitral valve replacement

Table 2 Aortic homograft replacement of the mitral valve (Harefield Hospital August 1969–August 1976) 377 patients, aetiology of mitral valve lesion

	No.	Percentage
Rheumatic	318	84.5
Floppy	42	11.0
Ischaemic	15	4.0
Congenital	2	0.5

RESULTS

Early and late mortality

There were 53 early deaths within the first 4 weeks after operation; an early mortality of 10.8% for the total number of patients. Seventy-five patients died within the follow-up period, which varied between 6 weeks and 7 years (an average of 48 months). There was a late mortality of 15.2%. The mortality figures for the single valve replacement with, or without, additional procedures is shown in Table 1. Actuarial analysis of survival (using the method described by Berksen and Cage[4]) is shown in Figure 4. The survival rate at 7 years was 71%. The number of patients at risk, who completed this period, was 108. The causes of late death are shown in Table 3. Of these 38 (7.7%) were due to cardiac causes, while 12 (2.4%) were non-cardiac and 25 (5%) were unknown.

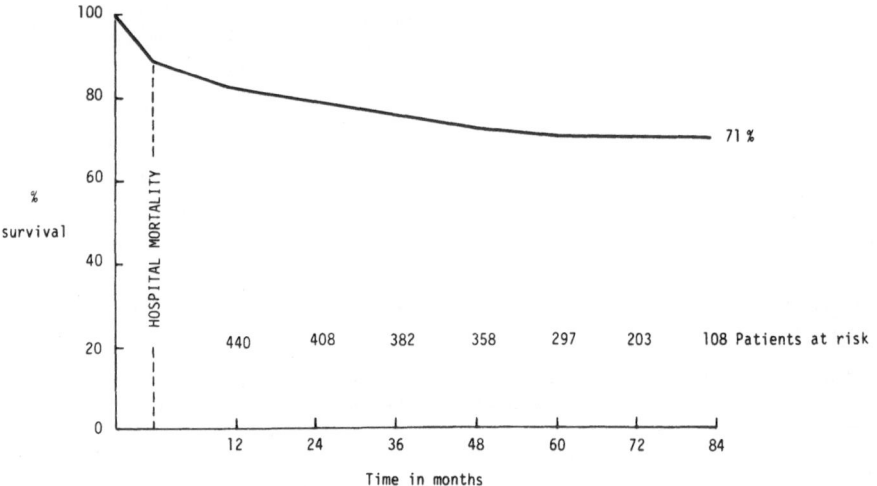

Figure 4 Aortic homograft replacement of mitral valve (Harefield Hospital August 1969–January 1977) 493 patients–mean follow up 48 months, actuarial survival for total MVR

Table 3 Aortic homograft replacement of the mitral valve (Harefield Hospital August 1969–January 1977) 493 patients, causes of late mortality

	No.	Percentage
A) CARDIAC		
Valve related complications	24	4.9
Congestive cardiac failure	9	1.8
Myocardial infarction	4	0.8
Pulmonary embolism	1	0.2
	38	7.7
B) NON-CARDIAC		
Renal failure	3	
Carcinoma of bronchus	1	
Carcinoma of colon	1	
Cerebrovascular accident	2	
Cerebral tumour	1	
Pneumonia	1	
Gastrointestinal haemorrhage	1	
Volvulus of sigmoid colon	1	
Road traffic accident	1	
	12	2.4
C) UNKNOWN	25	5.1

Valve failure

Failure of the homograft valve occurred in 16 patients (4.2%). Of these five (1.3%) were due to endocarditis and 10 (2.7%) to degenerative valve failure (Table 4). The incidence of valve failure as related to time and expressed as a percentage of patients at risk at different times after operation, is shown in Figure 5. Endocarditis tended to occur mainly during the first postoperative year with a smaller incidence over the next 5 years (also shown on Figure 5). Degenerative valve failure, resulting in calcification and stenosis or regurgitation (Figure 6), tended to occur after the third postoperative year (Figure 5). This latter complication occurred mainly in homografts taken from donors over the age of 70 years.

Table 4 Aortic homograft replacement of the mitral valve (Harefield Hospital August 1969–January 1977) 377 patients – follow-up 5–89 months – mean 47 months, mechanical valve failure

Complication		No.	Percentage
Endocarditis 5 ⟨ Fungal		2	0.5
Bacterial		3	0.8
Degenerative ⟨ Valve regurgitation		7	1.9
Valve stenosis		3	0.8
Valve distortion		1	0.2
TOTAL		16	4.2

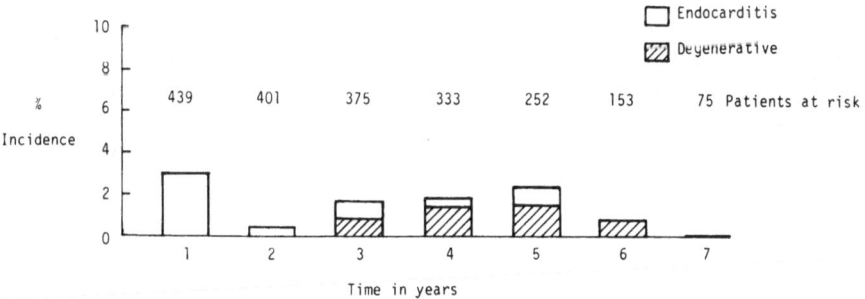

Figure 5 Aortic homograft replacement of mitral valve (Harefield Hospital August 1969– January 1977) 493 Patients–mean follow up 48 months, percentage incidence of valve failure with relation to time

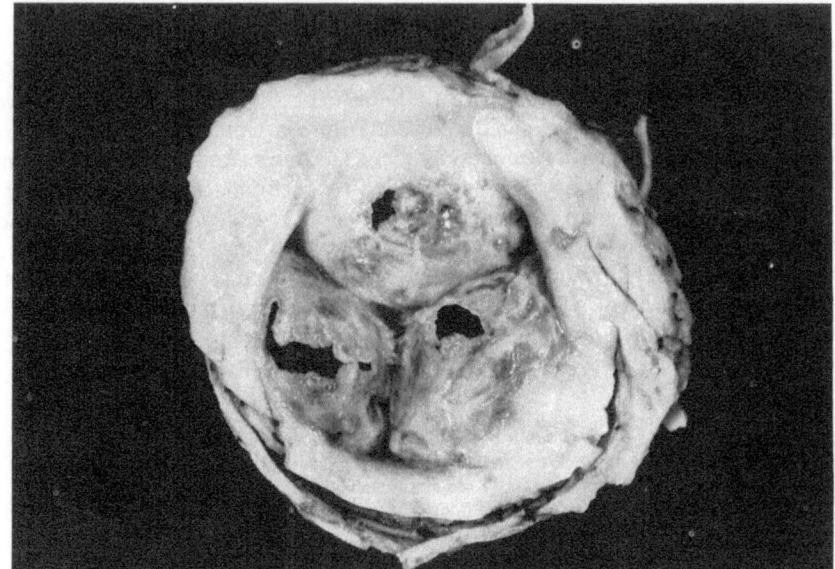

Figure 6   Degenerative valve failure

Thromboembolic complications

Anticoagulants were not used except if there was a specific indication, such as removal of clot from the left atrium or severe pulmonary hypertension and a low output state. Systemic embolism was encountered only on one occasion.

COMBINED HOMOGRAFT REPLACEMENT OF THE AORTIC VALVE AND AORTIC HOMOGRAFT REPLACEMENT OF THE MITRAL VALVE

Between August 1969 and October 1975, 116 patients underwent homograft replacement of the mitral and aortic valves. Additional procedures were performed in 15 of these patients (Figure 7). The age and sex distribution of these patients is shown in Table 5. The early and late mortality was similar to patients undergoing single valve replacement (Table 6). Mechanical valve failure occurred in seven patients (6%) and was due to fungal endocarditis in four (3.4%) and bacterial in one (0.1%), and valve degeneration in two patients (0.8%).

DISCUSSION

Analysis of our experience with the use of antibiotic-sterilized, unstented, aortic homograft valves for homograft replacement shows that this valve substitute gives satisfactory results for up to 7 years.

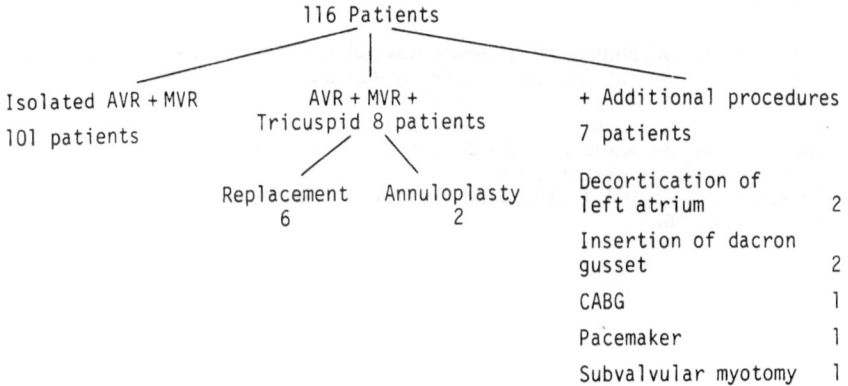

Figure 7 Combined aortic homograft replacement of aortic and mitral valves (Harefield Hospital August 1969–October 1975)

Table 5   Aortic homograft replacement of the mitral valve (Harefield Hospital August 1969–August 1976) 493 patients, age and sex distribution

Mitral valve replacement (377)	*Aortic and mitral valve replacement (116)*
Males 133 ⎫ Females 244 ⎭ mean age 50 years	Males 52 ⎫ Females 64 ⎭ mean age 48 years

Table 6   Combined aortic homograft replacement of aortic and mitral valves (Harefield Hospital August 1969–January 1977) 116 patients – mean follow-up 48 months, hospital and late mortality

		Early		*Late*		*Total*	
Operation	*No.*	*No.*	*Percentage*	*No.*	*Percentage*	*No.*	*Percentage*
MVR + AVR + additional procedure	116	16	13.8	14	12.0	30	25.5
Isolated MVR + AVR	101	12	11.9	13	12.8	25	24.7

AVR = aortic valve replacement
MVR = mitral valve replacement

The main advantages are freedom from thromboembolic episodes and better haemodynamic performance when compared to prosthetic or stented homografts. However, we believe that when compared to normal mitral valves they are relatively stenotic, particularly at fast heart rates and on exercise.

Infective endocarditis, involving the homograft, continues to carry a high mortality. The incidence of late, degenerative valve failure to date, has been relatively low, and appears to be related to the age of the donor.

Continued evaluation of the results of this valve substitute is required to define its performance for longer periods of time.

References

1. Yacoub, M. H. and Kittle, C. F., (1969). A new technique for replacement of the mitral valve by a semilunar valve homograft. *J. Thorac. Cardiovasc. Surg.*, **58**, 859
2. Yacoub, M. H., Knight, E. and Towers, M. K. (1973). Aortic valve replacement using fresh unstented homografts. *Thorax Chir.*, **21**, 451
3. Yacoub, M. H. and Kittle, C. F. (1970). Sterilisation of valve homografts by antibiotic solution. *Circulation*, **41** (Suppl. II), 19
4. Berksen, J. and Cage, R. P. (1956). Calculation of survival rates for cancer. *Proc. Staff Meet., Mayo Clinic*

8

Echocardiographic studies after mitral valve replacement

D. G. GIBSON

Echocardiography may be used to study patients after mitral valve surgery in two separate ways. The first of these, direct observation of the prosthesis[1] or homograft[2], has been valuable in determining its normal appearance and, in the case of mechanical prostheses, in detecting abnormalities of movement caused by degeneration or thrombosis. However, it is an approach with limitations, since records of this type may be totally normal in spite of severe malfunction. We have therefore found it more informative to direct our attention not primarily at the prosthesis, but at the effects of the prosthesis or homograft on the pattern of left ventricular wall movement during filling. Although direct inspection of the echocardiogram may give useful information, particularly in the presence of mitral paraprosthetic regurgitation[3], the value of the method can be considerably increased if a simple computing technique is used, and transverse left ventricular dimension, measured as the distance between the septum and posterior wall endocardium, is displayed continuously throughout the cardiac cycle.

The normal pattern of dimension change during diastole is shown in Figure 1, derived from the echocardiogram of a normal subject[4]. Here, the lowest trace represents changes in dimension with time, and the rate of change of dimension expressed in absolute units (cm/s) and in normalized terms (s^{-1}) at the top. The timing of mitral valve opening corresponds to minimum dimension. Following this, dimension increases rapidly at first, but during mid-diastole it changes little during the period of diastasis. This filling pattern is displayed even more clearly on the trace of rate of change of dimension with time. There is an early increase in the velocity of dimension increase, but within 200 ms, this trace has returned virtually to the baseline, marking the onset of the mid-diastolic period of diastasis. Using this curve, it is thus possible to describe the pattern of wall movement during filling in terms of the peak rate of increase of dimension and of the duration of the rapid filling period. The first of these is directly related to the peak rate of increase of volume, but an additional factor is ventricular size, since when the cavity is large a given rate of increase of volume causes a lower rate of increase of dimension than when it is normal. Angiographic studies have shown that this additional effect of cavity size is unimportant provided that end-diastolic dimension is less than 6 cm. Since a large left ventricle is relatively uncommon in mitral valve disease, this does not greatly restrict the use

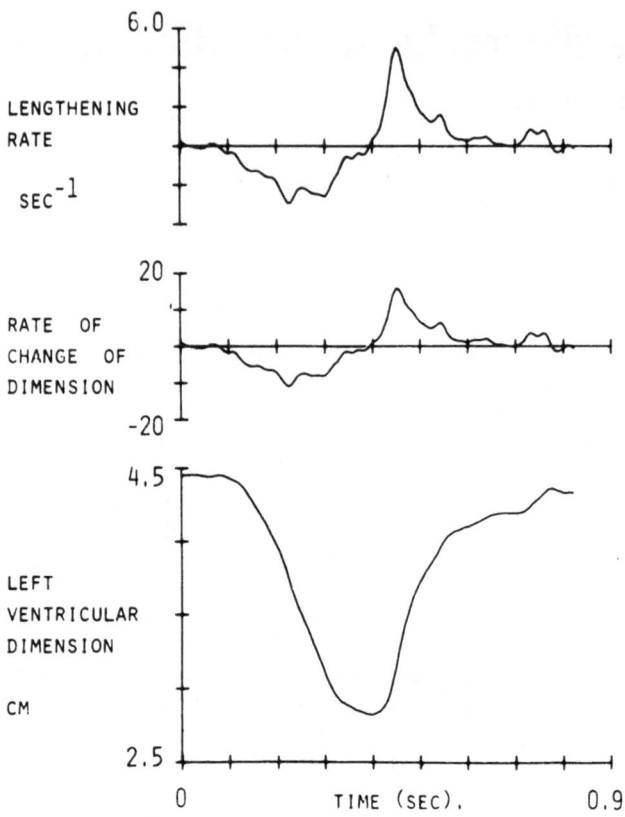

Figure 1 Normal left ventricular dimension and its rate of change during a single cardiac cycle

of the method. Rapid filling period also provides significant information about mitral valve performance, since overall cardiac function is unlikely to be significantly affected provided that the duration of diastole is greater than the rapid filling period. As heart rate increases, however, the duration of diastole is reduced, and if it becomes shorter than the rapid filling period, then inflow of blood into the left ventricle is either reduced, or maintained by increasingly large pressure gradients across the prosthesis. Rapid filling period thus gives an indication of the sensitivity of prosthetic function to tachycardia. In addition, angiography has shown that rapid filling period measured from transverse dimension is identical to that measured from the ventricular volume trace regardless of cavity size[5].

These ideas are illustrated in Figure 2, showing the computer output from a patient with a mitral Starr–Edwards prosthesis[3]. It is apparent that the peak rate of increase of dimension is less than normal, and that this low rate

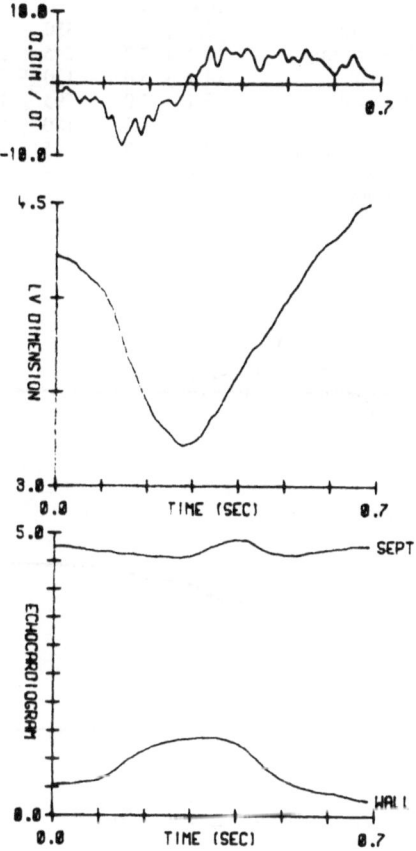

Figure 2   Changes in left ventricular dimension, from the echocardiogram of a patient with a mitral Starr–Edwards prosthesis

is maintained throughout diastole, with complete loss of the division into rapid early filling period and diastasis. Output from a patient with a Björk–Shiley prosthesis is shown in Figure 3, illustrating a more normal pattern. Values of peak rate of increase of dimension and rapid filling period from a variety of surgical procedures are given in Table 1. It is apparent that closed mitral valvotomy is associated with a significant improvement in filling pattern. The function of the Björk–Shiley prosthesis and the Hancock heterograft are remarkably similar in spite of the structural differences between the two, and that both give values significantly less abnormal than the

Table 1 Changes in left ventricular dimension after mitral valve surgery

Procedure	Peak diastolic dD/dt (cm/s)	Time to 20% Peak dD/dt (ms)
Normal	16.0 ± 3.2	160 ± 30
Mitral stenosis	7.2 ± 1.5	330 ± 65
Mitral valvotomy	10.4 ± 2.7	245 ± 55
Mitral repair	14.4 ± 5.0	170 ± 50
Starr–Edwards	7.4 ± 3.0	295 ± 110
Bjork–Shiley	10.5 ± 4.2	180 ± 80
Hancock heterograft	10.3 ± 3.7	245 ± 80

Mean values ± 1 SD

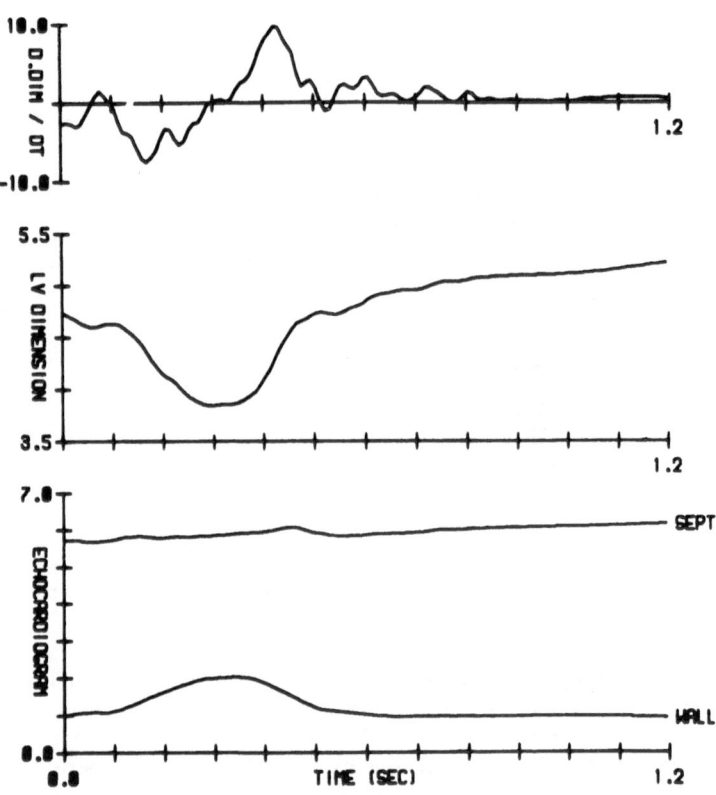

Figure 3 Changes in left ventricular dimension from a patient with a Björk–Shiley prosthesis

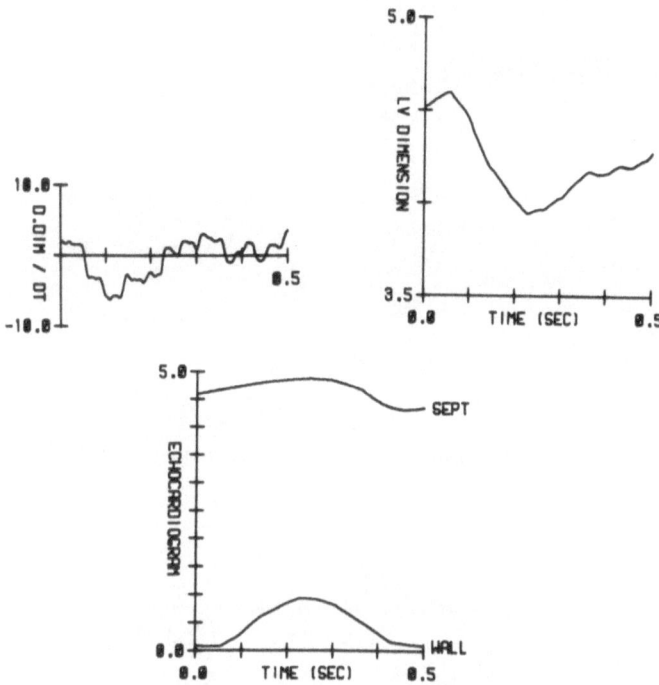

Figure 4   Changes in left ventricular dimension from the echocardiogram of a patient with an obstructed Björk–Shiley prosthesis

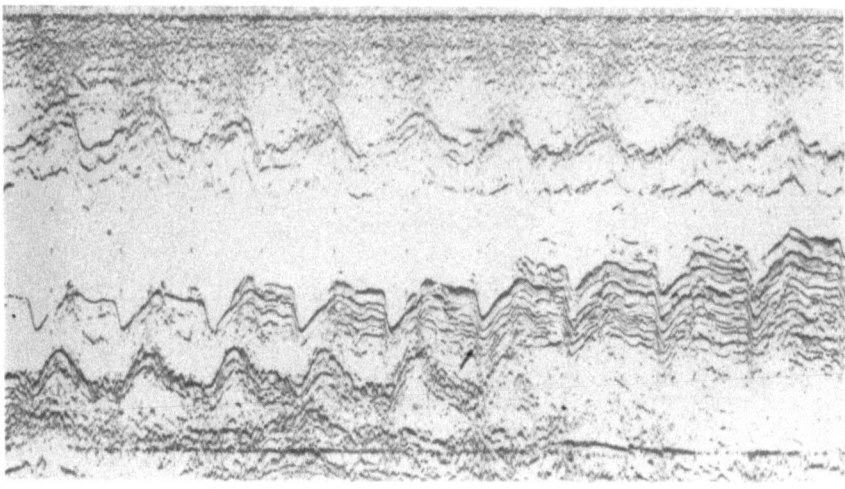

Figure 5   Slow scan from aortic root to left ventricular cavity, showing reduced movement of the disc of a Björk–Shiley prosthesis, due to thrombotic obstruction (compare Figure 4)

79

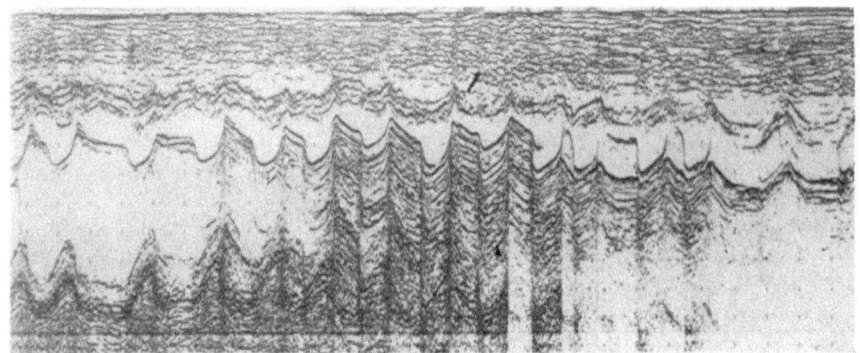

Figure 6 Slow scan from a patient with a normally functioning Björk–Shiley prosthesis

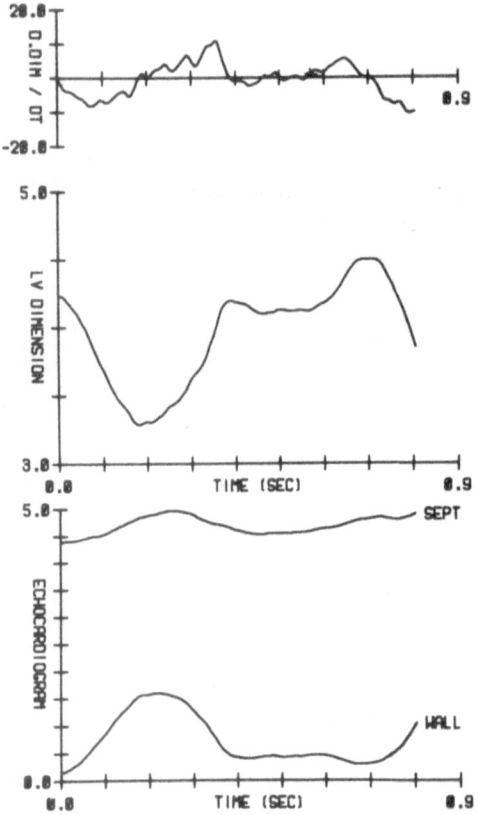

Figure 7 Changes in left ventricular dimension after treatment of patient with obstructed prosthesis with streptokinase

Starr–Edwards. Left ventricular filling after mitral valve reconstruction was virtually normal, both with respect to peak rate of dimension increase and rapid filling period. The reason for this is not clear, although recent studies with a complex three-dimensional finite element model of the left ventricle indicate that the presence of a rigid mitral ring is likely to have significant effects on the pattern of wall movement regardless of whether the valve is obstructive or not[6]. Nevertheless, these results provide the stimulus for further endeavours in the field of conservative mitral valve surgery.

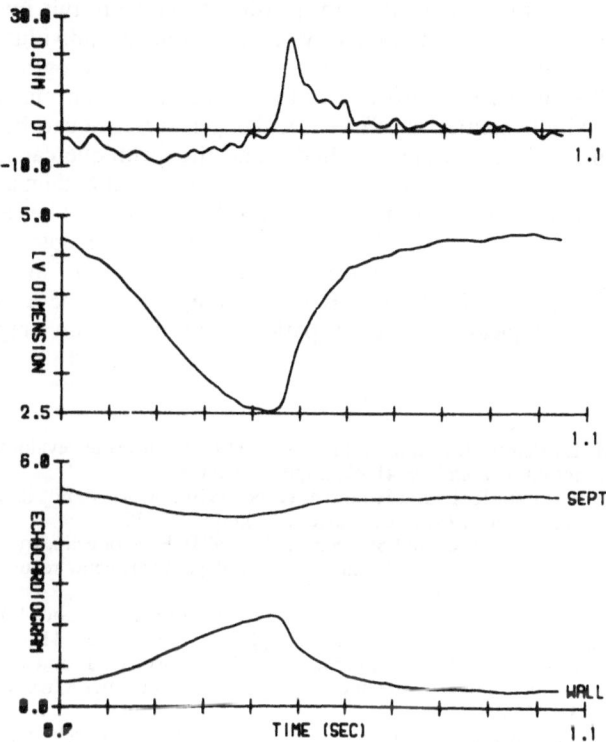

Figure 8 Changes in left ventricular dimension from the echocardiogram of a patient with a mitral Starr–Edwards paraprosthetic leak

The picture of left ventricular wall movement for any particular procedure given by this method is so consistent that departures can readily be recognized. Figure 4 shows the output from a patient who presented *in extremis* with an obstructed Björk–Shiley prosthesis; the filling pattern is clearly very abnormal. The underlying diagnosis was obvious clinically from loss of the valve clicks, and by observation of the prosthesis itself which showed impaired movement of the disc (Figure 5) compared to normal (Figure 6). Since it was not possible to proceed to immediate surgery, she was treated with streptokinase, and echocardiography was used to document progressive improvement in filling pattern over the next 24 h (Figure 7). Subsequently, mitral valve replacement was undertaken uneventfully.

Figure 8 shows the output from a patient in pulmonary oedema with a mitral Starr–Edwards prosthesis, who had a peak rate of increase of dimension of 30 cm/s, much greater than that seen with the normally functioning prosthesis. This indicated the presence of a paraprosthetic leak, which was confirmed at operation. A similar diagnosis has been made in 13 other cases.

There are now many thousands of patients who have undergone mitral valve replacement. Although postoperative cardiac catheterization is possible in selected groups of patients, it is not possible to perform this investigation on all of them, or on more than a very few occasions in individual patients. The present results show the potential value of echocardiography in this setting, in allowing various procedures to be compared, and malfunction to be detected. Abnormalities of left ventricular performance can be identified and analysed by closely related methods[7] and the technique can be used to assess the results of conservative procedures in individual patients, where the exact haemodynamic pattern of filling cannot be predicted. The technique is cheap, requiring only 2–3% of the capital and revenue costs of cardiac catheterization, totally safe, rapid and non-invasive, and can readily be performed on an outpatient basis. It therefore appears to be a satisfactory method of physiological follow-up of patients after mitral valve replacement.

References

1. Johnson, M. L., Paton, B. C. and Holmes, J. H. (1970). Ultrasonic evaluation of prosthetic valve motion. *Circulation*, **41–42**, Supp. II, page 3
2. Gianelly, R. E., Popp, R. L. and Hultgren, H. N. (1970). Heart sounds in patients with homograft replacement of the mitral valve. *Circulation*, **42**, 309
3. Miller, H. C., Gibson, D. G. and Stephens, J. D. (1973). Role of echocardiography and and phonocardiography in the diagnosis of mitral paraprosthetic regurgitation with Starr–Edwards prostheses. *Br. Heart J.*, **35**, 1217
4. Gibson, D. G. and Brown, D. J. (1973). Measurement of instantaneous left ventricular dimension and filling rate using echocardiography. *Br. Heart J.*, **35**, 1141
5. Sutton, M. G. St. J., Traill, T. A., Ghafour, A. S., Brown, D. J. and Gibson, D. G. (1977). Echocardiographic assessment of left ventricular filling after mitral valve surgery. *Br. Heart J.*, **39**, 1283
6. Vinson, C. (1977). Mechanical properties of the human left ventricle during diastole. (PhD thesis, Brunel University)
7. Gibson, D. G. (1978). Non-invasive study of left ventricular function. In D. Longmore (ed.) *Modern Cardiac Surgery* (Lancaster: MTP Press)

9

Haemolysis associated with prosthetic valves: cardiac haemolytic anaemia, red cell fragmentation syndrome

D. A. WATSON AND S. M. MANOHITHARAJAH

Haemolysis is a well-known complication following cardiac surgery. It was first documented in 1954 by Rose and co-workers following insertion of the Hufnagel prosthesis in the aorta[1]. The pathogenesis seemed obscure; at that time numerous postulates were made including an autoimmune mechanism, and interestingly some patients were treated with steroids and immuno-suppressive drugs and also had a splenectomy.

Although haemolysis is common, a haemolytic anaemia is uncommon. In the majority of patients the haemolysis is well compensated; erythropoiesis can be accelerated to ten times its average or normal capacity and maintain a reasonable haemoglobin. It is only when the haemolysis is excessive and persistent that erythropoiesis finally lags behind destruction of red cells leading to overt anaemia. This imbalance may become obvious sooner if the marrow becomes deficient in iron or folates.

It appears to occur with various types of aortic valves and also with mitral valve prosthesis. Significant haemolysis has been observed in patch repairs of ostium primum or endocardial cushion defects, in repair of aortic and mitral lesions and in tetralogy repair.

Why haemolysis takes place selectively, in some patients but not in others, is not quite clear. However, in cardiac haemolytic anaemia following the insertion of prosthetic devices, the existence of some form of haemodynamic defect has been present, and with valvular prostheses regurgitation around or through the prosthesis has been the most common finding. Observation and conjecture have pointed to turbulence, obstruction, pressure gradients, shearing forces, paravalvular leakage, bare Teflon, collision, crushing and size of valve as contributory factors to the haemolysis. A number of instances, however, have been reported in which overt haemolysis was present in the

MODERN CARDIAC SURGERY

Table 1 Incidence of overt and compensated haemolysis in both aortic and mitral ball valves and disc valves

Aortic valve	Overt*	Compensated
Aortic ball valve	127–5% 55–9% } 5–15% 54–11%	*72%/92%/90%
Disc valve (BS)	Uncommon (one case in Leeds)	35% (65%)
Mitral valve	*Overt*	*Compensated*
Mitral ball valve (SE)	*35–6% 14–7% } 5% 97–2%	⟋Mild 85% ⟍Moderate[2]
Disc valve (BS)	32–3%[3]	*35%/30%/15%[3]
Homograft	None	Normal red survival[2,3]

* The incidence of haemolysis reported in different centres.

absence of an obvious haemodynamic defect. Surface properties of prosthetic material could be of crucial importance because covering bare prosthetic patches with endocardium has minimized haemolysis[4]. In general all of these factors relate to only two aspects of the prosthesis – its surface characteristics and its function or dynamics.

The available evidence makes it most unlikely that patients who have developed haemolysis suffer from any intrinsic abnormality of the red cells. Red cell survival studies have clearly shown that the abnormality is due to an extracorpuscular defect.

Therefore haemolysis is intravascular due to mechanical fragmentation and it represents the sum of the contributing elements, which may vary individually but in the aggregate consist in the character and area of the impingement surface and the effective forces.

Investigations to determine the incidence and severity of haemolysis comprise estimation of haemoglobin, haematocrit, fragment count, reticulocyte count, LDH, haptoglobin, haemosiderin in the urine and red cell survival. Additional tests to exclude any other causes of haemolysis are direct Coombs' test, osmotic fragility, red cell enzyme screen, Hams' test and haemoglobin electrophoresis.

It is our practice to screen patients at the follow-up anticoagulant clinics with a haemoglobin estimation, blood film and test for haemosiderin in the urine.

TREATMENT

There is considerable evidence to support the prophylactic administration of iron supplements to the majority of patients with aortic and mitral ball valves and to any other patient with persistent haemosiderinuria[5,6]. In patients with excessive haemolysis and anaemia the standard régime is administration of iron, folates and blood transfusions. Reducing the work of the heart by reducing physical activities of the patient may be helpful.

84

HAEMOLYSIS ASSOCIATED WITH PROSTHETIC VALVES

In some patients blood transfusion actually restabilizes a vicious cycle of anaemia leading to cardiac failure, to increased red cell damage, to more haemolysis, to increased anaemia[7]. If these standard measures do not sustain an adequate haemoglobin level it may be obligatory to weigh the complications of long-term haemolysis and repeated blood transfusion against the risk of reoperation to correct any structural defect or valve replacement.

Avoidance of the problem at present lies in obtaining the best technical results from implantation. In the future avoidance lies in developing a valve material with the stability and inertness of the present hydrophobic materials but with surface characteristics more like those of endothelium.

References

1. Rose, J. C. Hufnagel, C. A., Freis, E. D., Harvey, W. P. and Partenope, E. A. (1954). The haemodynamic alterations produced by a plastic valvular prosthesis for severe aortic insufficiency in man. *J. Clin. Invest.*, **33**, 891
2. Donnelly, R. J., Rahman, A. N., Manohitharajah, S. M., Deverall, P. B. and Watson, D. A., (1973). Chronic haemolysis following mitral valve replacement. A comparison of the frame-mounted aortic homograft and the composite-seat Starr–Edwards prostheisis. *Circulation*, **48**, 16
3. Ahmad, R., Manohitharajah, S. M., Deverall, P. B., and Watson, D. A. (1976). Chronic haemolysis following mitral valve replacement. A comparative study of the Björk–Shiley, composite-seat Starr–Edwards and frame-mounted aortic homograft valves. *J. Thoracic Cardiovasc. Surg.*, **71**, 2
4. Sayed, H. M., Dacie, J. V., Handley, D. A., Lewis, S. M. and Cleland, W. P. (1961). Haemolytic anaemia of mechanical origin after open heart surgery. *Thorax*, **16**, 356
5. Donnelly, R. J., Rahman, A. N., Manohitharajah, S. M. and Watson, D. A. (1972). Anaemia with artificial heart valves. *Lancet*, **ii**, 283
6. Slater, S. D. and Fell, G. S. (1972). Intravascular haemolysis and urinary iron losses after replacement of heart valves by a prosthesis. *Clin. Sci.*, **42**, 545
7. Moisey, C. U., Manohitharajah, S. M., Tovey, L. A. D. and Deverall, P. B. (1972). Haemolytic anaemia in a child in association with congenital mitral valve disease. *J. Thoracic Cardiovasc. Surg.*, **63**, 5

10

Thromboembolism and valve failure: a multi-centre valve study

R. J. DONNELLY

In the practice of cardiac surgery there are a number of complications which cause emotional distress to the cardiac surgeon. These include air embolus and heart block at the time of surgery; after surgery it is probably thrombo-embolism, and particularly cerebral embolism, which provokes most disquiet. It is the attempt to overcome this problem which has been responsible for the plethora of heart valve substitutes appearing in the last 15 years or so and, indeed, the major impetus for the development of biological valves was an endeavour to reduce the risk of thromboembolism. The perfect valve sub-stitute has not yet arrived but, if it ever does, its first requirement will be a zero risk of thrombosis and embolus.

INCIDENCE OF THROMBOEMBOLISM

Major advances have been made in design and materials since the early prosthetic valves. Differing results, however, with the same valve models continue to be reported. In view of experience in recent years, there remains among cardiac surgeons a certain scepticism about claims made by manu-facturers with commercial interests and by surgeons whose reputation is tied to the results of some new or improved valve. Independent assessment is required but there are many difficulties in comparing results from different centres; these difficulties are compounded by the different statistical methods hitherto used in presenting results.

Some of these methods are unsatisfactory. For example a straight per-centage figure of a total patient population is sometimes given, with a com-ment that follow-up ranges from 6 months to 4 or 5 years. What does this mean in terms of risk to the individual patient? Even if the mean follow-up time is given, this is only an index of the quality of follow-up and does not mean that $x\%$ of patients are likely to have an embolus by y months of follow-up.

Similarly, the use of patient-months is unhelpful in determining risk to individual patients. Are four patients for 12 months at the same risk as 48 patients for 1 month? Clearly not. The use of patient-years has more value since the initial time unit is longer, but the same criticism applies although it is alleviated by the fact that the majority of embolic incidents may occur within the first 1–2 years.

Probably the most valid method of reporting the complications of valve replacement is on an actuarial basis, provided numbers are sufficient. In graphic form this demonstrates the percentage of patients who can be expected to be complication-free at determined time intervals after operation.

COMPARISON OF PROSTHETIC AND BIOLOGICAL VALVES

For most surgeons the major attraction of the prosthetic valve remains its durability, but there is no prosthetic valve which can be safely left in the mitral position without the administration of anticoagulants. There is little doubt that biological valves have a significant advantage with respect to the risk of thromboembolism. Only Starr has claimed parity in this respect for his cloth-covered valves, but anticoagulation remains necessary and this is an important consideration. There is a definite morbidity and mortality associated with the use of anticoagulants, estimated by Dr Shumway and his colleagues as 5.5% per patient-year and 0.9% per patient-year respectively. In addition, the lifestyle of the patient on anticoagulants is seriously disturbed. The requirement constantly to take his drugs is a reminder of his heart condition. A cardiac neurosis may be further promoted, even in the patient who is doing well, by the need regularly to attend hospital clinics for blood tests where he mingles with other cardiac patients, one or other of whom in time will fail to appear because he has died or suffered some complication. The cost of drugs, time off work and hospital transport must also be considered. The lifestyle of the patient with a satisfactory biological valve (or indeed of the patient with a satisfactory conservative procedure) is markedly different. If he is well he may be able more or less to forget his cardiac condition from one 6-monthly or yearly visit to the next, and the financial requirements of his condition are much reduced. There is some debate as to whether patients with biological valves in the mitral position should be anticoagulated during the early postoperative period. Although the risk of embolus is small, the evidence is that it is within the first 2 or 3 months that it is most likely to occur so that, unless there is a specific contra-indication, it would seem a wise precaution to anticoagulate patients during this period.

THROMBOEMBOLISM RISK FACTORS

We are not able at the moment clearly to identify all those patients at risk from thromboembolism. Why do some few patients and not others develop thrombus on their valve? Several factors may be implicated (Table 1). The valve type chosen obviously has a significant effect on the risk to the individual patient. Refinements in valve manufacture have reduced this risk, but

Table 1   Thrombeombolism—risk factors

1. Valve type–prosthetic
              –biological
2. Surgical technique–valve orifice
                     –suture material
                     –Teflon pledgets
3. Quality anticoagulant control
4. Patient factors–heart rhythm
                  –size left atrium
                  –calcification
                  –clot in left atrium
                  –?other factors

there still remains a difference in patient susceptibility. Surgical technique is important with the clean removal of any tissue which tends to encroach on the valve orifice. How important is the choice of suture material and is it necessary to attempt to bury the knots? Does a continuous suture have any advantage over an interrupted one? Is the use of Teflon pledgets, to buttress the sutures against cutting out, to be avoided?

The quality of anticoagulant control would appear to be of considerable importance and in this respect there is ample opportunity for individual patient variability. How closely is the dosage supervised? Do patients forget to take their tablets or do they run out and delay getting a new prescription? Is the anticoagulant stopped during teeth extractions or other surgical procedures? Many consider that it is dangerous to stop anticoagulants abruptly—that a rebound phenomenon occurs with an increased risk of thromboembolism. Finally what other patient factors are important? Heart rhythm; cardiac output, particularly in the early postoperative period; and the presence of calcification or clot in the left atrium at the time of surgery are probably significant. We know very little about other host factors which might be implicated.

MULTICENTRE VALVE STUDY

In an attempt to answer some of these questions, the members of the Cardiac Surgical Research Club have initiated a multi-centre valve study. The scope of this study is not limited to thromboembolism. Our aim is to look at the

Table 2   Cardiac surgical research club (Multicentre valve study)

1. Cambridge – English
              – Milstein
2. Cardiff – Breckenridge
3. Leeds – Deverall
         – Watson
4. Liverpool – Donnelly
5. Newcastle – Blesovsky
6. Sheffield – Smith
7. Southampton – Monro

results of valve replacement with particular reference to thromboembolism, haemorrhage, valve failure and late mortality. At the moment the surgeons named in Table 2 are taking part, but we would welcome the contributions of any other surgeons who wish to join the study; there are considerable personal advantages in so doing in terms of ongoing computerization, tabulation, analysis and ready availability of individual surgical follow-up and results.

Patients are admitted to the study as follows: all patients who undergo aortic and/or mitral and/or tricuspid valve replacement except:

1. those patients who die before hospital discharge (i.e. we are not looking at operative mortality);
2. those patients who are not suitable for follow-up (e.g. they come from another country where follow-up cannot be guaranteed).

On discharge from hospital preoperative and operative details are completed on appropriate forms and returned to the author in Liverpool to be transcribed on to optical mark sheets for reading by computer at the University of Liverpool Computer Laboratories. At yearly intervals following surgery reminders are sent out to the appropriate surgeons requesting follow-up information. Event-free or incident sheets are returned by them for further computerization.

Results for the group as a whole or for individual surgeons are available at 48 hours' notice. Systems of analysis are still being programmed but these will include actuarial tables for embolus, haemorrhage, valve failure, re-operation and late mortality according to valve type and position. It is intended also to relate these to preoperative patient features, to surgical technique and to choice and control of anticoagulants.

The study is in its second year and is now beginning to gather momentum as yearly follow-up information becomes available. Over 700 patients have so far been admitted to the study, and follow-up is now available in 300. Following mitral valve replacement information is available at 12 months in 157 patients, and the incidence of thromboembolism, valve failure and late mortality for the various valve models is shown in Table 3. Numbers are generally small and in most groups mean little. However, in 32 patients with

Table 3   Cardiac surgical research club (Multicentre valve study)

	Total number		Embolus (%)	Valve failure (%)	Late mortality (%)
	Inserted	Followed-up for 12 months			
Starr–Edwards 6120	73	32	6.25	6.25	3.1
Starr–Edwards 6400	8	3	33.3	0	0
Björk–Shiley	214	108	7.4	6.5	11.1
Lillehei–Kastor	23	3	66.6	0	66.6
Hancock	29	11	0	18	18
Carpentier–Edwards	4	0	0	0	0

Mitral valve replacement – 12-month follow-up.

the early Starr–Edwards model the incidence of thromboembolism is 6.25%
at 12 months, compared with 7.4% for the Björk–Shiley mitral valve. No
embolus has occurred in 11 patients with a Hancock pig valve.

MITRAL VALVE REPLACEMENT WITH BJÖRK–SHILEY VALVE

If we look more closely at the results at 12 months of mitral valve replacement
with the Björk–Shiley pyrolite-disc prosthesis, out of 108 patients, 7.4% have
suffered a thromboembolic incident and these have all occurred within the
first 6 months (Table 4). Eight patients were affected. Thrombosis of the valve
occurred in two, a retinal embolus in one and cerebral emboli in five. Three
of these eight patients died.

Table 4 Cardiac surgical research club (Multi-centre valve study)

108 patients	3 Months	6 Months	9 Months	12 Months
Embolus (%)	4.6	7.4	7.4	7.4
Valve failure (%)	1.9	5.6	5.6	6.5
Late mortality (%)	6.5	10.2	10.2	11.1
Incident (%)	10.2	19.5	19.5	21.3

12-month follow-up after mitral valve replacement with Björk–
Shiley prosthesis.

Valve failure was suffered by 6.5% of the patients. These included the two
patients with thrombosis of the valve, three others with infection and two
with paravalvular leaks. All underwent reoperation and four of these died.
Of those patients who left hospital, 11.1% died within 1 year, the four at
reoperation already mentioned plus one with haemorrhage into the myocardium, two with cerebral embolus, one with paravalvular leak, two with
associated heart disease and two with unknown cause – 12 patients in all. By
12 months a total of 21.3% of patients had suffered a complication of some
kind. The early results of this study do not mean a great deal at this stage but
will gain in significance with the passage of time. We expect to have useful
information on the performance of different valve types, to relate these to
individual patient and surgeon differences and to provide a service to the
busy cardiac surgeon by providing for him an ongoing and always up-to-date
analysis of his surgical results.

Acknowledgment

This work was supported by a grant from the National Heart Research
Fund.

11

Mitral valve replacement

E. B. STINSON

In our area of the world replacement of the mitral valve has become a widely accepted therapeutic procedure since 1960 when Starr and Harken independently successfully first replaced mitral valves and established the concept of functional rather than anatomical repair of mitral valve disease. It is evident from other experience presented in this volume that there remains a proper role for reconstruction of the mitral apparatus, but at our institution we encounter perhaps a somewhat different population of patients. In less than 5% of cases at our institution does autologous tissue lend itself to haemodynamically acceptable plastic revision. This may be due in part to the age distribution of patients whom we have treated, since the average age in our series has been 56 years and has ranged up to 89 years. This is in contrast to most other series in which average patient age has usually ranged between 40 and 50 years.

To begin to address the subject of surgical treatment of mitral valve disease I would like to summarize preoperative factors that have proved, in analysis of our experience, to be significant correlates of early and later postoperative survival and function. Between 1963 and mid-1975, a total of 897 patients underwent mitral valve replacement at Stanford. This total number includes patients undergoing concomitant cardiac procedures,

Table 1. **Primary aetiology of mitral valve lesion**

Rheumatic	695
Myxomatous degeneration	112
Ischaemic mitral disease	54
Infective endocarditis	8
Prosthetic valve dysfunction	16
Miscellaneous	12
TOTAL	897

except for simultaneous replacement of another cardiac valve. The aetiological classification of underlying disease in these patients is shown in Table 1. In approximately 700 patients the primary disease was rheumatic valvulitis, in 112 myxomatous degeneration of the mitral apparatus was present, and in 54 patients primary ischaemic disease was distinguished as the cause of mitral valve dysfunction. These latter patients are considered separately from those in whom coronary artery disease was present as a separate process, incidental to the primary mitral valve lesion.

Early postoperative mortality rates were then calculated on the basis of primary aetiological classification as shown in Table 2. These data illustrate

Table 2 Perioperative deaths according to primary aetiology of mitral valve lesion

	Patients	No.	Percentage
Rheumatic valvular disease			
without coronary artery disease	634	43	6.8
with coronary artery disease	61	18	29.5
Myxomatous degeneration			
without coronary artery disease	93	5	5.4
with coronary artery disease	19	4	21.0
Ischaemic mitral disease	54	10	18.5
Infective endocarditis	8	4	50.0
Prosthetic valve dysfunction	16	0	0
Other	12	2	16.7
TOTAL	897	86	9.6

the extremely unfavourable impact of either incidental or primary coronary artery disease. In patients with rheumatic valvulitis without associated coronary disease the operative risk over the past 12 years has been 6.8%, but rises to nearly 30% in patients with associated coronary disease. Similar, although slightly lower, mortality figures apply to patients with degenerative (myxomatous) mitral lesions. In patients with purely ischaemic mitral valve dysfunction the operative risk has been 18.5%.

Similarly, the influence of underlying aetiology of mitral valvular disease on long-term postoperative survival is shown in Figure 1. Only the largest subgroups are included, that is, those with rheumatic valvulitis, myxomatous degeneration, or ischaemic mitral valve dysfunction. At 5 years postoperatively patients with rheumatic disease exhibit a survival rate of 70%, including operative mortality, whereas those with myxomatous disease sustain a survival rate of approximately 54%, and those with complicated coronary artery disease and ischaemic mitral valve dysfunction show a survival rate of only 32%. Indeed, the 1-year mortality rate of 51% for the latter patients was three times higher than that for the other two groups. After the first postoperative year, however, the survival curves for all three groups are generally parallel, suggesting the operation of an early selection process that may necessitate different curve-fitting techniques to characterize postoperative survival according to underlying aetiology. It should be noted

94

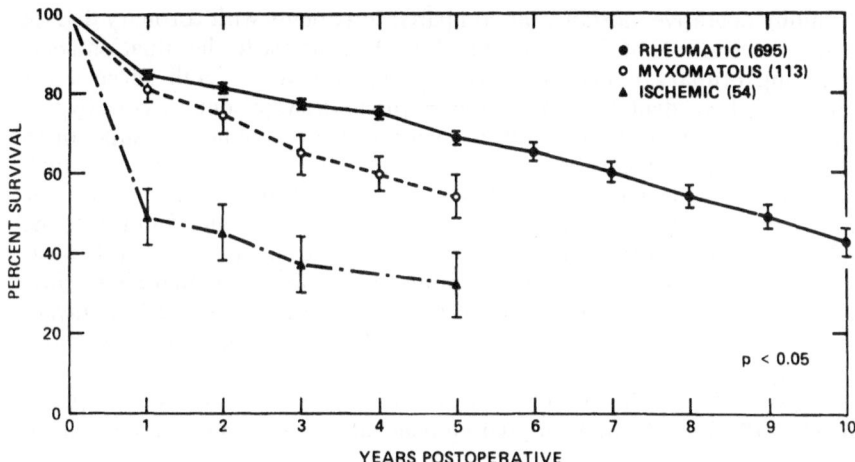

Figure 1 Long-term postoperative survival, calculated by the actuarial method, for patients undergoing mitral valve replacement. Operative mortality is included. Patients are categorized according to the primary underlying aetiological disease process. Vertical bars indicate standard error

in passing that concomitant aortocoronary bypass grafting had no discernible benefit on overall long-term survival in those patients with ischaemic mitral disease.

The dominant influence of coronary artery disease is further analysed in Figure 2, in which the overall patient group was dichotomized on the basis of the presence or absence of coronary disease, regardless of whether this was primary or incidental to mitral valve dysfunction. Survival rates at 5 years postoperatively are similar to those illustrated previously, in that patients without coronary disease show a survival rate of approximately 70%, again

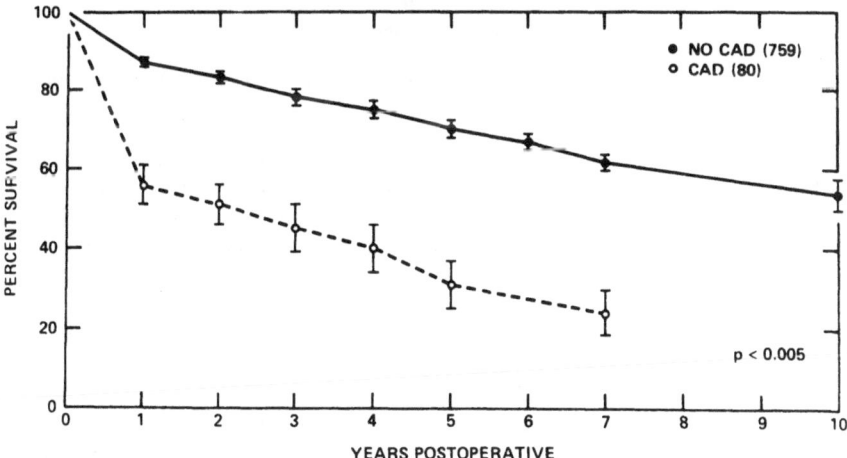

Figure 2 Long-term postoperative survival after mitral valve replacement for patients with and without coronary artery disease

including operative mortality, as compared to patients with coronary disease whose survival rate at 5 years is only 31 %. In contrast to the situation characterizing primary ischaemic heart disease, however, overall survival for patients with incidental coronary disease who underwent simultaneous bypass grafting at the time of mitral valve replacement was significantly superior to that of patients with coronary lesions for which bypass grafting was omitted.

Aside from the correlations that can be established independently for underlying aetiology of mitral valve disease, we have also examined the influence of the predominant type of functional lesions on overall postoperative survival. In part, this recapitulates the preceding analysis because of the nearly uniform association of some disease processes such as myxomatous degeneration or ischaemic mitral valve dysfunction with mitral regurgitation, as opposed to stenosis or mixed functional lesions. Nevertheless, as shown in Figure 3, it is apparent that the 5-year survival rate of approximately 70% for patients with predominant mitral stenosis or mixed stenosis

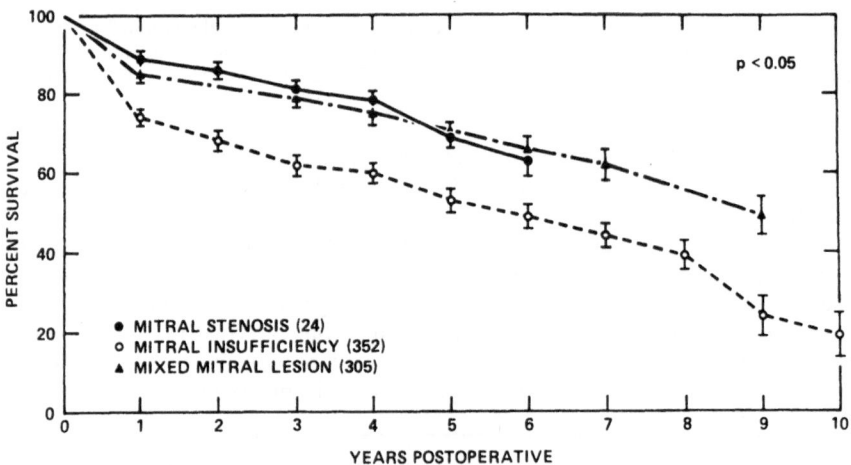

Figure 3 Long-term postoperative survival after mitral valve replacement, according to the predominant type of functional valve lesion

and regurgitation is significantly higher than the 53% survival rate for patients with isolated mitral regurgitation. This remains true even after exclusion of the 54 patients with primary ischaemic disease of the mitral apparatus. These statistics lend some support to the concept that patients with chronic left ventricular overload generally come to operation with more severe degenerative changes in the myocardium than patients with chronic left ventricular pressure overload or left ventricular inlet obstruction. This has been established for patients with aortic valve lesions, and it would seem likely that the same factor is operative in patients with mitral valve disease.

Additional preoperative variables that are significantly predictive for elevation of early postoperative mortality include patient age greater than 60 years, classification in NYHA functional Class IV, a cardiac index less than 2 l/min/M², elevation of left ventricular end-diastolic pressure above

12 mmHg, and increases in pulmonary artery systolic and mean pressures above 50 mmHg and 30 mmHg, respectively. The correlation of such features with increased operative risk is not surprising, but many previous reports have failed to establish statistically significant relationships for these factors because of limitation of data base. The large number of patients available for the present analysis permitted the derivation of statistically meaningful correlations with these factors, but this does not imply that such are highly dependable for patient selection. Their greater importance lies in patient counselling and establishment of prognosis.

Correlates of late postoperative survival are identical except for the disappearance of pulmonary artery pressures as significant predictors, probably because of the reversibility of vasoactive pulmonary hypertension.

Overall, therefore, the principal causes of morbidity and mortality after mitral valve replacement are related to the state of preoperative left ventricular function and patient age. There are also, however, significant differences in long-term results according to the type of valve replacement device that is utilized. Rates of prosthesis-related complications were further studied in the same population of 897 patients described above. For purposes of this discussion attention need be directed only toward currently relevant valve substitutes, including the bare strut model 6120 Starr–Edwards prosthesis, fresh aortic allograft valves, and glutaraldehyde-preserved porcine aortic valve xenografts. The primary descriptors of valve performance that are discussed include thrombogenic potential and valve durability.

Actuarial curves illustrating the time-related incidence of thromboembolism after mitral valve replacement with Starr–Edwards or xenograft valves are shown in the centre panel of Figure 4. We have employed a rigorous definition of thromboembolism so as to include all new neurological deficits occurring postoperatively, whether transient or permanent, as well as all episodes of peripheral or arterial insufficiency of an acute nature unless proved to be non-embolic in nature. This stringency of definition is important if one is to avoid bias. It is apparent from Figure 4 that the incidence of thromboembolism after xenograft replacement of the mitral valve is significantly lower than with Starr–Edwards prostheses. It is also important to note that 16 of the 24 embolic events contributing to the curve characterizing xenograft valves, or 67%, occurred within the first 3 months after operation. These data support our current practice of short-term anticoagulation after isolated xenograft valve replacement, limited to the first 3 postoperative months, unless intercurrent thromboembolic complications have developed.

Comparison of thromboembolism rates after mitral valve replacement with fresh, stented aortic allografts versus porcine xenografts has shown the allograft valve to be inferior by a difference of borderline statistical significance. Interestingly, curves describing thromboembolic events after mitral valve replacement with these two types of tissue valve substitutes begin to diverge only after the first postoperative year. This observation is consistent with the time-course of degenerative changes observed in allograft valves. Five years postoperatively 72% of patients are free of thromboembolism after aortic allograft replacement of the mitral valve, as opposed to 89% of patients receiving porcine xenograft valves.

These data may be summarized in a somewhat different fashion by calculating linearized rates of thromboembolism, defined as the ratio of the total number of thromboembolic events to total patient-years in analysis, multiplied by 100 in order to convert to a percentage figure. For Starr–Edwards, fresh aortic allograft and xenograft replacement of the mitral valve, linearized thromboembolism rates are 10.9% per patient-year, 7.3% per patient-year, and 4.1% per patient-year, respectively. The latter figure is skewed by

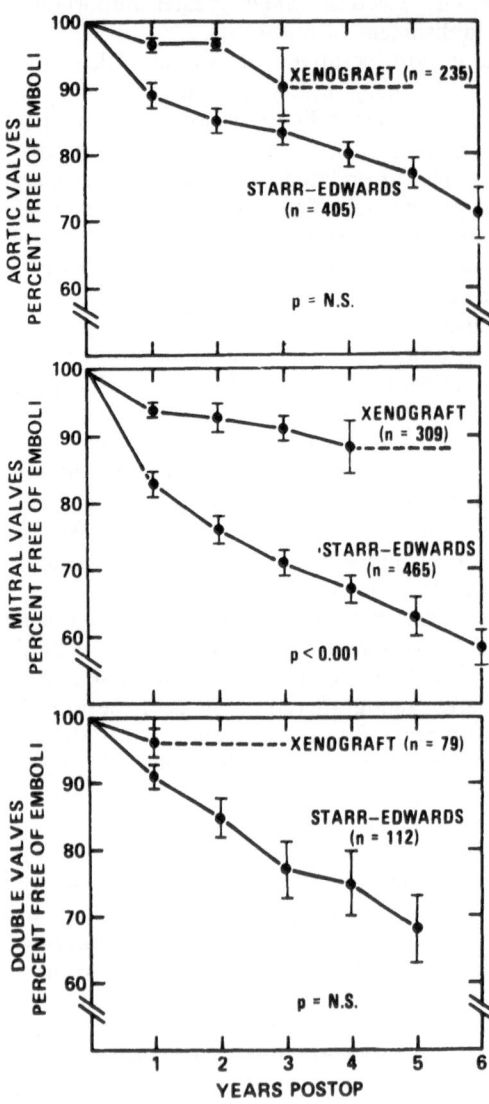

Figure 4 Thromboembolism rates, calculated by the actuarial method, after mitral valve replacement with a porcine aortic valve xenograft or a Starr–Edwards model 6120 prosthesis are illustrated in the centre panel

an uneven distribution of events in time, as mentioned earlier. It should further be noted that the fatal thromboembolism rate for Starr–Edwards mitral prostheses is 1.0% per patient-year in our experience, as contrasted to 0% for both types of tissue valve substitutes.

Long-term durability of tissue valves has appropriately been a feature of prominent concern in regard to mitral valve replacement. In our analyses we have utilized multiple criteria for the diagnosis of valve failure, including

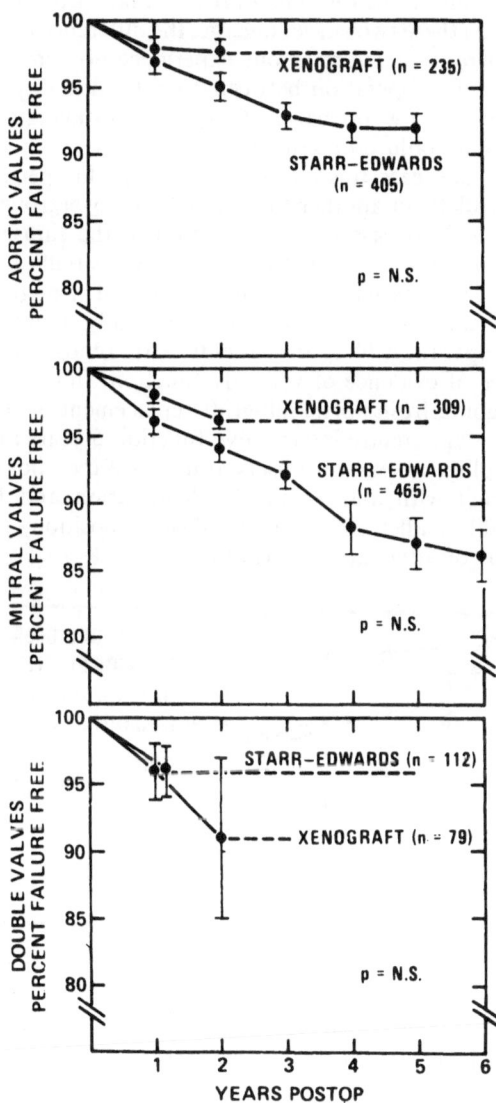

Figure 5 Time-related valve failure rates after mitral valve replacement with a porcine aortic valve xenograft or Starr–Edwards model 6120 prosthesis are illustrated in the centre panel. No statistically significant difference between the actuarial curves is present

the postoperative development of a murmur characteristic of valvular regurgitation (unless proved by angiography to be periprosthetic without any central leaflet component) thrombotic valvular occlusion, multiple embolic episodes leading to reoperation, infective endocarditis leading to reoperation or death, and haemodynamic valvular dysfunction confirmed by cardiac catheterization and requiring reoperation or resulting in death. On the basis of these criteria the actuarial curves shown in the centre panel of Figure 5, comparing valve failure rates for xenograft and Starr–Edwards valves, were developed. Although these two curves diverge, the difference is not statistically significant, and there is therefore in our experience no demonstrable difference up to 5 years after operation between overall durability, as defined, of xenograft versus Starr–Edwards valves. Only three instances of what may be termed primary tissue failure of xenograft valves have been encountered in our experience. In one case this consisted of idiopathic perforation of one of the xenograft leaflets, in another there was tissue overgrowth of a 27 mm xenograft, and in a third case fibrin deposition in the sinuses of the valve occurred in a patient with an idiopathic generalized vasculitis.

Comparison of the long-term durability record of xenograft valves with that of fresh aortic allograft valves has shown a highly significant difference. At 5 years after operation 97% of patients with xenograft valves can be expected to be free of evidence of valve dysfunction. In contrast, only 40% of patients undergoing fresh aortic allograft replacement of the mitral valve can expect to enjoy apparently intact valve function 5 years after operation. The primary pathological features observed in recovered allograft specimens have been consistent with non-specific biodegradation and have included dissolution of viable leaflet components, fibrin deposition, mineralization, and scattered areas of attenuation or rupture.

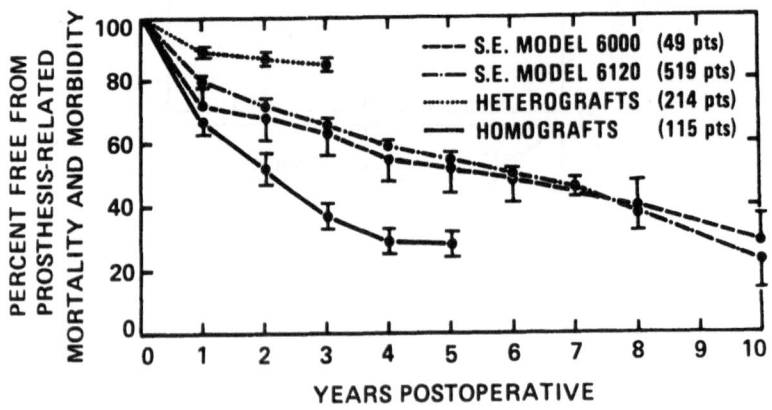

Figure 6 Actuarial curves illustrating the percentage of patients free of any prosthesis-related death or complication as a function of time postoperatively

Another feature that is important in the comparative evaluation of mechanical versus biological mitral valve substitutes is the morbidity associated with long-term oral anticoagulation. Indefinite anticoagulation is required for all types of mechanical intracardiac prostheses and the attendant hazards of such a regimen should be incorporated into analysis of late postoperative results. In our experience anticoagulation after mitral valve replacement with Starr–Edwards valves has been associated with an incidence of non-fatal haemorrhage of 5.5% per patient-year and an incidence of fatal haemorrhage of 0.9% per patient-year. These statistics are similar to the risks of long-term anticoagulation described in many other studies.

Finally, we have developed what we have termed composite morbidity and mortality actuarial curves for each of the valve types that we have utilized over the past 12 years at our centre. These curves are illustrated in Figure 6. Each curve represents the percentage of patients free of any prosthesis-related death or complication (including anticoagulant-related haemorrhage) as a function of time. Despite the unequal data sets, it is apparent that patients with xenograft (heterograft) valves have enjoyed superior overall results, at least within the constraints of follow-up periods now exceeding 5 years.

In summary, thorough evaluation of the operative treatment of mitral valve disease by valve replacement incorporates many factors related both to patient characteristics and the type of valve substitute utilized. The current results observed after mitral valve replacement with porcine xenografts justify, I believe, earlier operative intervention before patients have reached the stage of Class IV disability associated with advanced left ventricular dysfunction. Finally, I would promote the concept that refinements in technology and materials in the field of valve replacement have brought us to the point at which it is inappropriate to group together all the aetiological causes of valve dysfunction in the analysis of results of operative treatment. As a minimal gesture, for instance, the presence or absence of associated coronary artery disease should be taken into account and individual sub-groups of patients analysed accordingly.

12

Antimicrobial treatment of allograft valves

W. H. WAIN

The introduction by Barratt-Boyes and Roche[1] of fresh allograft valves for valve replacement used an antibiotic mixture as an alternative antimicrobial treatment to the chemical sterilization with ethylene oxide described by Longmore et al.[2]. That antibiotic mixture was not satisfactory in this hospital and Lockey et al.[3] described another mixture, 'B'. This was changed to mixture 'C' in 1974 after extensive work by Waterworth et al.[4]. However, mixture 'C' was found to be unsuitable because of the occurrence of resistant *Pseudomonas* spp. and of *Candida* spp. and it was changed in 1975 to the mixture described by Yacoub et al.[5]. This was changed again in 1976 to include nystatin as the antifungal agent instead of amphotericin B.

During 1976 the use of antibiotic mixtures was re-examined and a new mixture, Danynm, was introduced[6]. All these changes are listed in Table 1, together with the formulations of the different mixtures. The results using

Table 1 Composition of different antibiotic mixtures used at the National Heart Hospital, 1970–1977 (g/l)

Date of Use	1970	1972	1974	1975	1976	1976
Mixture and author	(A) Barratt-Boyes (1964)	(B) Lockey (1972)	(C) Waterworth (1974)	Yacoub (1973)	Hanynm Wain (1977)	Danynm Wain (1977)
Benzyl penicillin	0.03		1.00			
Methicillin		10.00				
Carbenicillin				10.00	10.00	10.00
Cephaloridine				10.00	10.00	0.04
Neomycin				5.00	5.00	1.00
Kanamycin	1.00					
Gentamycin		4.00	1.00			
Streptomycin	1.00					
Erythromycin		6.00				
Polymixin B			0.01	0.70	0.70	0.70
Nystatin		0.50	0.50		0.50	0.50
Amphotericin	0.025			0.25		

Table 2 Effectiveness of different antibiotic mixtures

Date of use	Mixture	Number of valves treated	Number of valves growing fungi	Number of valves growing bacteria
1970	Barratt-Boyes	66	8 (12%)	23 (35%)
1971	Lockey	416	10 (2%)	0
1974	Waterworth	196	55 (28%)	55 (28%)
1975	Yacoub	230	35 (15%)	0
1976	Hanynm (Wain)	233	5 (2%)	0
1976	Nydanm (Wain)	100	13 (13%)	2 (2%)
1976	Danynm (Wain)	240	2 (1%)	4 (2%)

these mixtures are presented in Table 2, together with the results of an experimental mixture, Nydanm, in which the low concentration of nystatin, 0.5 M unit, (0.1 g) per litre was insufficient to control the fungal contamination.

The occurrence in 1975 of gentamycin-resistant *Pseudomonas* spp. and of *Candida* spp. in valves treated with the mixture 'C' of Waterworth et al.[4], resulted in the re-introduction of routine microbiological screening of all biological tissues intended for clinical use. The necessity for such screening in antibiotic-treated tissues has been emphasized by the isolation from Danymn-treated valves of two *Candida* spp. with unusually low sensitivities to nystatin and two bacterial isolates with resistance to some of the antibiotics present in Danynm[6].

Anyanwu et al.[7] reported an incidence of 1% of miliary tuberculosis in patients with allograft valve replacements. The Center for Disease Control, Atlanta, USA, has reported 14 isolates of *Mycobacteria* spp. from glutaraldehyde-treated porcine xenograft valves[8]. The screening technique described by Wain et al.[6], will not detect *Mycobacteria*. Although there have been no cases of miliary tuberculosis in patients receiving allograft valve replacements from this hospital, a survey of 150 untreated valve tissues was made in order to assess the extent of mycobacterial contamination. In that survey, all examinations for acid-fast bacilli and all cultures for *Mycobacteria* spp. at 8 weeks were negative. Nevertheless a routine screening for *Mycobacteria* spp. has been introduced for all antibiotic-treated biological tissues.

In the present procedure, the allograft valve or other biological tissue is trimmed and prepared under clean but non-sterile conditions using a fresh set of sterile instruments for each valve to reduce cross-contamination. Four pieces of the trimmings, 10 × 3 mm are retained and treated in 30 ml Danynm at the same time as the valve is treated in 250 ml Danynm. The antibiotic/nutrient medium mixture is made up by mixing:

Tissue culture medium 199 (× 10 strength)	88 ml
Heat-inactivated newborn calf serum	70 ml
4.4% sodium bicarbonate (to adjust the pH to 7.4)	100 ml
Cephaloridine 400 mg	
Carbenicillin 10 g	
Polymixin B 5 M units	
Neomycin sulphate 0.7 M units	
Sterile distilled water	to 1000 ml

This mixture retains its antibacterial effectiveness for at least 7 days in the dark at 4 °C[6]. The antifungal agent, nystatin, is less stable and 1 M unit, (200 mg) is added to 400 ml of the antibiotic/nutrient medium mixture to prepare Danynm just before it is used to treat the valve and trimming samples.

The valve and trimming samples, in separate bottles of Danynm, are kept at room temperature for 24 h to allow growth-dependent antibiotics, such as penicillin, to be effective. The valve is then stored at 4 °C in the dark until microbiological clearance has been received from tests made on three of the samples. They are transferred individually into glucose broth for aerobic bacteria, into Brewers medium (thioglycollate broth) for anaerobic bacteria; and into Sabourauds broth for fungi. The three samples are cultured for 9 days at 37 °C. After 3 days, and again after 6 days, they are subcultured onto appropriate solid media and the plates are cultured at 37 °C for 3 days. All the cultures are examined daily for visible growth, and the absence of any detectable growth after 9 days is used as the basis for declaring the valve to be suitable for clinical use. The fourth sample of valve tissue is cultured for *Mycobacteria*. It is transferred from Danynm to 4% NaOH for 20 min at room temperature. After centrifugation the pellet is extensively diluted, centrifuged again and the pellet inoculated onto a Löwenstein–Jensen slope and cultured at 37 °C for 8 weeks. The culture is examined at weekly intervals and a culture report at 8 weeks is attached to the valve documentation. The valve is stored for clinical use for up to 8 weeks from the date of preparation.

A 7-year follow-up of 247 patients with antibiotic-treated allograft valves in this hospital has shown an annual incidence of infective endocarditis of 0.92%[9]. This may be compared with that of 0.98% per annum for 4760 prosthetic heart valves over a 10-year period reported by Wilson[10]. This incidence of 0.92% together with the experimental results of Wain et al.[6], and the 7-year experience reported in this paper, endorse the practice of using antibiotics to treat contaminated tissue for subsequent surgical use, provided that there is adequate microbiological screening.

References

1. Barratt-Boyes, B. G. and Roche, A. H. G. (1969). A review of aortic valve homografts over a six and one-half year period. *Ann. Surg.*, **170**, 483
2. Longmore, D. B., Lockey, E., Ross, D. N. and Pickering, B. N. (1966). The preparation of aortic valve homografts., *Lancet*, **2**, 463
3. Lockey, E., Al-Janabi, N., Gonzalez-Lavin, L. and Ross, D. N. (1972). A method of sterilizing and preserving fresh allograft heart valves. *Thorax*, **27**, 398
4. Waterworth, P. M., Lockey, E., Berry, E. M. and Pearce, H. M. (1974). A critical investigation into the antibiotic sterilization of heart valve homografts. *Thorax*, **29**, 432
5. Yacoub, M., Knight, E. J. and Towers, M. (1973). Aortic valve replacement using fresh unstented homografts *Thoraxchirurgie*, **21**, 451
6. Wain, W. H., Pearce, H. M., Riddell, R. W. and Ross, D. N. (1977). A re-evaluation of the antibiotic sterilization of heart valve allografts *Thorax*, **32**, 740
7. Anyanwu, C. H., Nassau, E. and Yacoub, M. (1976). Miliary tuberculosis following homograft valve replacement. *Thorax*, **31**, 101
8. FDA (1977). *Morbidity and Mortality Report, Feb. 1977: isolation of* Mycobacteria *species from porcine heart valve prostheses*, pp. 42–43. Center for Disease Control

9. Ross, D. N., Martelli, V. and Wain, W. H. (1978). Allograft and autograft valves used in aortic valve replacement. In M. Ionescu (ed.). *Tissue Heart Valves*. (London: Butterworths)
10. Wilson, W. R. (1977). In R. J. Duma (ed.). *Infections of Prosthetic Heart Valves and Vascular Grafts*. (Baltimore: University Park Press)

Section III
Endocardial cushion

13

Anatomy of the common atrioventricular canal

F. E. DE SALAMANCA, M. UGARTE AND M. QUERO

The present work is based on an anatomical study of 54 specimens from the anatomical collection of Clinica Infantil La Paz, Madrid, showing endocardial cushion defects.

Cases with important dominance of either ventricle (single ventricle and related anomalies) and/or visceral heteroataxia were excluded.

EMBRYOLOGY OF THE AURICULOVENTRICULAR VALVES

The endocardial cushions form the margins of the primitive atrioventricular canal[1,2], connecting the primitive atria and ventricle. Later, this canal undergoes rightward displacement towards the bulbus cordis[3], so the right part of the atrioventricular canal lies over the right ventricle. In this process the atrioventricular canal incorporates a new element on its anterior-right aspect, probably derived from the dextrodorsal bulbar ridge[2]. The anterior and posterior endocardial cushions fuse, dividing the primitive common atrioventricular canal into right and left atrioventricular orifices.

We suggest the origin of the atrioventricular valves as shown in Figure 1.

(a) Anterior component of anteroseptal mitral leaflet. Derives from the anterosuperior endocardial cushion.

(b) Posterior common leaflet. This represents the incomplete development of the posteroinferior endocardial cushion and its subsequent failure to divide into the posterior component of the anteroseptal mitral leaflet and the septal tricuspid leaflet[1,2].

(c) Left and right lateral leaflets. The left lateral cushion later becomes the posterior mitral leaflet in cases of ostium primum atrial septal defect and in normal hearts, while the right one becomes the posterior tricuspid leaflet[2].

(d) Anterior tricuspid leaflet. This is generally thought to be of conal origin[2,5,6].

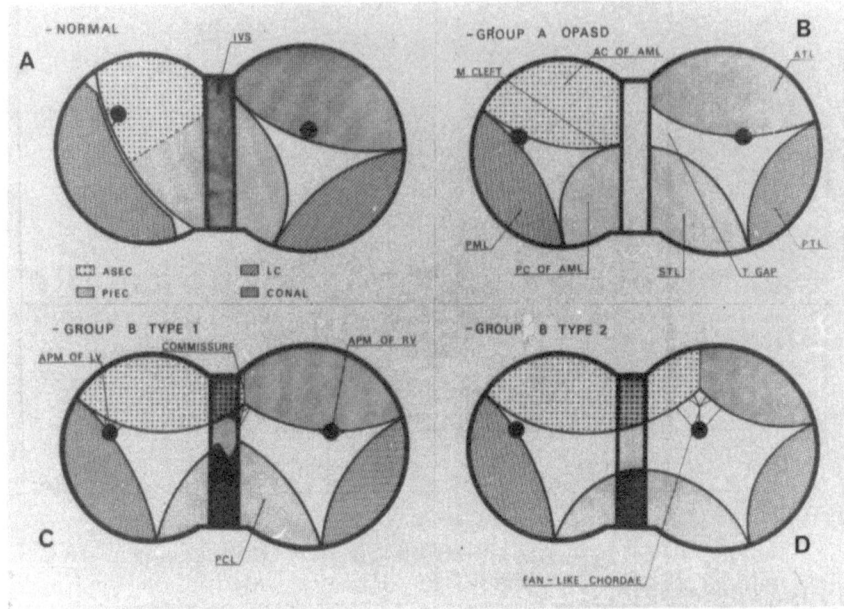

Figure 1 Diagrammatic representation of anatomical components of atrioventricular valves in normal heart and in different types of endocardial cushion defect. (a) Upper left: normal heart. Anterosuperior endocardial cushion (ASEC) converts wholly into anterior component of anteroseptal mitral leaflet (AC of AML). Posteroinferior endocardial cushion (PIEC) converts into posterior component of anteroseptal mitral leaflet (PC of AML) and septal tricuspid leaflet (STL). Posterior mitral leaflet (PML) and posterior tricuspid leaflet (PTL) are developed from left and right lateral cushions (LC), respectively. Anterior tricuspid leaflet (ATL) is considered to be of conal origin. (b) Upper right: partial form (ostium primum atrial septal defect—OPASD). Existence of fibrous continuity between AC of AML and PC of AML, though cleft is present between them (M CLEFT). STL is smaller than usual and there is gap (T GAP) between it and ATL, where normal anterior tricuspid commissure should be. (c) Lower left: complete form, less severe cases. AC of AML joins ATL forming a commissure which is attached by short chordae tendinae to crest of interventricular septum (IVS). Medially located fissure tending to divide posterior common leaflet (PCL) into two halves. (d) Lower right: more severe cases. Commissure between AC of AML and ATL is inserted into anterior papillary muscle of the right ventricle (APM of RV) and is located more to the right than in the less severe cases because of straddling of AC of AML over IVS towards right ventricle and to smaller sized ATL. APM of RV in these cases may be located more medially than usual. In all types of endocardial cushion defects anterior papillary muscle of left ventricle (APM of LV) is usually laterally displaced with respect to normal heart

ANATOMY OF ENDOCARDIAL CUSHION DEFECTS

Endocardial cushion defect specimens show, as a common feature, a deficiency of the posterior smooth septum[7], and the posterior ventricular wall (Figure 2).

The degree of deficiency is similar in partial and complete forms[8], as measured in our series. Normal ratio of outflow and inflow tracts is 1 : 1 versus 1 : 0.75 in endocardial cushion defect specimens.

The atrioventricular valves show a defective (partial form) or absent (complete form) fusion of the anterior and posterior elements (Figure 1b, c and d).

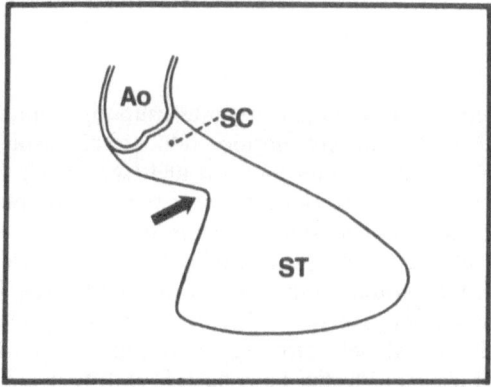

Figure 2 Diagrammatic frontal view of interventricular septum and aortic root. Ao: Aorta; SC: conal septum; ST: trabeculated septum. Posterior smooth septum is absent. Goose-neck appearance is suggested

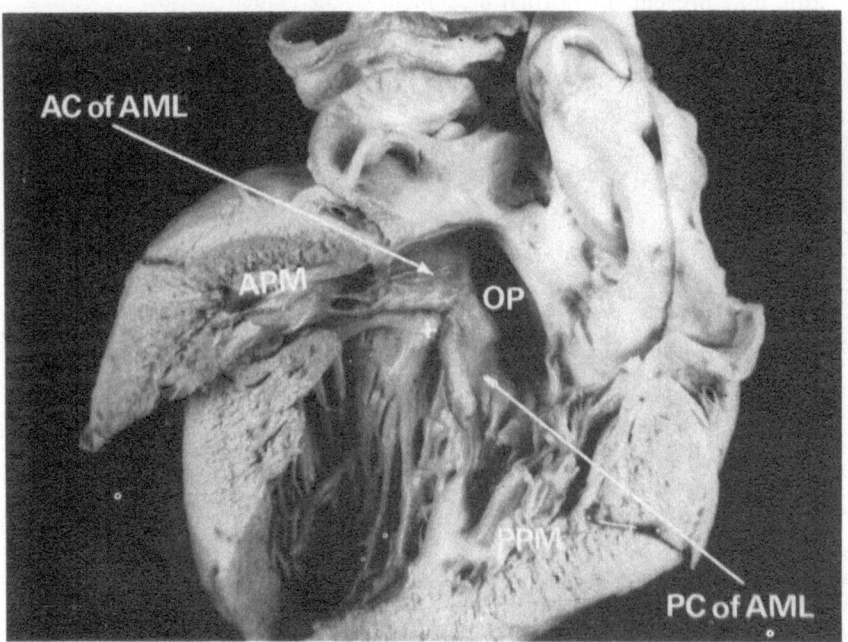

Figure 3 Left ventricular view of partial form case. Ostium primum (OP) and cleft (X) between anterior (AC of AML) and posterior (PC of AML) components of anteroseptal mitral leaflet. Upward displacement of anterior papillary muscle (APM) and increased mass of posterior group of papillary muscles (PPM). Interatrial septum is basically intact

The interatrial septum may be normal, deficient or absent. Frequent patent foramen ovale and ostium secundum-type defects are found[8,9]. The ostium primum defect is functionally an interatrial defect, but anatomically is a ventricular septal defect with low implantation of the auriculoventricular valves. The interatrial septum is not affected by the malformation (Figure 3).

Partial forms

There is incomplete fusion between the anterosuperior endocardial cushion and the left half of the posteroinferior endocardial cushion (Figure 1b). There is a cleft in the anteroseptal mitral leaflet (see Figure 3). The size and shape of the anterior and posterior halves of the anteroseptal mitral leaflet vary widely. The anterior tricuspid leaflet is normal. The septal tricuspid leaflet is underdeveloped; it does not attain the anterior tricuspid leaflet to form a commissure as would be the case in normal hearts. Thus, there is a gap of valvular tissue between them (Figure 4). This gap is by no means a continuation of the mitral cleft, although its origin is somewhat similar. No clefts in the septal tricuspid leaflet have been found by us.

Redundant valvular tissue and rolled rims of the leaflets are common, especially in the cleft anterior mitral leaflet. The presence and length of chordae tendinae anchoring the rims of the cleft to the interventricular septum may prevent the normal movement of the leaflet[4,10,11].

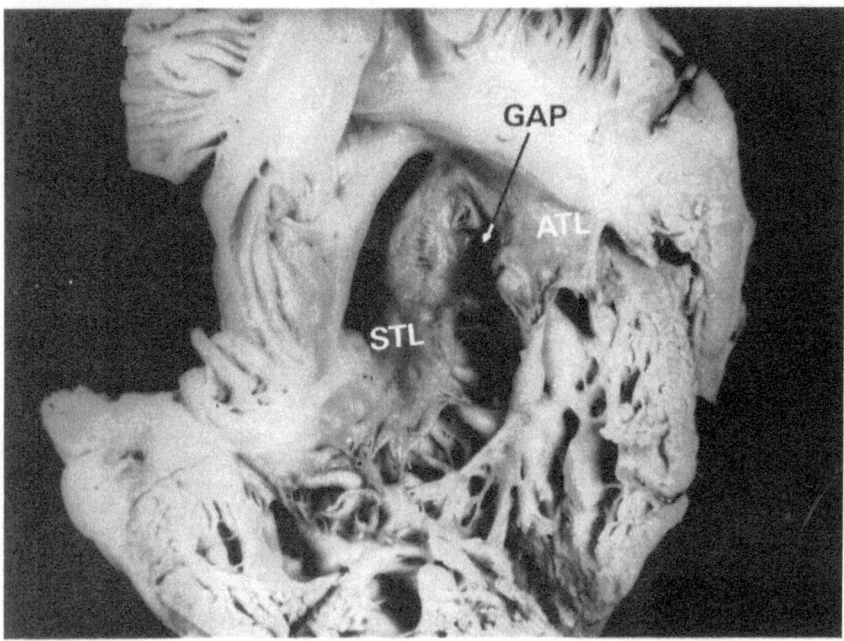

Figure 4 Right ventricular view. Wide gap between ATL and STL (anterior and septal tricuspid leaflets)

The papillary muscles are usually displaced, both laterally and upwards; often they fuse, originating parachute auriculoventricular valves, 9.3% in our material (Figure 5).

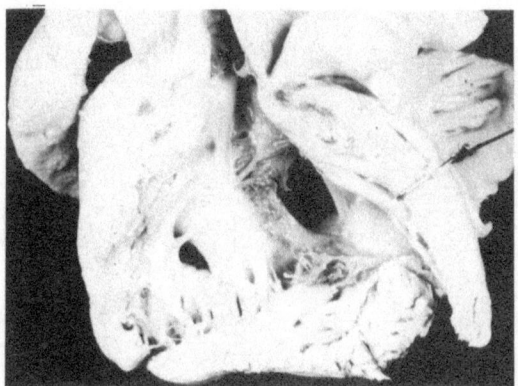

Figure 5 Parachute left atrioventricular valve; single group of papillary muscles

Accessory orifices exist in 62% of our specimens. They are formed by incomplete fusion of valvular components (Figure 6). The fusion line is easily recognizable and the rim of the orifice is supported by chordae tendinae. The orifices occur most often between posterior and lateral components.

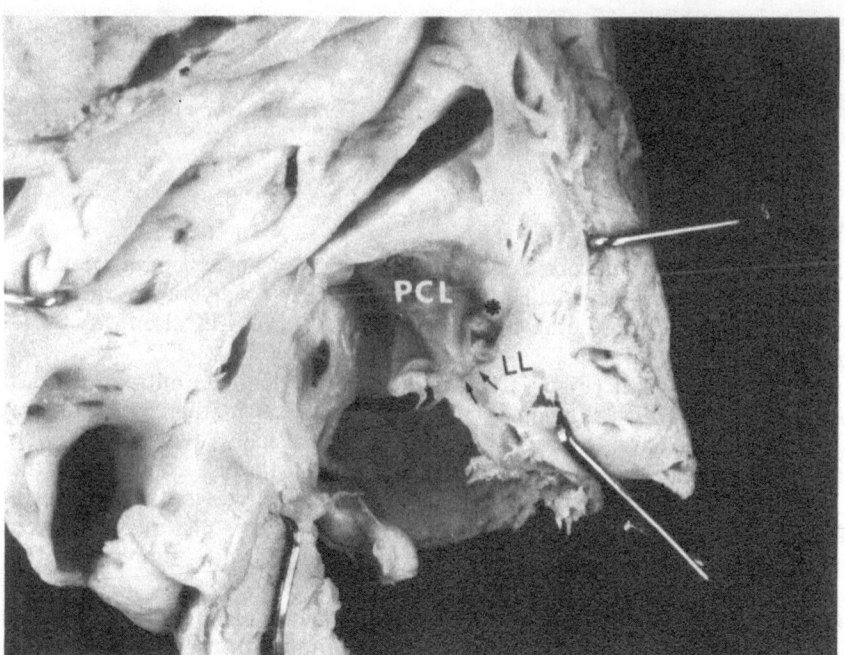

Figure 6 Left atrial view; accessory atrioventricular orifice (*). Fusion line (arrows) between posterior common leaflet (PCL) and left lateral leaflet (LLL)

The insertion of both the anterior and posterior halves of the anteroseptal mitral leaflet to the interventricular septum is defective, leaving significant ventricular septal defects in 29% of our partial form specimens (Figure 7).

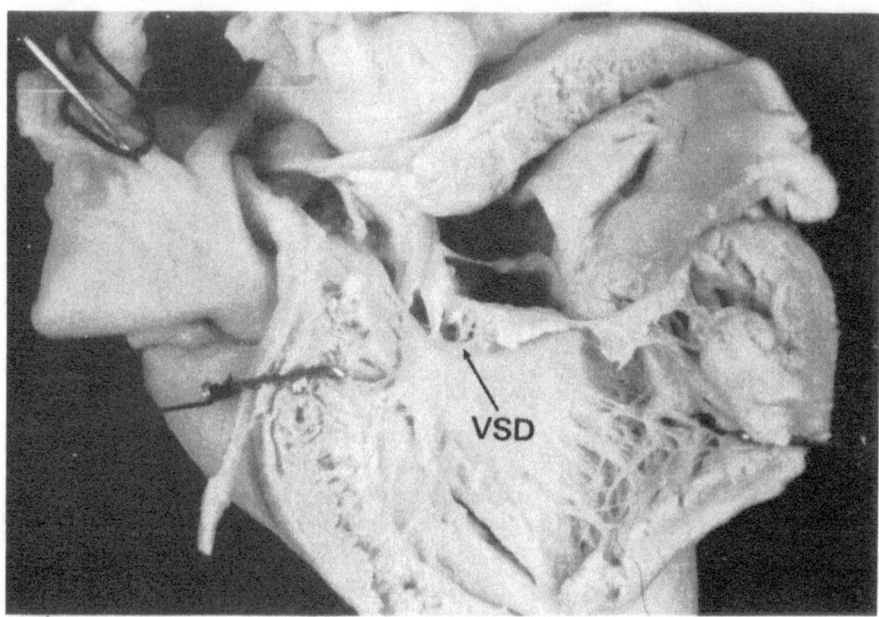

Figure 7 Left ventricular view of partial form case. Deficient insertion of AC of AML to IVS. Ventricular septal defect (VSD)

Complete forms

There is no medial fibrous continuity between the anterior and posterior elements of the atrioventricular canal; thus there is a single atrioventricular orifice, but there is no common atrioventricular valve. Mitral and tricuspid elements are recognizable.

In less severe cases (Figures 1c and 8) the anterior left (mitral) valvular element inserts on its medial side into the crest or the right side of the interventricular septum. This insertion is usually defective, leaving significant ventricular septal defects. It joins, by means of a commissure, the right anterior (tricuspid) valvular element, whose size is fairly normal. Previously reported criteria for the identification of commissures have been used[12–14], especially the presence of fan-like chordae supporting the commissure.

The posterior common leaflet shows partial division into left and right halves, as would be the case in partial forms and normal hearts. In some cases the size of this leaflet is almost normal, hiding its tip below the anterior valvular elements. Only close examination shows that there is no fibrous

114

continuity between anterior and posterior elements. Those cases look similar to partial forms.

The presence of anomalous papillary muscles, accessory orifices and redundant valvular tissue is common, as in partial forms.

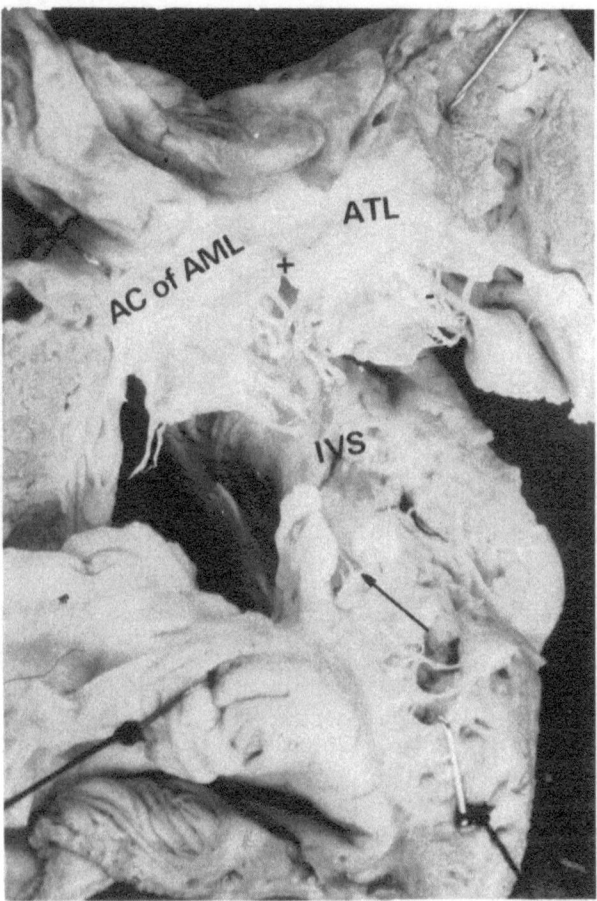

Figure 8 Less severe complete form case, viewed from above. Commissure (*) between anterior component of anteroseptal mitral leaflet (AC of AML) and anterior tricuspid leaflet (ATL) is inserted by means of short chordae tendinae into top rim of interventricular septum (IVS). Fissure (arrow) in posterior common leaflet divides it into two halves of roughly similar size

In the more severe cases (Figures 1d and 9) the anterior left (mitral) element does not insert into the interventricular septum, straddles over it and inserts into the anterior papillary muscle of the right ventricle. To the right it joins, by means of a commissure, the anterior tricuspid leaflet, which is smaller than a normal one. In some cases the mitral element extends far to the right, and the tricuspid element is hypoplastic, giving the appearance of an anterior common undivided leaflet. The posterior common leaflet is generally undivided and not attached to the interventricular septum.

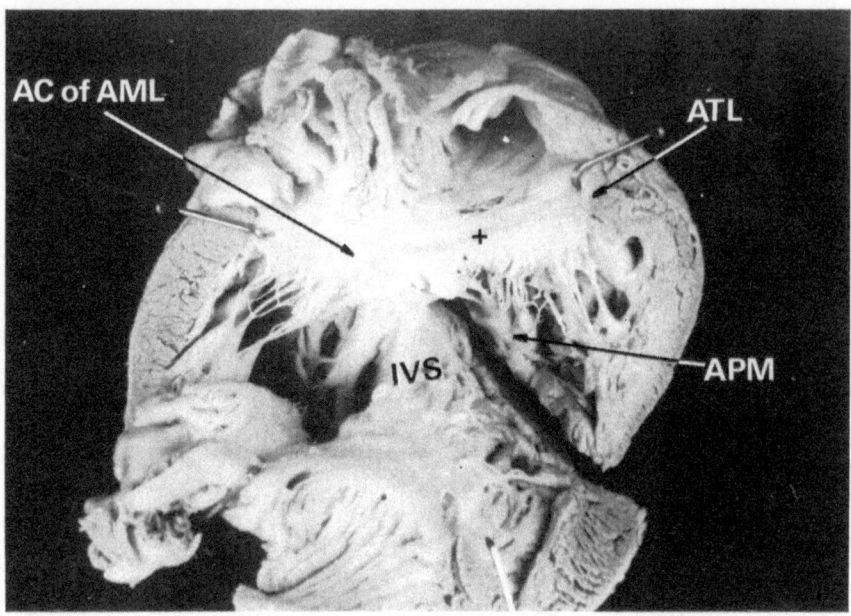

Figure 9. More severe complete form. Commissure (*) between straddling anterior component of the anteroseptal mitral leaflet (AC of AML) and anterior tricuspid leaflet (ATL) is displaced to the right, being clearly contained in right ventricle and anchored by means of fan-like chordae to anterior papillary muscle of the right ventricle (APM)

In contrast to the remaining endocardial cushion defect specimens, the anterior papillary muscle of the right ventricle is medially displaced. This may be due to the fact that it supports a valvular element from the left ventricle.

COMMENTS

In the common atrioventricular canal, the valvular apparatus is always composed of two elements on its anterior side – a left or mitral one and a right or tricuspid one – separated by a commissure. The component situated to the right of the commissure is an anterior tricuspid leaflet whose size may vary. The component situated to the left of the commissure or mitral component may insert on its medial side into the interventricular septum or into the anterior papillary muscle of the right ventricle. On its lateral side it always inserts into the anterior papillary muscle of the left ventricle.

Early in the life of the embryo the anterosuperior endocardial cushion is found straddling the interventricular septum; it later rotates and shifts towards the left ventricle to become the anterior component of the anteroseptal mitral leaflet[1], and fuses with the posterior component developed from the posteroinferior endocardial cushion. If the anterior component of the anteroseptal mitral leaflet is displaced towards the left ventricle, as in the normal heart, but is only partially fused to the posterior component, a cleft in the anteroseptal mitral leaflet will result (partial form). If the anterior component of the anteroseptal mitral leaflet is shifted towards the left ventricle but has not fused to the posterior component, its medial side will insert into the crest of the interventricular septum and the commissure joining it to the anterior tricuspid leaflet will necessarily be located over the interventricular septum (less severe complete forms). If the anterior component of the anteroseptal mitral leaflet is not shifted towards the left ventricle nor has fused to the posterior component developed from the posteroinferior endocardial cushion, it will insert on its medial side into the anterior papillary muscle of the right ventricle, thus giving the false appearance of an anterior common leaflet. Nevertheless, careful inspection will reveal that, to the right of this anterior component, joined to it by a commissure, there exists an anterior tricuspid leaflet, however small. In such cases the commissure is located in the right ventricle.

The underdevelopment of the anterior tricuspid leaflet in those cases may be the result of the fact that, since the anterosuperior endocardial cushion is abnormally located, the anterior tricuspid leaflet cannot so easily develop from the dextrodorsal conus swelling, and a lesser amount of endocardial tissue of conal origin is able to reach the atrioventricular ring.

Thus, we consider that the concept of a divided or undivided anterior common leaflet[15,16] must be re-examined and that we should think in terms of an anterior component of the anterior mitral leaflet attached to the interventricular septum or to the anterior papillary muscle of the right ventricle, straddled over the interventricular septum. The division, usually described in the anterior common leaflet, is really a commissure between the anterior (mitral) left component and the anterior (tricuspid) right component, of conal origin.

Endocardial cushion defects are a continuous spectrum of anomalies, the anatomy of which depends on the horizon on which the growth of the posteroinferior endocardial cushion is stopped and the degree of displacement of the anterosuperior endocardial cushion towards the right ventricle.

References

1. Grant, R. P. (1962). The embryology of the ventricular flow pathways in man. *Circulation*, **25**, 756
2. Van Mierop, L. H. S. (1969). Endocardial cushion defects. In F. H. Netter (ed.) *The Ciba Collection of Medical Illustrations, Vol. 5: Heart*, p. 139. (New York: Ciba)
3. Quero, M., Perez Martinez, V. M., Maitre Azcarate, M. J., Merino Batres, G. and Moreno Granados, F. (1973). Exaggerated displacement of the atrioventricular canal towards the bulbus cordis (rightward displacement of the mitral valve). *Br. Heart J.* **35**, 65
4. Al Omeri, M., Bishop, M., Oakley, C., Bentall, H. H. and Cleland, W. P. (1965). The mitral valve in endocardial cushion defects. *Br. Heart J.*, **27**, 161
5. Odgers, P. N. B. (1938). The development of the pars membranacea septi in the human heart. *J. Anat.*, **72**, 247

6. Tenckhoff, L. and Stamm, S. J. (1973). An analysis of 35 cases of the complete form of the persistent common atrioventricular canal. *Circulation*, **48**, 416
7. Goor, D., Lillehei, C. W. and Edwards, J. E. (1968). Further observation on the pathology of the atrioventricular canal malformations. *Arch. Surg.*, **97**, 954
8. Ugarte, M., Enriquez de Salamanca, F. and Quero, M. (1976). Endocardial cushion defects. An anatomical study of 54 specimens. *Br. Heart J.*, **38**, 674
9. Wakai, C. S. and Edwards, J. E. (1956). Developmental and pathologic considerations in persistent common atrioventricular canal. *Proc. Staff Meetings Mayo Clin.*, **31**, 487
10. Sommerville, J. (1966). Clinical assessment of the function of the mitral valve in atrioventricular defects related to the anatomy. *Am. Heart J.*, **71**, 701
11. Frater, R. W. M. (1965). Persistent common atrioventricular canal: Anatomy and function in relation to surgical repair. *Circulation*, **32**, 120
12. Lam, J. H. C., Ranganathan, N., Wigle, E. D. and Silver, M. D. (1970). Morphology of the human mitral valve. I. Chordae tendinae: a new classification. *Circulation*, **41**, 449
13. Ranganathan, N., Lam, J. H. C., Wigle, E. D. and Silver, M. D. (1970). Morphology of the human mitral valve. II. The valve leaflets. *Circulation*, **41**, 459
14. Silver, M. D., Lam, J. H. C., Ranganathan, N. and Wigle, M. D. (1971). Morphology of the human tricuspid valve. *Circulation*, **43**, 333
15. Rastelli, G. C., Kirklin, J. W., and Titus, J. W. (1966). Anatomic observations on complete form of persistent common atrioventricular canal with special reference to atrioventricular valves. *Mayo Clin. Proc.*, **41**, 296
16. Rastelli, G. C., Ongley, P. A., Kirklin, J. W. and McGoon, D. C. (1968). Surgical repair of the complete form of persistent common atrioventricular canal. *J. Thoracic Cardiovasc. Surg.*, **55**, 299

14

Conducting tissue in complete atrioventricular canal malformations

J. L. WILKINSON, AUDREY SMITH AND R. H. ANDERSON

In order to understand the abnormalities which occur in the conducting system in atrioventricular canal malformations, it is desirable first to review the normal features of the atrioventricular node, bundle of His and bundle branches.

Reference to Figure 1 will demonstrate that the atrioventricular node extends through the mid-portion of the atrial septum, just above the atrioventricular annulus. The atrioventricular bundle perforates through the

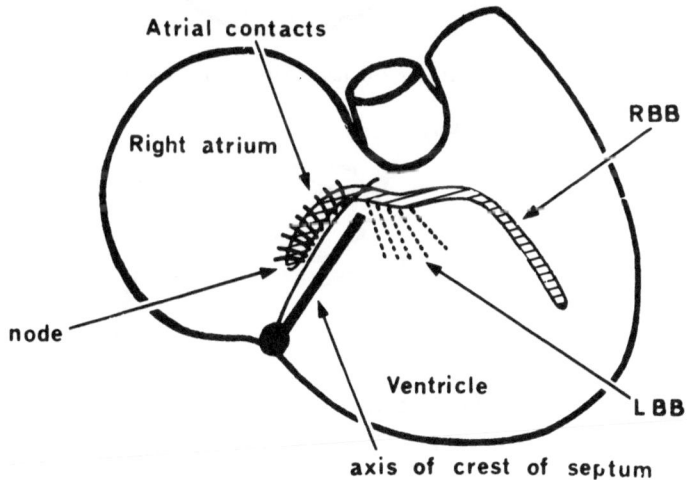

Figure 1 Diagrammatic view of the septal structures and specialized atrioventricular conducting pathways of the normal heart as viewed from the right side. Abbreviations: RBB = right bundle branch, LBB = left bundle branch

fibrous annulus in a relatively anterior position. It runs a short course along the crest of the muscular interventricular septum in close relation to the membranous septum. It then bifurcates into the fan-like left bundle branch and the cord-like right bundle branch. The origin of the left bundle branch is in mid-septal position, so that the length of its anterior and posterior divisions, which traverse the septal surface towards the anterior and posterior walls of the heart, is approximately equal.

By contrast a similar view of a heart with an atrioventricular canal defect shows several abnormal features (Figure 2). Marked deficiency of the posterior part of the ventricular septum[1,2] is associated with posterior deviation of the atrioventricular node and of the perforating bundle[3,4,5]. The node itself is smaller than normal and histologically has reduced atrial input fibres[5].

The bundle pursues an abnormally long course on the crest of the muscular septum before bifurcating[5], but despite this the origin of the left bundle branch is markedly posteriorly displaced[3,4,5]. In addition the left bundle

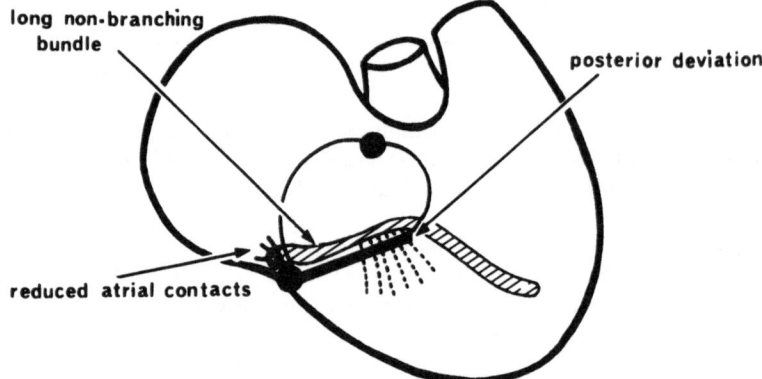

Figure 2   Similar diagram to Figure 1 in heart with atrioventricular canal defect

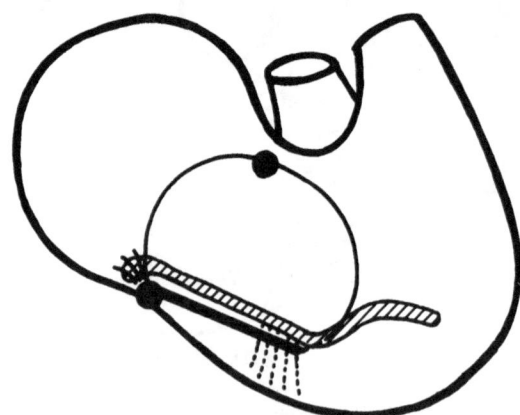

Figure 3   Similar diagram to Figures 1 and 2 with more severe deficiency of posterior septum

arises over a wide area along the crest of the septum[3,5] in the inferior rim of the defect, and the bundle then continues forwards anteriorly to become the right bundle branch[5]. The posterior displacement of the origin of the left bundle branch results in marked shortening of its posterior division, whilst its anterior division is abnormally prolonged. This leads to premature activation of the posterobasal portion of the left ventricle which has been demonstrated electrophysiologically, and probably accounts for the classic electrocardiographic abnormality[6,7].

In cases with severe deficiency of the posterior septum the bundle descends steeply down the posteroinferior rim of the defect (Figure 3)[5].

The surgical considerations relating to the abnormal conducting system in atrioventricular canal defects are:

1. The abnormal position of the atrioventricular node.
2. The long and vulnerable descending bundle in the posteroinferior rim of the defect and on the crest of the septum.
3. The bifurcating bundle on the inferior rim of the defect.

Despite its abnormal position the atrioventricular node is related to the same landmarks as in the normal heart. It lies at the apex of the triangle of Koch, being posterior to the insertion of the tendon of Todaro, immediately above the atrioventricular annulus and between the ostium of the coronary sinus and the atrioventricular annulus[5] (Figures 4 and 5).

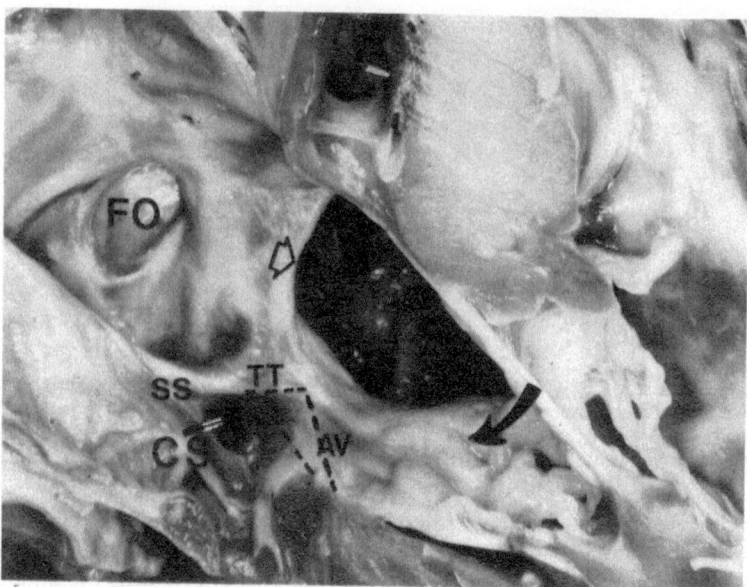

Figure 4 Photograph of specimen showing right-sided view of atrioventricular canal defect with landmarks of triangle of Koch (same specimen as Figures 5 and 6). Abbreviations: FO = fossa ovale, CS = ostium of coronary sinus, SS = sinus septum, TT = tendon of Todaro, AV = atrioventricular annulus. Open arrow indicates lower border of atrial septum, closed arrow indicates common posterior leaflet

From Figure 5 it can be seen that the node, although normally related to the markers of the triangle of Koch, is posteriorly displaced to such an extent that it lies below the ostium of the coronary sinus rather than anterior to it.

As such it is frequently more a part of the posterior atrial wall than of the interatrial septum[5]. From the node the bundle descends steeply down the posteroinferior rim of the defect and continues anteriorly as the right bundle branch.

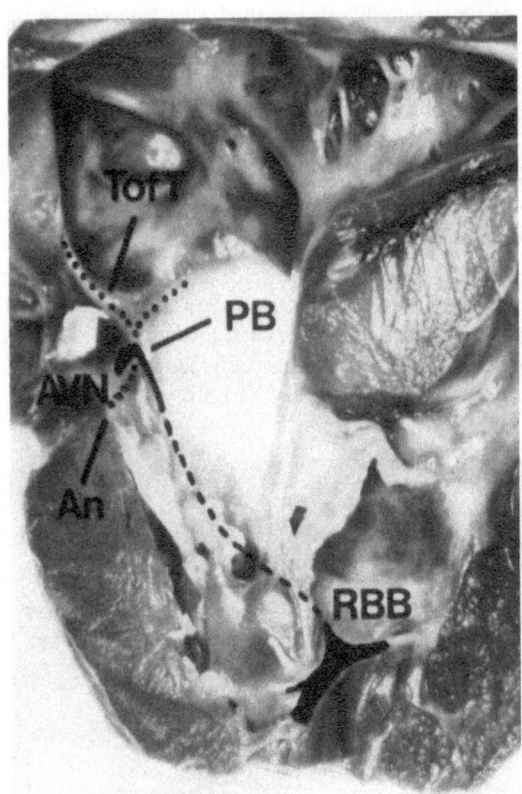

Figure 5 Right-sided view of septal structures in specimen with atrioventricular canal defect with conducting system superimposed. The tendon of Todaro (T of T) and atrioventricular annulus (An) are indicated. Other abbreviations: AVN = atrioventricular node; PB = perforating bundle; RBB = right bundle branch

The abnormal distribution of the left bundle branch is illustrated in Figure 6, where the marked asymmetry of the divisions of the left bundle can be clearly seen, the posterior fascicles being abnormally short while the anterior pathways are long.

The abnormal anatomy of the conducting system and its proximity to the defect mean that it is especially vulnerable to surgical trauma. During much of its course the main bundle lies on the crest of the ventricular septum in a subendocardial position. Moreover, the position of the atrioventricular node and perforating bundle is such that in continuing a suture line from the right side of the ventricular septum onto the atrial septal rim of the defect the conducting pathway has to be crossed. A means of avoiding this is to take the line of sutures around the posterior rim of the ostium of the coronary sinus— leaving the latter draining to the left atrium.

Whilst the distribution of conducting tissue described here has been found to be relatively constant in most of the hearts studied histologically, in some unusual situations where atrioventricular discordance or situs ambiguus have occurred, abnormal anterior nodes and connections have also been found in association with atrioventricular canal defects[5].

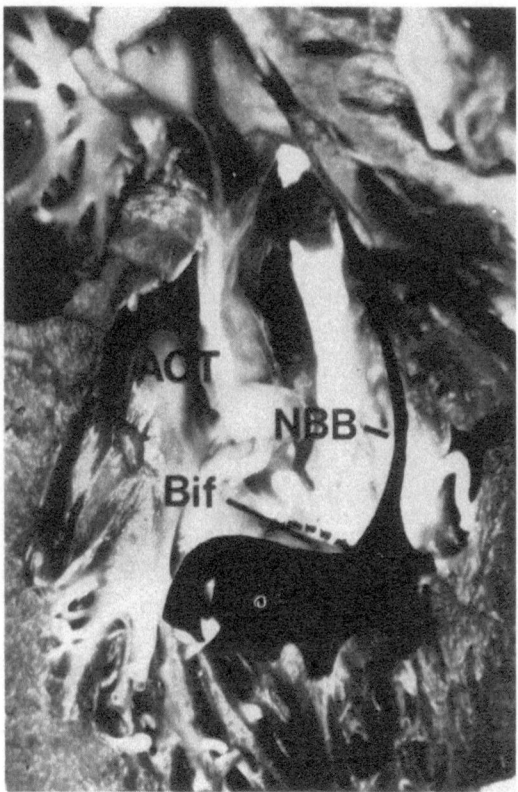

Figure 6 View of left side of defect from same specimen as Figure 5, with conducting pathways superimposed. Abbreviations: NBB = non-branching bundle; Bif = bifurcation; AOT = aortic outflow tract

References

1. Goor, D., Lillehei, C. W. and Edwards, J. E. (1968). Further observations on the pathology of the atrioventricular canal malformation. *Arch. Surg.*, **97**, 954
2. Ugarte, M., Salamanca, F. E. and Quero, M. (1976). Endocardial cushion defects. An anatomical study of 54 specimens. *Br. Heart J.*, **38**, 674

3. Feldt, R. H., Du Shane, J. W. and Titus, J. L. (1970). The atrioventricular conduction system in persistent common atrioventricular canal defect. Correlation with electrocardiogram. *Circulation*, **42**, 437

4. Lev, M. (1958). The architecture of the conduction system in congenital heart disease: 1. Common atrioventricular orifice. *Arch. Path. (Chicago)*, **65**, 174

5. Thiene, G. and Anderson, R. H. (19—). The conducting tissues in atrioventricular canal malformations. *Proceedings of European Symposium on Paediatric Cardiology, 1977*. (Edinburgh: Churchill Livingstone) (in preparation)

6. Boineau, J. P., Moore, E. N. and Patterson, D. F. (1973). Relationship between the ECG, ventricular activation, and the ventricular conduction system in ostium primum ASD, *Circulation*, **48**, 556

7. Durrer, D., Roos, J. P. and Van Dam, R. T. (1966). The genesis of the electrocardiogram of patients with ostium primum defects (ventral atrial septal defects). *Am. Heart J.*, **71**, 642

15

Atrioventricular canal: surgical anatomy and repair

C. LINCOLN

There are three major anatomic abnormalities in the heart of patients with complete atrioventricular canal which influence the outcome of the surgical repair. These are:

1. deficiency of the posterior base of the heart;
2. malalignment between atrial and ventricular septa;
3. malformation of the mitral and tricuspid valves.

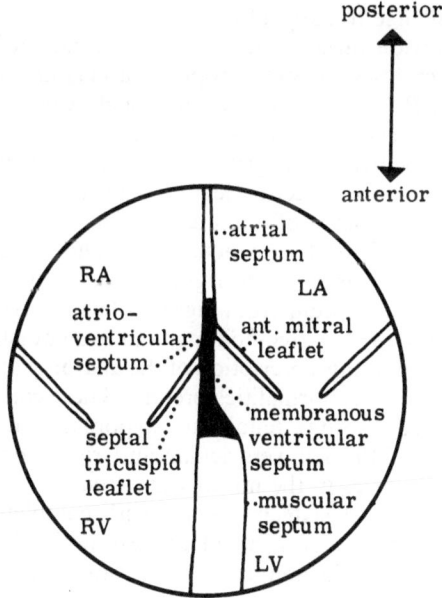

Figure 1   Diagrammatic representation of complete atrioventricular canal defect

In simplistic terms there is a deficiency of the vital structures at the centre of the heart: by that is meant that the lower part of the atrial septum is absent, the upper part of the ventricular septum is absent, and the mitral and tricuspid valve leaflets are grossly deformed due to abnormal morphogenesis (Figure 1).

SURGICAL ANATOMY

If the left ventricular inflow and outflow tracts are measured there is marked shortening of the left ventricular inflow tract, and narrowing of the left ventricular outflow tract, in most hearts. The ventricular and atrial septa form an angle of 15° to one another in the normal heart. In addition, the ventricular septum lies at 45° in relation to the frontal plane. Commonly, in patients with complete atrioventricular canal the ventricular septum has rotated anteriorly so that it lies parallel to the frontal plane, and the angle between the ventricular and atrial septum is 50°. Failure of fusion of the conus contribution to the lateral cushions form the anterior leaflet of the tricuspid valve and the superior endocardial cushion to the lateral cushion form the anterior leaflet of the mitral valve, together with failure of fusion with the lateral cushions with the inferior endocardial cushion reduce the posterior leaflet of the mitral and tricuspid valve. This is the variation in anatomy which occurs in the valve leaflets of this condition.

When considering surgical repair it is the malalignment between the atrial and ventricular septa, and the wide variation from patient to patient in the complexity of the malformation of the mitral and tricuspid valve leaflets, which gives the challenge to surgical repair.

Although there is wide variation from patient to patient in the complexity of the leaflet abnormalities, Rastelli proposed a classification of this defect into three types: A, B, and C, and although such a classification has been criticized on morphogenetic grounds, for the surgeon it is a convenient classification around which to describe the surgical repair. In the Rastelli type A defect the common anterior leaflet is partly divided, and there is chordal attachment to the crest of the interventricular septum. In type B the anterior common leaflet is partly divided, but its chordal attachment comes from a papillary muscle based in the right ventricle, the chordae therefore crossing the crest of the septum from right to left. In type C the anterior common leaflet is undivided, is free-floating, and is unattached to the crest of the septum. In addition to this description of the anatomy of the valve leaflets, there are frequently other abnormalities present. These can be seen as scanty valve tissue, shortened chordae tendineae, hypoplasia of the mitral valve tissue, abnormalities of the left ventricular and right ventricular papillary muscles, and double orifices in the mitral valve tissue.

In a consecutive series of sixteen patients with complete atrioventricular canal who have undergone treatment at the Brompton Hospital, the wide variation in the anatomy of the abnormal valves can be seen. It is also evident that in all the ventricular septum is lying parallel to the frontal plane (Figures 2–5).

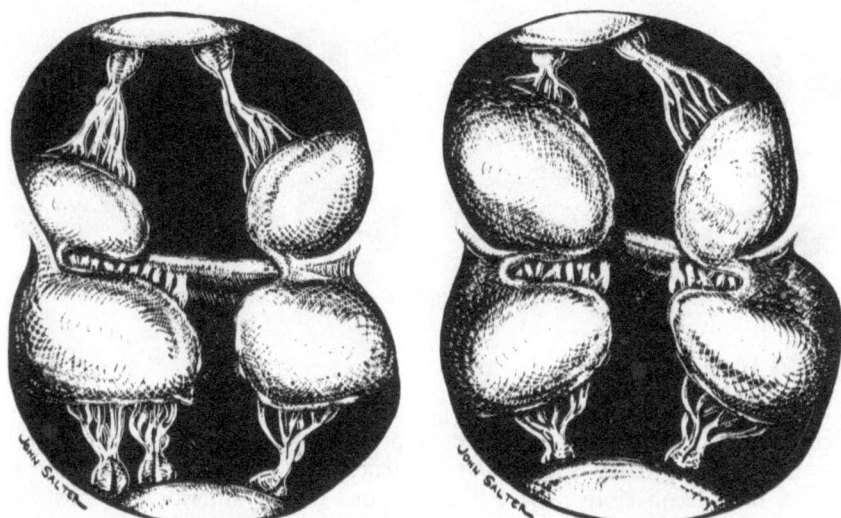

Figure 2 Type A Rastelli defect showing most favourable cusp tissue for repair

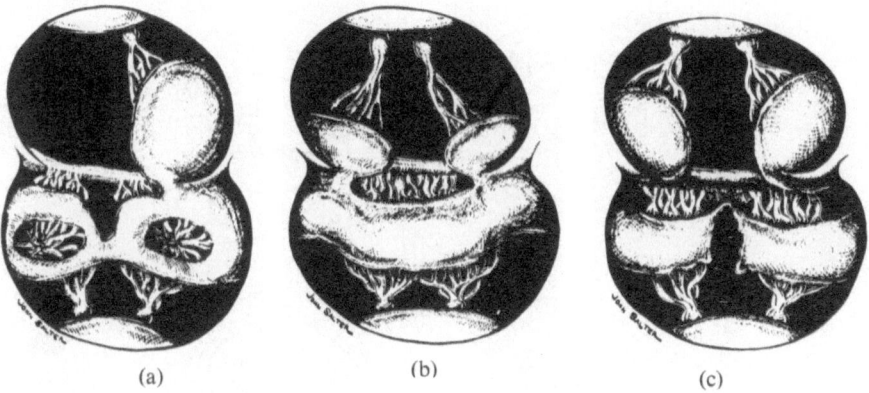

(a) (b) (c)

Figure 3 Type A variations; complete atrioventricular canal (a) showing double orifice. All show partial fusion of the components of mitral valve leaflets

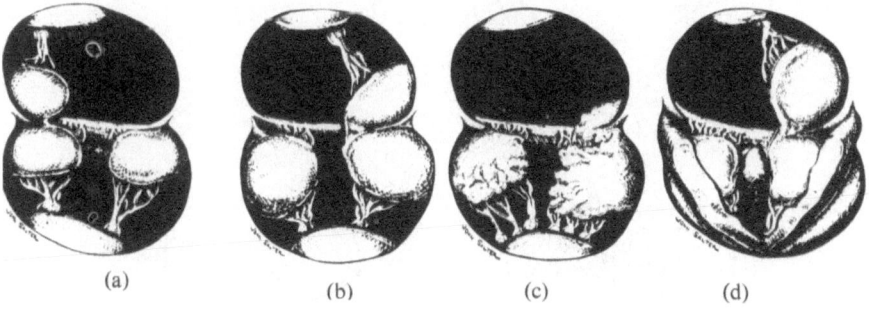

(a) (b) (c) (d)

Figure 4 Type A; complete atrioventricular canal. In (c) note extreme dysplasia of cusp tissue

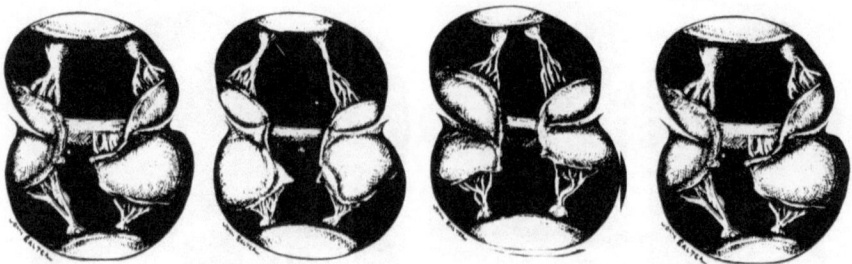

Figure 5 Type C; complete atrioventricular canal

SURGICAL REPAIR

'Newer concepts in anatomy, diagnosis, and surgical repair of persistent common atrioventricular canal' were reported by Rastelli and others in 1968. In this, the ventricular–atrial septa deficiencies are made good by the use of a sheet of Dacron cloth. The mitral portions of the anterior and posterior common leaflets are approximated, and the reconstructed anterior mitral leaflet is sutured to the patch, as is the reconstructed septal leaflet of the

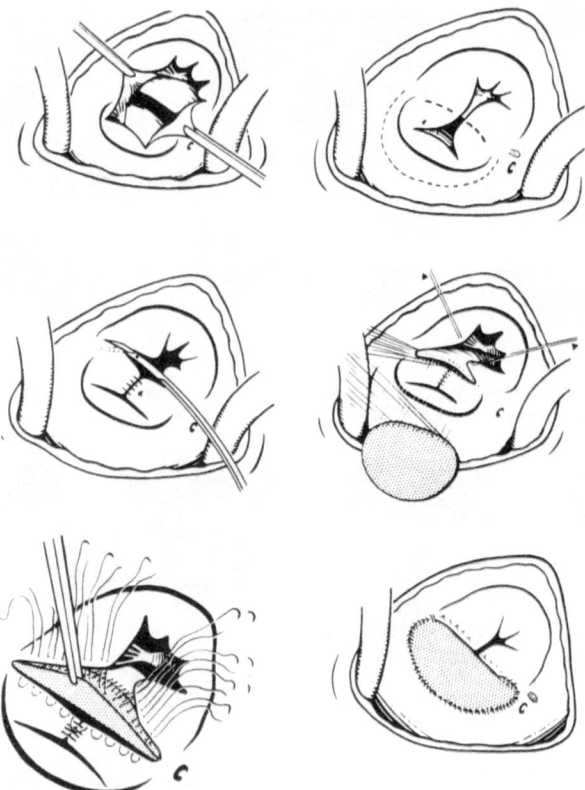

Figure 6 Repair of complete atrioventricular canal as suggested by Rastelli

128

tricuspid valve. The upper part of the patch is then sutured to the inferior aspect of the rim of the atrial septum. This classical repair has gained wide acceptance (Figure 6).

Complications of this complex surgery are:

1. Damage to the atrioventricular conducting tissue; this can be avoided by using intracardiac His bundle identification and, in addition, keeping the suture-line in the right ventricle well back from the crest of the septum.
2. Residual mitral incompetence due to inadequacy of the repair of the cleft of the septal leaflet of the mitral valve. Occasionally this can be haemo-dynamically unimportant.
3. Haemolysis, which is usually transient.
4. Catastrophic dehiscence of the repair with massive mitral and tricuspid incompetence, together with a residual ventricular septal defect.

More recently, we have adopted a two-patch technique, whereby the ventricular component of the Dacron patch is sutured to the under-surface

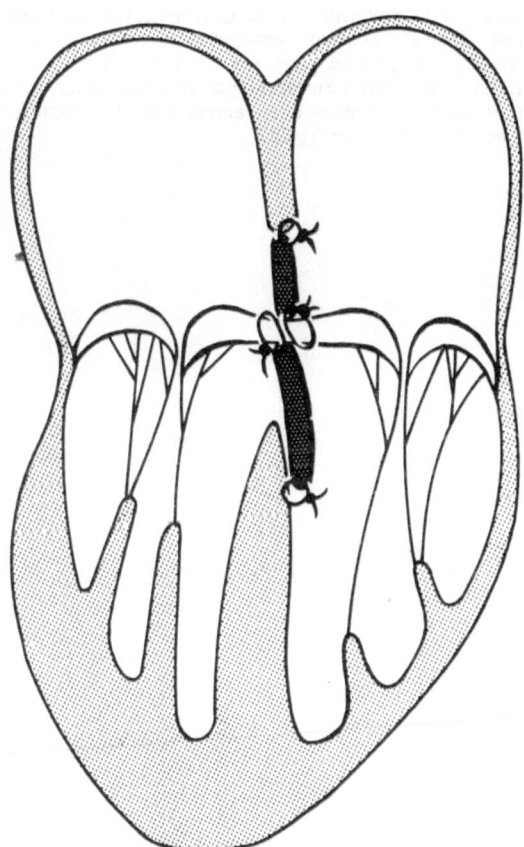

Figure 7 Repair of complete atrioventricular canal using separate patches to close the ventricular and atrial septal defects

of the common leaflets, and a separate superior or atrial patch is sutured to the upper surface of the anterior common leaflets. This has the advantage of avoiding the incising of the valve tissue, which in infants and small children is extremely friable and thin (Figure 7).

CONCLUSION

It is nearly always possible to repair the complex abnormalities in this form of congenital heart disease, and it is rarely necessary to resort to valve replacement. Such is the variation from patient to patient in the valve leaflet malformation that rigid classification is difficult. The use of a two-patch technique may confer added security to the repair, particularly in infants and young children.

Bibliography

Tenckhoff, L. and Stamm, S. J. (1973). An analysis of thirty-five cases of the complete form of persistent common atrioventricular canal. *Circulation*, **48**, 416

Rastelli, G. C., MacAlistair, B. D. and McGoon, D. C. (1968). Newer concepts in anatomy, diagnosis and surgical repair of persistent common atrioventricular canal. *Proceedings of the Fifth European Congress of Cardiology, Athens*, pp. 83–86

Pacifico, A. D. and Kirklin, J. W. (1976). Surgical repair of complete atrioventricular canal with anterior common leaflet attached to an anomalous right ventricular papillary muscle. *J. Thorac. Cardiovasc. Surg.*, **65**(5), 727

16

Correction of complete atrioventricular canal in infancy

J. STARK

Correction of complete atrioventricular canal in children was put on a solid basis by the work of the Mayo Clinic group[1]. The results of surgery in older children are improving[2,3]. However, a number of patients with this lesion present early in infancy and die in intractable heart failure. The survivors are at risk of early development of pulmonary vascular obstructive disease.

Pulmonary artery banding used to be the only palliation available, and the results varied. High mortality and morbidity in some centres led to abandoning the procedure and trying medical therapy only. Our experience with pulmonary artery banding for complete atrioventricular canal is shown in Table 1. Between 1957 and 1973, 29 infants had pulmonary artery banding. In two, associated coarctation of the aorta was present. The operation was indicated only when congestive heart failure was intractable to maximum medical treatment. There were eight deaths (mortality rate of 27%). In addition, there were four late deaths (14%) 5–18 months postoperatively.

Table 1 Pulmonary artery banding
for complete atrioventricular canal
1957–1973

Total 28 infants		
Hospital deaths	8	(28%)
Late deaths	4	
Total:	12	(43%)

These results of pulmonary artery banding were better than the results reported from several other centres, but the mortality rate was still high. The most likely explanation for these poor results is the fact that mitral incompetence is often present, and the pulmonary artery banding can only be effective in patients with predominantly left-to-right shunt at ventricular

131

level. Banding does not help in patients with severe mitral incompetence; in these patients it can cause deterioration. Because of these results of pulmonary artery banding, and because of the improvements achieved in the treatment of other complex congenital heart defects in infancy[4,5] we decided in 1975 to perform total repair in all symptomatic infants with complete atrioventricular canal, irrespective of age or weight.

Both cardiopulmonary bypass and the technique of deep hypothermia and circulatory arrest were used. In general, we prefer cardiopulmonary bypass, so that placement and tying of the crucial stitches can be done on a beating heart, thus checking and avoiding injury to the conducting mechanism. As the position of the conducting mechanism is relatively constant in patients with atrioventricular canal, we have not used intraoperative mapping. The technique of deep hypothermia and circulatory arrest is preferred for very small and sick infants. The operative technique used was the one suggested by Rastelli[1] with minor technical modifications. There are various possibilities in placing the stitches in the area of the atrioventricular node. They can be placed on the right side of the septum and the area of the bundle of His crossed with fine superficial stitches.

Alternatively, the stitches can be placed on the right side of the septum and then to the right of the coronary sinus, thus leaving the coronary sinus to drain to the left atrium. The conducting mechanism is thus safely avoided, and from the experience with the Mustard operation, we know that this small venous admixture is negligible.

In patients with common anterior or posterior leaflet, it is important to divide the leaflet in such a way as to leave a good and competent mitral valve. If necessary one can 'borrow' some tissue from the tricuspid portion of this leaflet. Residual tricuspid valve incompetence is less important than incompetence of the mitral valve. It is also important to reattach the leaflets on the patch at a level of the hypothetical upper margin of the ventricular septum. The stitches attaching the valve to the patch can be buttressed with small pledgets either of Teflon or pericardium. It has been reported from several centres that the suture of the valve to the patch can become disrupted. It is also an experience of various centres that the pledgets placed on these stitches are not a 100% guarantee that this will not happen. We ourselves prefer to use small pledgets of pericardium. In our series, only one

Table 2 Atrioventricular canal repair in infancy

Name	Age (months)	Type	Result	Comment
L.C.	2	C	Died after 24 days	PAB and PDA at 1 month Hypoplastic MV
L.W.	5	C	Well 2 years	——
A.L.	4	A	Well 17 months	Atrioventricular dissociation 10 days
V.N.	4	A	Well 8 months	Diaphragmatic hernia repaired— 4 months
A.C.	8	B	Well 2 months	Reoperation (VSD) 13 days

PAB = pulmonary artery banding; PDA = persistent ductus arteriosus; MV = mitral valve; VSD = ventricular septal defect.

out of five patients had a disruption of the suture line, but this was the disruption at the ventricular septum, not the leaflets from the patch.

Table 2 shows our results of correction of complete atrioventricular canal in infancy. In the first infant, persistent ductus arteriosus ligation and pulmonary artery banding failed to improve the severe heart failure. Complete repair was therefore undertaken. This was technically feasible, but the patient died 27 days after correction in chronic congestive heart failure. There was evidence of residual mitral incompetence. Since the policy of early correction of severely symptomatic infants with atrioventricular canal was adopted in 1975, we have operated upon four additional infants without mortality (Table 2).

Table 3 shows the results collected from recent literature.

Table 3   Repair of complete atrioventricular canal in infancy

Author	Year	No.	Died
Culpepper et al.[6]	1974–76	8	2
Berger et al.[2]	1975–76	16*	3
Mair et al.[7]	1972–75	5	1
Great Ormond Street Hospital for Sick Children	1973–77	5	1
TOTAL:		34	7 (20%)

* Children less than 2 years.

In conclusion, repair of complete atrioventricular canal in infancy remains a challenging operation which is often lifesaving. We hope that the more aggressive approach and increased experience will result in better survival of patients with complete atrioventricular canal.

References

1. Rastelli, G. C., Ongley, P. A., Kirklin, J. W. and McGoon, D. C. (1968). Surgical repair of the complete form of persistent common atrioventricular canal. *J. Thoracic Cardiovasc. Surg.*, **55**, 299
2. Berger, T. J., Kirklin, J. W., Pacifico, A. D. and Kouchoukos, N. T. (1977). Surgery for complete atrioventricular canal under 2 years of age. *Am. J. Cardiol.*, **39**, 302 (abstract)
3. McMullan, M. H., Wallace, R. B., Weidman, W. II. and McGoon, D. C. (1972). Surgical treatment of complete atrioventricular canal. *Surgery*, **72**, 905
4. Kirklin, J. W. (1973) *Advances in Cardiovascular Surgery*. (New York and London: Grune and Stratton Inc.)
5. de Leval, M. and Stark, J. (1974). Open heart surgery during the first year of life. *Acta Chirurg. Belg.*, **73**, 481
6. Culpepper, W., Kolff, J., Reprogle, R. and Arcilla, R. (1977). Correction of complete atrioventricular canal defect during infancy. *Am. J. Cardiol.*, **39**, 293 (abstract)
7. Mair, D. D. and McGoon, D. C. (1977). Surgical correction of atrioventricular canal during the first year of life. *Am. J. Cardiol.*, **39**, 293 (abstract)

17
The results of repair of complete atrioventricular canal

(A British multi-centre study)

D. K. C. COOPER

INTRODUCTION

No one cardiac surgical centre in the United Kingdom has a large experience of patients with complete atrioventricular canal. The results of total correction of this anomaly have been collected from five separate centres* and are presented here.

CLINICAL MATERIAL

Fifty-three patients underwent total correction of complete atrioventricular canal between January 1970 and February 1977 inclusive (23 males, 30 females). Eight patients had Down's syndrome. Details of the age at operation, which ranged from 2 months to 15 years, and the Rastelli classification can be seen in Table 1. There were rather more Type C lesions in this series than in most previously reported groups.

Table 1   Complete atrioventricular canal defects (British Multi-centre Study)

	Age at operation – Rastelli type – mortality					
	< 1 year	1–5 years	6–10 years	> 10 years	Total	Mortality
A	6 (3)*	18 (7)	8 (3)	3 (0)	35 (13)	37%
B	1 (0)	0	0	0	1 (0)	0%
C	2 (1)	7 (4)	5 (3)	1 (0)	15 (8)	53%
Not clear	1 (1)	1 (0)	0	0	2 (1)	50%
TOTAL	10 (5)	26 (11)	13 (6)	4 (0)	53 (22)	42%

Figures in parentheses show the number of patients who died

* Brompton Hospital (Mr Lincoln); Hospital for Sick Children (Mr Stark and Mr de Leval); Leeds (Mr Deverall); Liverpool (Mr Hamilton); Southampton (Mr Ross and Mr Monro).

ASSOCIATED HEART ANOMALIES

Sixteen of the 53 patients (30%) had either gross abnormalities of the left side of the common atrioventricular valve or one or more serious associated anomalies in addition to the basic complete atrioventricular canal. These lesions, together with more minor concomitant anomalies, which were common, are listed in Table 2, and the mortality associated with total correction is indicated.

Table 2   Complete atrioventricular canal defects (British Multi-centre Study)

Associated heart anomalies	
PDA	5
PFO or ASD (secundum)	10
Common atrium	2
Additional VSD	3 (1 died)
RVOTO	5 (3 died)
Hypoplastic LV	3 (all died)
DORV	2 (both died)
Systemic venous drainage abnormalities	7 (2 died)
Gross abnormalities of 'mitral valve'	9 (7 died)
Dextrocardia	1

PDA = persistent ductus arteriosus; PFO = persistent foramen ovale; ASD = atrial septal defects; VSD = ventricular septal defects; RVOTO = right ventricular outflow tract obstructions; LV = left ventricle; DORV = double outflow right ventricle

In the nine patients where 'gross' abnormalities of the left side of the common atrioventricular valve were present, these consisted mainly of poor development of the leaflets, accessory orifices, and of hypoplasia of the 'mitral' valve ring in this region.

In three patients additional ventricular septal defects were present, and in two of these the defects were multiple.

Left ventricular outflow tract obstruction was present in several patients, but was associated with the abnormal position and movement of the left side of the atrioventricular valve, which is an integral feature of complete atrioventricular canal.

PREVIOUS SURGERY

Fifteen patients (28%) had undergone previous pulmonary artery banding, and in three of these a persistent ductus arteriosus had been ligated at the same operation. Two patients had undergone shunt procedures for associated right ventricular outflow tract obstruction, and in one further patient a preductal coarctation and a persistent ductus arteriosus had been corrected at a previous operation.

OPERATIVE PROCEDURES

Total correction of the atrioventricular canal was attempted by the Rastelli[1,2] type of repair in 52 cases. In the remaining patient the situation was found to be inoperable by the presence of a double outlet right ventricle, and no operative repair was performed. Two patients required subsequent mitral valve replacement for severe mitral regurgitation, one at the same operation, and the other at a second operation during the same admission. Björk–Shiley valve prostheses were inserted in both cases. Prosthetic material, most commonly some form of dacron, was used to close the atrioventricular septal defect in 46 patients; in four pericardium and in one a combination of pericardium and dacron was used. In one case the nature of the patch was not stated, and in the inoperable case no patch was inserted.

Cardiopulmonary bypass, moderate hypothermia, and intermittent cross-clamping of the aorta was used in the majority of cases (44). This enabled sutures placed in areas close to the conducting tissue to be tied down with the heart beating. In six infants and three young children, however, deep hypo-termia with circulatory arrest was the method of myocardial protection chosen.

RESULTS OF OPERATION

Out of the 53 patients 21 died before leaving hospital; one died at home 6 weeks after operation, and one further patient died suddenly on the 16th postoperative day, 2 days after discharge from hospital, giving a total perioperative mortality of 42%. Follow-up of the survivors has been from 1 month to $5\frac{1}{4}$ years. There have been no late deaths. The mortality in relation to the Rastelli classification and the age at operation is shown in Table 1.

There is little difference in mortality in relation to age except in the very small group of children operated on when over 10 years of age. The mortality was slightly higher following repair of Rastelli Type C lesions than Type A, but this difference is not statistically significant.

Of the 15 patients who had undergone previous pulmonary artery banding, seven died at subsequent correction (47% mortality); this is not significantly different from the mortality in those who did not undergo previous pulmon-ary artery banding. (No details were sought regarding the mortality associated with pulmonary artery banding itself in this condition.)

If those patients with the more complex and severe associated anomalies are excluded, the mortality in the remaining 'simple' cases falls to 20% (six of 30 patients). This group contains those with a persistent ductus, a persistent foramen ovale, additional atrial septal defects or common atrium, those with systemic venous drainage abnormalities, and the one case of dextrocardia, but excludes those who had undergone previous pulmonary artery banding. The mortality in the more 'complex' cases was 70% (16 of 23 patients). If those having previous pulmonary artery banding are included in the 'simple' group, the percentage mortality does not significantly alter (simple group 27% — ten of 37, complex group 75% — 12 of 16).

MAJOR POSTOPERATIVE COMPLICATIONS AND CAUSES OF DEATH

There were several postoperative complications, such as bleeding and atelectasis, which are common to all open-heart procedures in children. There were also five deaths related to similar non-specific postoperative complications, one case each of Gram-negative septicaemia, brain abscess, inhalation pneumonia, respiratory insufficiency (?infection, ?mitral regurgitation) and a ventilatory accident. It was uncertain what part mitral regurgitation played in the demise of the patient with respiratory insufficiency.

The postoperative complications and deaths related to the more specific problems of total correction of complete atrioventricular canal are listed in Table 3.

Table 3   Complete atrioventricular canal (British Multi-centre Study)

Major postoperative complications and causes of death

Low output state =	20 (7 died)
Atrioventricular valve stenosis or regurgitation:	
mild	18
severe	7 (5 died)* (2 required valve replacement, one of whom died).
Atrioventricular conduction defects:	
transient	6
permanent	5 (4 died)*
Haemolysis =	4
LVOTO =	3 (all died)
Recurrence of VSD =	3 (2 required reoperation)

* Two patients are included in both of these groups
LVOTO = left ventricular outflow tract obstruction; VSD = ventricular septal defect

In at least three of the seven deaths associated with a low output state, mitral regurgitation would appear to have played some part. In those listed as atrioventricular valve stenosis or regurgitation, mitral regurgitation was by far the commonest complication. In the mild cases it remains of minimal clinical significance, and although an apical systolic murmur is still present at routine follow-up, the majority of patients require no form of medication.

Left ventricular outflow tract obstruction can result from operative repair of complete atrioventricular canal and was considered to be a major factor in the death of three patients, in one of whom a Björk–Shiley valve prosthesis had been inserted in the mitral ring. In one of the two cases where associated double outlet right ventricle was seen, an attempt to correct the situation failed, with death resulting from left ventricular outflow tract obstruction within a few hours of the operation.

In the six patients in which transitory conduction problems were encountered postoperatively, first-degree heart block occurred in one patient, a nodal rhythm in two, and complete atrioventricular dissociation in three. In one of these three the heart block was intermittent. All three required artificial pacing; sinus rhythm resumed spontaneously within 10 days.

In one further patient there were no conduction defects after correction of the lesion, but the repair broke down necessitating a second operation for repair of the ventricular septal defect and insertion of a Björk–Shiley valve prosthesis; after the second operation complete atrioventricular dissociation was present, but the ventricular rate was 70 per min and has remained so; the child has made a satisfactory recovery.

In four patients atrioventricular conduction defects were present postoperatively and remained so until the death of the patient. In three, complete atrioventricular dissociation was present, and in two of these cases was associated with significant mitral regurgitation. In the fourth patient sudden cardiac arrest occurred 1 hour after discontinuation of bypass; 2:1 heart block had persisted during this period.

Table 4 compares the results of those operations performed before 1975 with those performed subsequently. There has been no statistically significant improvement in the results of surgery. This may, in part, be accounted for by the larger number of infants and young children in the later period, though there were relatively more 'complex' cases in the earlier period.

Table 4 Complete atrioventricular canal (British Multi-centre Study)

(Mortality related to year of operation)		
	Total	Died	Percentage Mortality
< 1975	23	10	43
1975–1977	30	12	40
TOTAL	53	22	42

CONCLUSIONS

In a series of 53 infants and children undergoing total correction of complete atrioventricular canal, 30% had serious associated cardiac anomalies which were a major factor in accounting for the high hospital mortality of 42%. There have been no late deaths. Severe mitral regurgitation, postoperative left ventricular outflow tract obstruction, and complete heart block remain major complications of the operation and accounted for a high proportion of the deaths in this series.

References

1. Rastelli, F. C., Ongley, P. A. and Kirklin, J. W. et al.: (1968). Surgical repair of the complete form of persistent common atrioventricular canal. J. Thoracic Cardiovasc. Surg., 55, 299
2. McGoon, D. C. (1973). Complex congenital malformations: surgery for complete form of atrioventricular canal. In J. W. Kirklin (ed.) Advances in Cardiovascular Surgery, pp. 45–56. (New York: Grune and Stratton)

18

Anatomy and conducting tissue in partial atrioventricular canal defects

J. L. WILKINSON, AUDREY SMITH AND R. H. ANDERSON

Partial atrioventricular canal defects, or ostium primum ASDs, are in most respects very similar to complete atrioventricular canal defects in regard to both anatomy and conducting pathways.

The distinguishing feature of partial defects is the presence of separate mitral and tricuspid valves, which implies of course that fusion between the anterior and posterior endocardial cushion has occurred. The posterior part of the ventricular septum is markedly deficient[1,2], as in complete defects, but the fused mitral and tricuspid annuli are attached to the crest of the septum and there is, therefore, no interventricular component to the defect. The atrial component of the defect resembles that of complete defects, being bordered above by the crescentic free margin of atrial septum (Figure 1). Again there is a marked reduction in the ratio of length of inflow tract to that of outflow tract of the left ventricle[2,3] (see Figure 5).

The mitral and tricuspid valves are almost invariably abnormal. In the case of the tricuspid valve the characteristic finding is that of a markedly abnormal and hypoplastic septal leaflet. This is usually rolled over and tethered to the ventricular septum directly along its 'free' margin with very short or absent chordae (Figure 1). It frequently does not have chordal attachments to the medial papillary muscle (of Lancisi) and the area of the commissure between it and the anterior cusp is characterized by a 'gap' (Figure 1).

The gap has been regarded in the past as a 'cleft' — analogous with that present in the mitral valve. Recent work has suggested that it is related entirely to hypoplasia of the posterior endocardial cushion, as the anterior cushion does not contribute to the tricuspid valve[2].

The ostium of the coronary sinus is related to the posterior margin of the defect (Figure 2) and the landmarks of the triangle of Koch are readily identifiable as in complete defects.

The defect in the mitral valve takes the form of a cleft in the anteroseptal leaflet which extends from the free margin of the cusp towards the valve

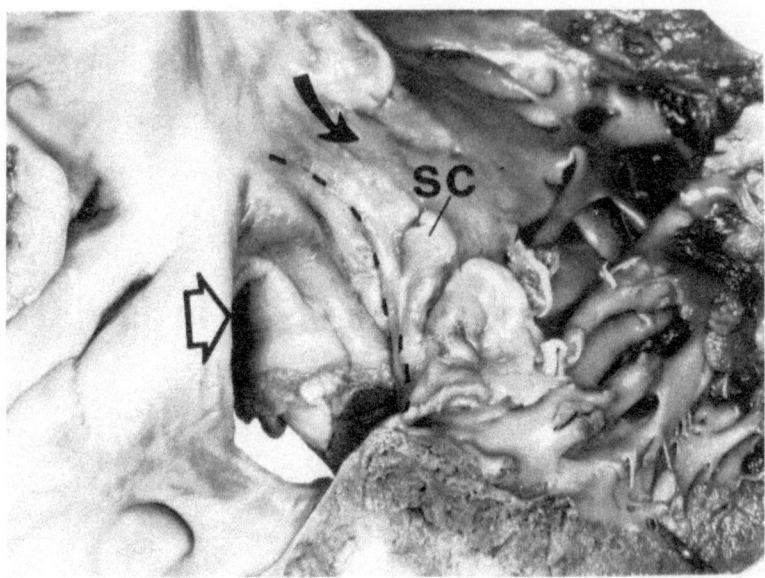

Figure 1 Right-sided view of partial atrioventricular canal defect. The hypoplastic septal cusp of tricuspid valve and the 'gap' are well seen. Key: SC = septal cusp of tricuspid valve; open arrow indicates upper margin of defect (atrial septum); broken line indicates lower margin of defect; closed arrow indicates 'gap'

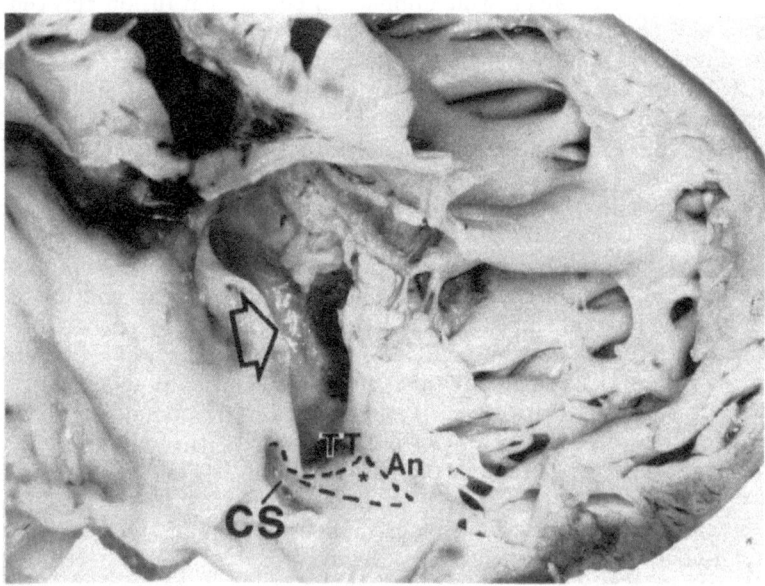

Figure 2 View of the coronary sinus area in a specimen with a partial atrioventricular canal defect with the landmarks of the triangle of Koch indicated. The position of the atrioventricular node within the triangle is indicated by an asterisk. Key: CS = ostium of coronary sinus; T.T. indicates line of tendon of Todaro; An = atrioventricular annulus. The open arrow indicates the upper margin of the defect as in Figure 1

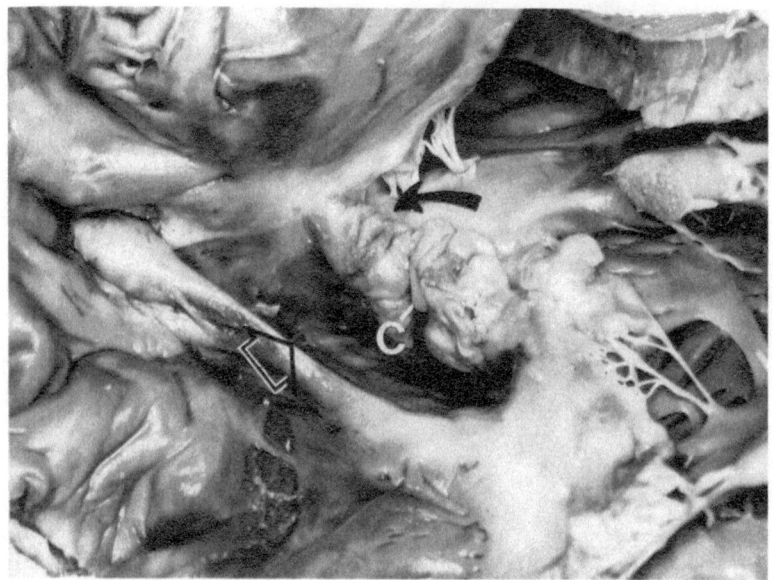

Figure 3 Right-sided view of partial atrioventricular canal defect showing tricuspid 'gap' and cleft mitral valve. Key: C = cleft in septal cusp of mitral valve; closed arrow indicates 'gap'; open arrow indicates upper margin of defect (see Figure 1)

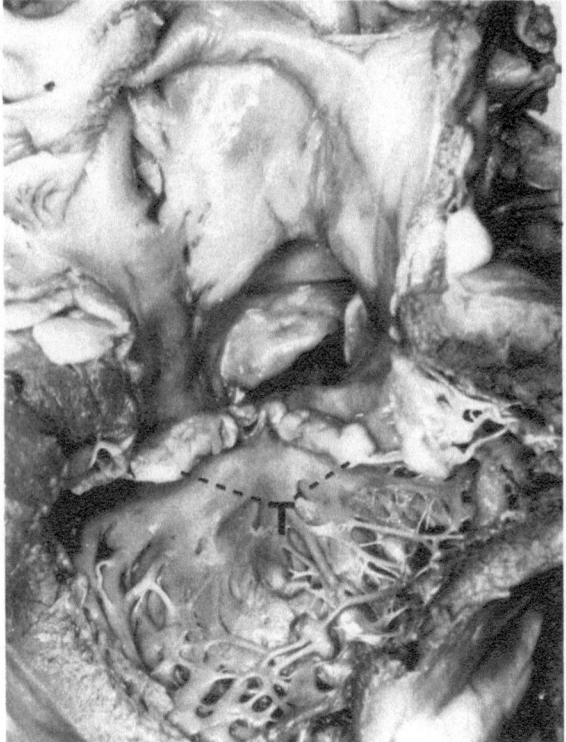

Figure 4 View of cleft mitral valve from the left side with the left atrium and left ventricle opened. Note the thickened edges of the cleft and the 'tubercles' (T)

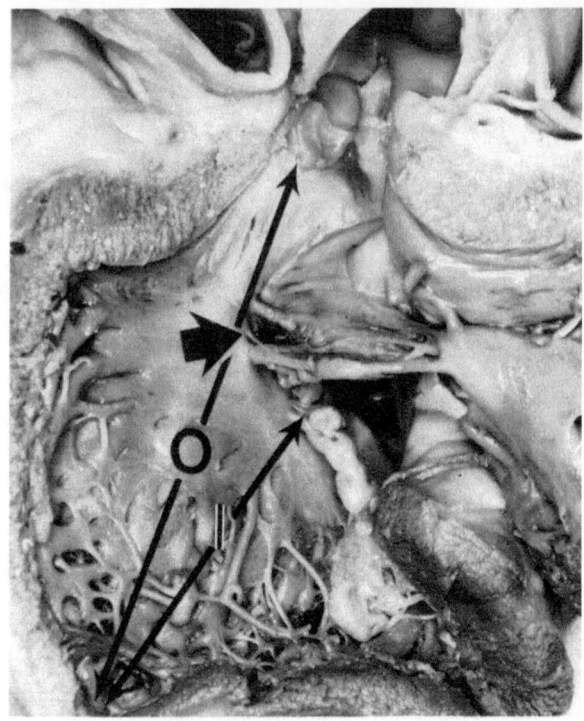

Figure 5 View of the left ventricular aspect of the ventricular septum showing downward and forward displacement of the mitral valve annulus (arrowed) and shortening of the posterior septum. Key: O = outflow diameter (apex—aortic valve); I = inflow diameter (apex—crest of posterior septum)

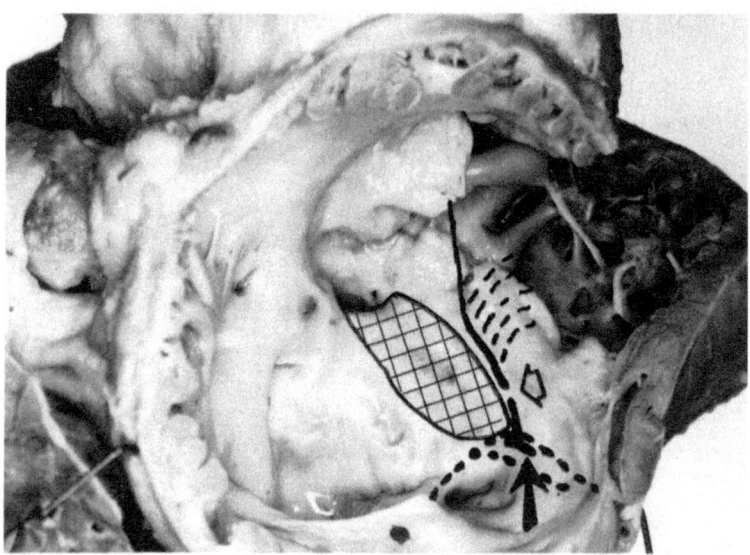

Figure 6 Right-sided view of an operated partial atrioventricular canal defect with disposition of conducting pathways superimposed. The node (closed arrow) lies within the triangle of Koch (dotted lines). An interruption in the main bundle (open arrow) was related to an area of fibrosis close to a suture in the posteroinferior corner of the patch (cross-hatched). The right bundle branch (solid line) arises as a continuation of the main

annulus. The extent of the cleft is variable but in most cases it extends right up to the annulus (complete cleft). The cleft is readily apparent when viewing the mitral valve through the atrial septal defect (Figure 3) but the anatomy is better demonstrated by a left-sided view (Figure 4).

The edges of the cleft are usually thickened and rolled over and the free margin of the cusps at the extremity of the cleft are frequently marked by small tubercles. These are useful markers for the surgeon as the points on the free margin of the cusp segments which should be approximated.

Other abnormalities of the mitral valve occur with a relatively high frequency, notably double orifice and parachute-type deformities with fusion of the papillary muscles[2].

The relative shortening of the left ventricular inflow tract and the downward and forward displacement of the mitral annulus are well seen in Figure 5.

The displaced mitral annulus and reduced inflow tract:outflow tract ratio is probably responsible for the characteristic 'gooseneck' seen angiographically. This can be readily understood by reference to Figure 5.

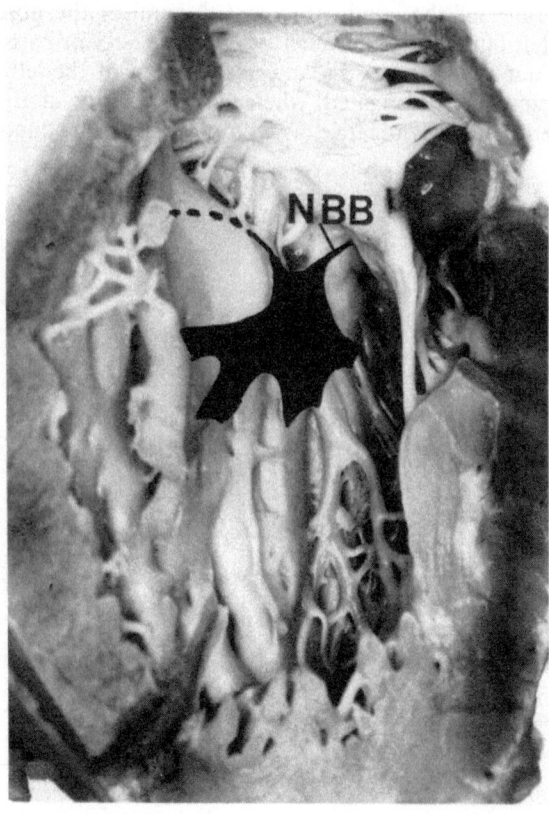

Figure 7 Left-sided view of same specimen as Figure 6 with disposition of left bundle branch indicated. Note relatively short course of the posterior division. The right branch is indicated by dotted line. Key: NBB = non-branching bundle

The conducting pathways in primum defects are similar in all essentials to those seen in complete atrioventricular canal defects (see Chapter 14) as illustrated in Figures 6 and 7.

ELECTROPHYSIOLOGICAL CONSIDERATIONS

Various theories have been proposed to explain the abnormal 'superior' axis of the electrocardiogram in atrioventricular canal defects.

Early activation of the posterobasal part of the left ventricle has been demonstrated by epicardial mapping[4,5] and has been attributed to posterior displacement of the left bundle branch[4,6].

Hypoplasia of the anterior division of the left bundle has also been cited[7].

Deficiency of the posterior septum and free wall[3] might in itself account in part for the 'asymmetry' of activation.

Dilatation of the left ventricle due to mitral incompetence has also been considered, but since the superior axis is present even in cases without a cleft mitral valve[1] and persists following correction, this explanation is untenable.

Recent studies of the conducting tissue[8] confirm the posterior displacement of the left bundle and the deficiency of the posterior part of the ventricular septum, but suggest that the anterior division of the left bundle branch is not hypoplastic but elongated, whereas the posterior division is markedly foreshortened. The asymmetric anatomy of the left bundle divisions is

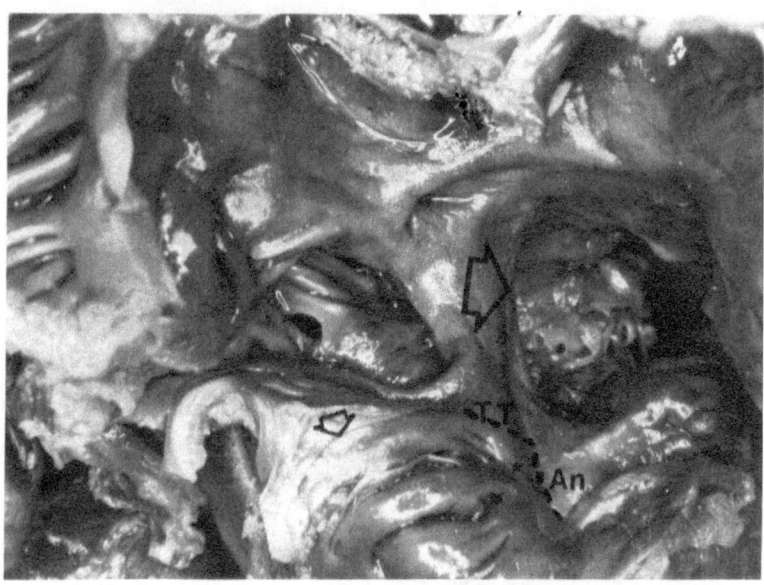

Figure 8 View of atrioventricular canal defect with absent coronary sinus. The valve of the inferior vena cava (small arrow) runs down towards the atrioventricular annulus (An) indicating the position of the tendon of Todaro (T.T.) and the atrioventricular node (asterisk); the large open arrow indicates the upper margin of the defect

probably sufficient to account for markedly asymmetric activation of the left ventricle and the resulting abnormal axis.

The occasional occurrence of common atrium in association with atrioventricular canal defects, and of absence of the coronary sinus ostium as a marker of the atrioventricular node make it desirable for the surgeon to be familiar with other possible markers. If the inferior vena cava is present and its 'valve' can be identified this may be used as a marker of the tendon of Todaro (Figure 8). Alternatively, the position of the posterior 'crest' of the ventricular septum, where it reaches the atrioventricular annulus also indicates the likely site of the node which lies on the atrial side of the annulus immediately above this point.

References

1. Goor, D. and Lillehei, C. W. (1975). In *Congenital Malformations of the Heart*, p. 143 (New York: Grune and Stratton)
2. Ugarte, M., Salamanca, F. E. and Quero, M. (1976). Endocardial cushion defects. An anatomical study of 54 specimens. *Br. Heart J.*, **38**, 674
3. Goor, D., Lillehei, C. W. and Edwards, J. E. (1968). Further observations on the pathology of the atrioventricular canal malformation. *Arch. Surg.*, **97**, 954
4. Boineau, J. P., Moore, E. N. and Patterson, D. F. (1973). Relationship between the E.C.G., ventricular activation, and the ventricular conduction system in ostium primum ASD. *Circulation*, **48**, 556
5. Durrer, D., Roos, J. P. and Van Dam, R. T. (1966). The genesis of the electrocardiogram of patients with ostium primum defects (ventral atrial septal defects). *Am. Heart J.*, **71**, 642
6. Lev., M. (1958). The architecture of the conduction system in congenital heart disease: 1. Common atrioventricular orifice. *Arch. Pathol. (Chicago)*, **65**, 174
7. Feldt, R. H., Du Shane, J. W., Titus, J. L. (1970). The atrioventricular 'conduction' system in persistent common atrioventricular canal defect. Correlations with electrocardiogram. *Circulation*, **42**, 437
8. Thiene, G. and Anderson, R. H. (1978). The conducting tissues in atrioventricular canal malformations. In *Paediatric Cardiology 1977*. (Edinburgh: Churchill Livingstone) (In preparation)

19

Surgery for ostium primum atrial septal defect

J. K. ROSS

This chapter is concerned only with the surgical technique of the repair of ostium primum atrial septal defect (ASD) and associated atrioventricular valve abnormalities. It does not, therefore, deal with diagnosis; selection for surgery; the place, if any, for palliation in infancy; or the late results. In the past 10 years I have repaired over 40 of these defects with two hospital deaths. My interest and experience with this abnormality dates from 1959, and I owe much to Dr Frank Gerbode and Sir Thomas Holmes Sellors, both considerable contributors to the surgical management of ostium primum ASD, for all they taught me.

The management of the mitral valve will be considered first, and secondly the management of the septal defect.

THE MITRAL VALVE

The cleft mitral valve

The decision to suture the cleft is not difficult if the valve has been shown to be regurgitant preoperatively. In the occasional case when there is little or no regurgitation the decision is more difficult. On the two occasions when I have left the cleft alone, in one the valve remained competent, and in the other regurgitation developed later. In valves without regurgitation that have had their clefts sutured, regurgitation has not been created in any instance; therefore I favour routine closure of the cleft. I have, incidentally, had one case of classical primum ASD with no cleft of the mitral valve.

The technique of suturing is important. A suture placed at the apex of the cleft and lifted up (see Figure 1) allows matching up of the two halves of the leaflet. The repair is always started at the septal end and carried towards the free margin of the cusp. The sutures should be passed from the ventricular to the atrial surface of the cleft margin, because in this way the in-curved margins may be rolled outwards on the needle-point. This reduces the risk of

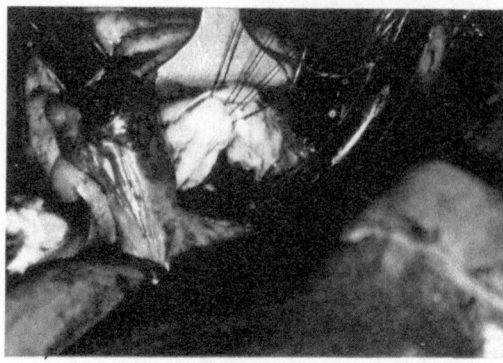

Figure 1 The mitral valve through the left atriotomy showing the cleft with the suture at the edge of the cleft

taking too much cusp tissue (which is the case when the suturing is done the opposite way) which causes shortening of the cusp by turning in more tissue. The suture line is made with serial interrupted 4/O or 5/O material, double-armed, and continued until the nodule is reached on the free margin of the cusp at the point of chordal insertion.

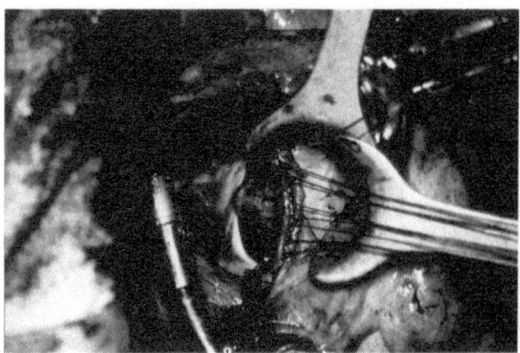

Figure 2 Closure of the septral defect using a pericardial graft

The repair must then be tested. As with all conservative procedures on the mitral valve, this can only be done satisfactorily with the heart beating, and therefore with tone in the papillary muscles. At this point in the operation, therefore, aortic root perfusion with a single coronary cannula is started, and a left ventricular vent is put in. If enough blood can be persuaded to enter the left ventricle by distorting the aortic root and creating aortic regurgitation, this may be sufficient to test the valve. If not, blood is introduced up the left ventricular vent using the second coronary cannula (see Figure 3). This method, taking great care not to over-distend the left ventricle and avoiding coronary air embolism by tripping the mitral valve as the left ventricle fills, allows proper inspection of the valve with the heart beating, and the clamp on

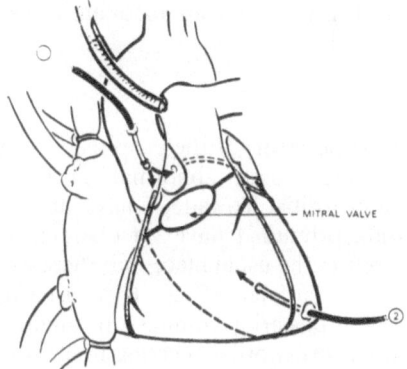

Figure 3 The left ventricular vent used as a perfusion cannula to test the repair of the mitral valve

the aorta preventing cerebral air embolism. Extra sutures are added if required, and the test repeated until a satisfactory result has been achieved.

Double mitral orifice

This unusual finding is commonly associated with some regurgitation, and in the cases that I have seen, the regurgitation has been limited to one of the two orifices. (see Figures 4a and b). The functional state of the valve can only be precisely demonstrated by testing the valve before attempting repair. The regurgitation may be controlled by repairing the cleft in the usual way, and although I have not had to do this, the lesser orifice (if it is the regurgitant one) may have to be closed altogether. It goes without saying that the single remaining orifice or the sum of the two orifices post repair must be adequate and not stenotic – if this cannot be achieved this could be an indication for valve replacement.

In one case the accessory orifice was found in the left half of a classically

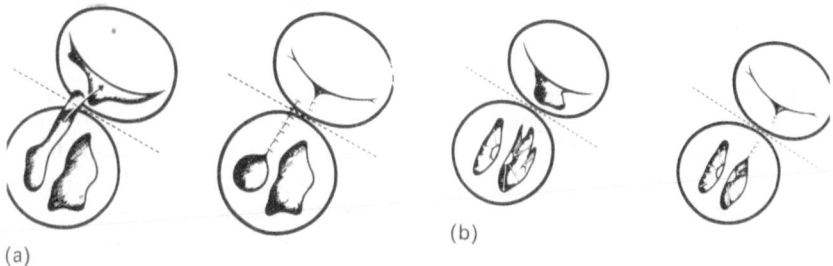

(b)

(a)

Figure 4 (a and b) Examples of double mitral valves orifice. The oblique dotted line represents the plane of the atrial septum

cleft anterior leaflet. On testing after routine suture of the cleft, there was no leak from either orifice, so the lesser one was left alone. Both orifices were individually stenotic, but together gave an adequate valve area.

Valve replacement

Valve replacement may be necessary if the cusp tissue is grossly deficient, if the chordal attachments are grossly abnormal, or if the valve has been affected by bacterial endocarditis. To date, I have had to replace only one valve in the oldest ostium primum I have yet operated on – a 59-year-old woman. The valve was cleft in the usual place, but there were no commissures and the valve had a roughly circular orifice. The posterior papillary muscle was inserted into where the posterior commissure ought to have been, and from this arose many very short chordae 'herring-bone' fashion, and attached to both cusps. There was no chordal support where the antero-lateral commissure should have been, and suture of the cleft would clearly have made the valve stenotic. Her post-operative X-ray shows the prosthetic valve clearly demonstrating the rotational abnormality in this condition (see Figure 5).

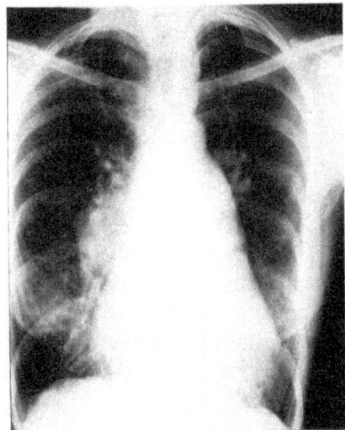

Figure 5 Post-operative X-ray of the prosthetic valve showing the abnormal rotation of the atrio-ventricular plane

To end my comments on the management of the valve – for some time I have been slightly uneasy about the repair when it gets to the free margin of the cusp, because often there is a small V-shaped notch which remains, however carefully the cleft is sutured. I wonder whether we should be trying something different here, and suggest one answer might be to borrow the plastic surgeons' approach to a cleft in another place. (See Figure 6a and b). The tricuspid valve has not presented any particular problem at operation or postoperatively – it is occasionally worth repairing if deficient and offering itself for suture.

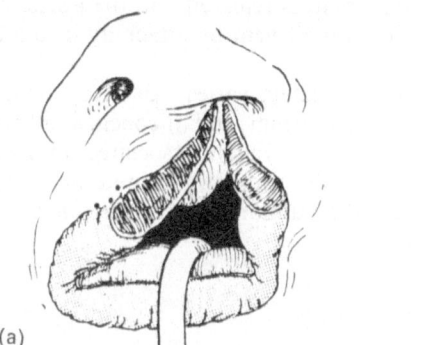
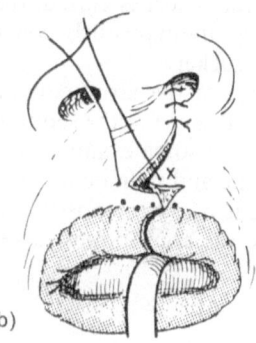

(a)

(b)

Figure 6 (a and b) Plastic repair used for hare lip. This technique of edge advancement might be suitable for avoiding the notch in the free margin when repairing the mitral valve. (Reproduced from *Plastic Surgery* by R. Battle, by kind permission of the author and Butterworths Ltd.)

MANAGEMENT OF THE SEPTAL DEFECT

The material used for closing the defect is one of personal choice, but I have always used the pericardium, and have had only one recurrent defect which was associated with important residual regurgitation. The risk of haemolysis due to a residual regurgitant jet striking a fabric patch was pointed out some years ago by W. P. Cleland, and if fabric is used there is much to be said for covering the left side of the patch with pericardium. If there is an associated secundum ASD this is usually closed by direct suture.

The technique of closure of the septal defect is only interesting where it applies to the area in the region of the conduction mechanism between the margin of the tricuspid valve and the right end of the septal defect rim. At this point I must admit to having no experience of bundle mapping. This distance is very variable, and in older adults can be considerable. Some make the suture line traverse away towards the coronary sinus and then back again, much as in the corresponding part of a Mustard procedure, but I have no first-hand experience of this method. If the right end of the free margin of the defect is grasped with dissecting forceps and lifted up, a ridge is developed which leads to the point where the inferior aspect of the repair ends on the tricuspid valve. If superficial but adequate bites are taken with the needle in the line of this ridge, it is possible to avoid damage to the conduction tissue. On occasions, this dangerous angle may be closed by taking more than one bite in purse-string fashion – again keeping the line of the needle track in the plane of the septum, and using this stitch to anchor the corner of the patch.

The next question is whether or not this part of the operation should be done with the heart beating, or in arrest. If the testing method described has been used for the valve, it is convenient to keep the heart beating for the first part (i.e. the difficult part) of the septal repair, but if the coronary sinus return or the movement makes it difficult to sew accurately, it is best to stop perfusing the aortic root briefly, place the few key sutures, and then re-start the heart to make sure the conduction mechanism is intact.

Once the defect is closed, the aortic clamp is released and the aortic root cannula is simultaneously converted into an air vent by attaching it to a low pressure sucker.

The size of the atrial component of the defect varies from very small to complete absence of the septum or common atrium, and in conclusion I want to show you some examples of this, (see Figure 7a–e). Associated anomalies of systemic and pulmonary venous return are common, but in no instance to date has it proved impossible to deflect the pulmonary and systemic venous return to the appropriate valve orifice.

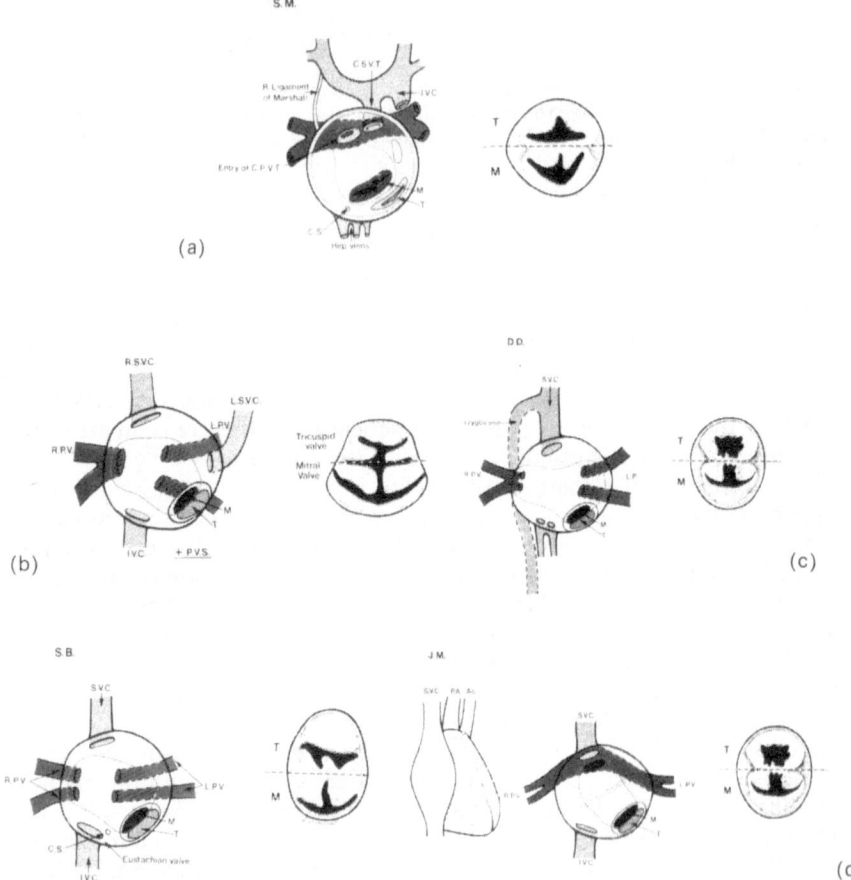

Figure 7 (a–e)   This series of diagrams shows the findings in five examples of common atrium. In each case the diagram on the right shows the configuration of the A-V valves with the dotted line indicating the plane of the atrial septum. A wide variety of venous returns may be encountered in this condition as the diagrams indicate

20

Endocardial cushion: partial A-V canal – long-term results

Å. SENNING

The atrioventricular (A-V) canal is a relatively rare congenital cardiac malformation in our surgical series. This defect of the endocardial cushion has shown all variations from the so-called ostium primum atrial septal defect (ASD), where there exists a fibrous continuity between the anterior superior endocardial cushion and the posterior–inferior endocardial cushion, to the total A-V canal with a ventricular septal defect (VSD) and free floating valves without attachment between the A-V valves and the intraventricular muscular septum. The partial form with an ASD and 'splits' or defects in the mitral and tricuspid valves has the valves fixed to the interventricular septum. Included in our series are patients with an unusually small VSD. The presence of a VSD and the fixation of the valves near this VSD makes the limitation to a total A-V canal uncertain.

SURGICAL MATERIAL

Our material consists of 68 patients. Thirty-two had associated anomalies; nineteen showed a ventricular septal defect; ten had a large foramen ovale defect that had to be closed; two had a sub-valvular aortic muscular stenosis; and one had a partial anomalous pulmonary venous return. Figure 1 shows the age distribution among the first 47 patients. Twenty-two were 1–10 years old at the time of operation, only one was 6 months of age. Twenty-three were between 11 and 50 years in this series. Twelve patients had a systolic pulmonary artery pressure above 50 mmHg. The degree of pulmonary hypertension did not seem to increase with age.

SURGICAL TECHNIQUE

When suturing the cleft mitral valve, the sutures are placed about 3–6 mm away from the thickened margin in order to narrow the valve orifice and to

155

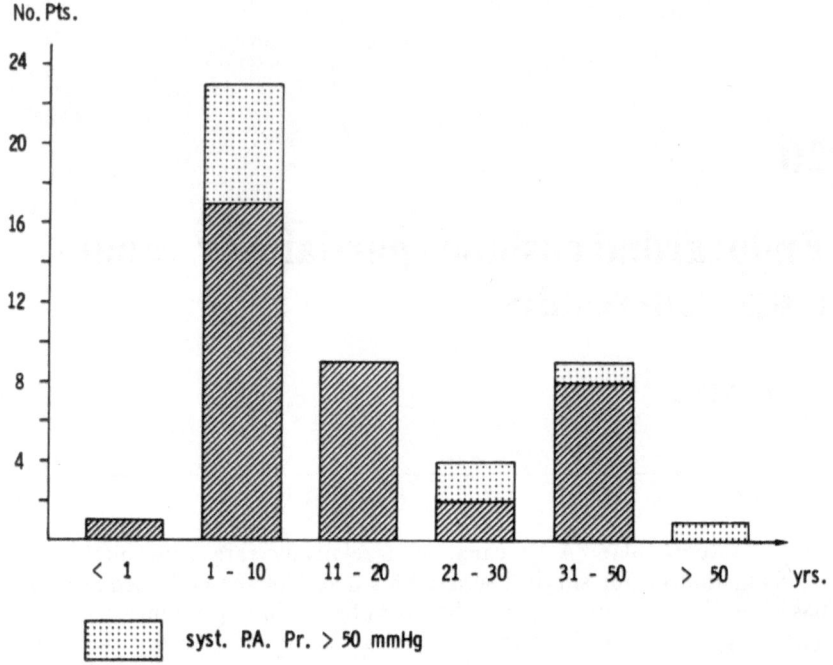

syst. P.A. Pr. > 50 mmHg

Figure 1 Age distribution of 47 patients undergoing surgery for endocardial cushion defect

elongate the subvalvular supporting mechanism. No chordae are cut. The intra-atrial septal defect is closed with a patch sutured at the top of the ridge between the tricuspid and mitral valves following the annulus on the mitral side and to the left of the rim of the atrial septum. The VSD when present, is closed with the aid of either a teflon felt or a small Dacron patch.

RESULTS

In three patients only was an ASD closed without reconstruction of the mitral valve (Table 1). In 47, an additional valvular repair was necessary. There were two early and two late deaths. Eighteen patients had in addition to the valvular repair and the closure of the ASD a closure of a small VSD.

Table 1 Patients undergoing partial A-V canal and outcome

			Deaths	
	No. of patients	Reoperations	Early	Late
ASD closure	3			
ASD closure + valvular repair	47	(2)	2	2
ASD + VSD closure + valvular repair	18			
TOTAL	68	(2)	2	2

ASD = atrial septal defect
VSD = ventricular septal defect

156

The cause of early death (Table 2) was a low postoperative output in one patient, who was more than 50 years of age with pulmonary hypertension, and arrhythmia in the other patient. Suicide was considered to be the cause of late death in one patient; the other one died at reoperation for replacement of the insufficient mitral valve. Autopsy showed a myocardial infarction and an overseen VSD.

Table 2 Patients undergoing partial A-V canal – cause of death

Early: postoperative low output	1
arrhythmia	1
Late: suicide	1
Reop: (MI + VSD) Myoc. Inf.	1
TOTAL	4

MI = mitral insufficiency
VSD = ventricular septal defect
Myoc. Inf. = myocardial infarction

FOLLOW-UP

Mitral valve function

At follow-up 7 months to 14 years postoperatively (Figure 2), the function of the mitral valve was studied in the first 48 patients. Twenty-seven had no

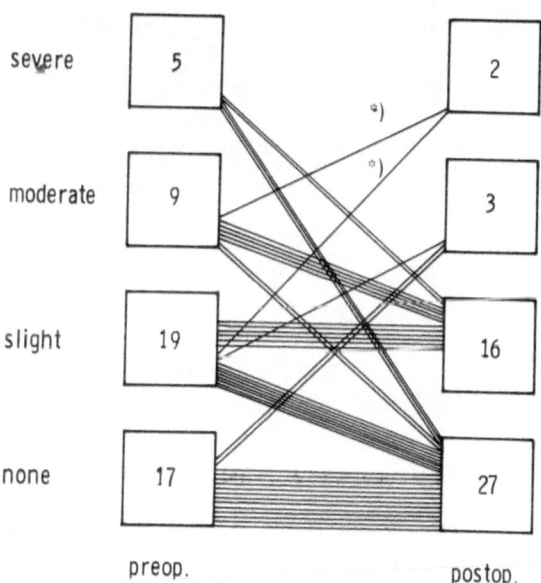

severe 5   2

*)

*)

moderate 9   3

slight 19   16

none 17   27

preop.   postop.

* Mitral Valve Replacement

Figure 2 Follow-up of 48 patients after partial A-V canal – degree of mitral regurgitation. Mean follow-up = 3.2 years

157

regurgitation, 16 had a slight and three a moderate insufficiency. Two patients, both adults, needed a mitral valvular replacement because of severe insufficiency.

Shunts

Two patients showed a 20% left-to-right shunt at the last follow-up. In three patients the shunt was estimated to be 30% and in another three between 40 and 60% (Figure 3).

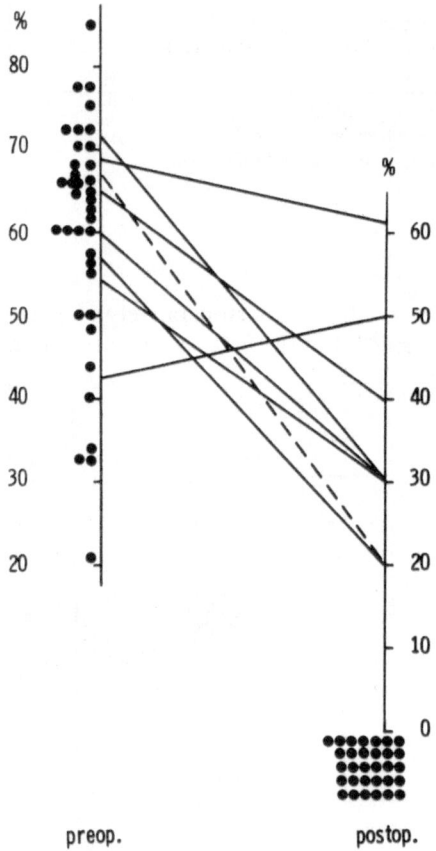

preop.　　　　　　　postop.

Figure 3 Follow-up of patients after partial A-V canal – degree of left-to-right shunt. Follow-up on 40 patients; mean follow-up = 3.3 years

Arrhythmias

In 37 patients the ECG was closely controlled. The mean follow-up was 3.3 years. There were 27 patients with a normal PQ time. Three had pre-operative and postoperative first degree A-V block. There was a second degree A-V block in one patient. A right bundle branch block was present in 19 patients and a partial bundle branch block in six. One patient had a total A-V block preoperatively and needed a pacemaker. At reoperation the total A-V block had disappeared and the rhythm varied between sinus and nodal rhythm.

Cardiothoracic ratio

In 37 patients the cardiothoracic ratio was measured 1 year postoperatively and 2–12 years postoperatively (Figure 4). With the exception of the two reoperated patients with severe mitral insufficiency and patients with moderate insufficiency and shunts the cardiothoracic ratio became significantly smaller than preoperatively. The ratio decreased from 0.58 to 0.48.

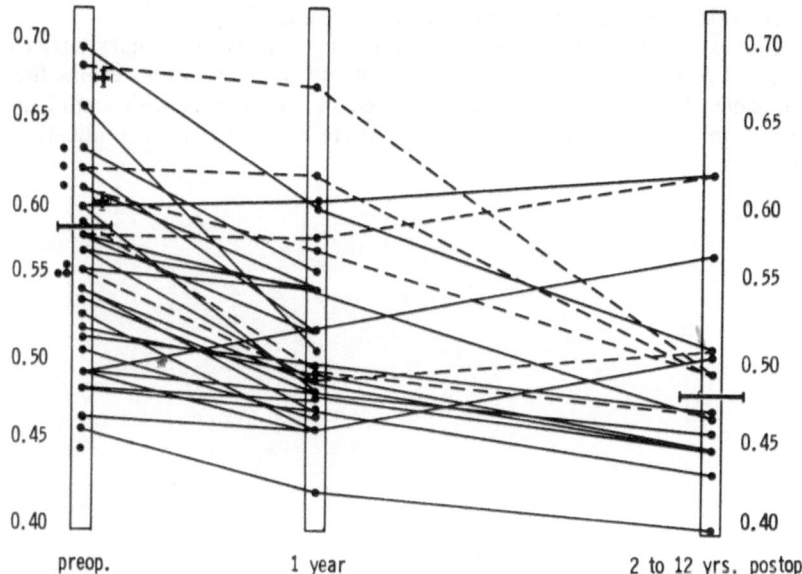

Figure 4   Follow-up of patients after partial A-V canal – cardiothoracic index. Follow up on 33 patients; mean follow-up = 3.1 years

Classification according to New York Health Authority (NYHA)

This classification is inadequate since about 50 % of the patients were children less than 10 years of age. Thirty-seven patients were classified at follow-up. One patient with pulmonary hypertension is still in class III, six patients with mitral insufficiency or shunts are considered to be class II and 29 are class 1. Among those are five who had pulmonary hypertension at operation.

DISCUSSION

Usually the partial type of endocardial cushion defect can be completely corrected. The main problem is still the mitral insufficiency. With this we think it is important to suture the valve in such a way that the subvalvular supporting mechanism is elongated at the same time as the valvular orifices are diminished. The reconstruction has not produced mitral stenosis and it has not occurred during follow-up in this series. On the other hand mitral insufficiency persisted postoperatively in some patients. Two of them have been reoperated for replacement of the mitral valve. In none of the cases was tricuspid insufficiency or stenosis caused by the operation.

A series of left-to-right shunts is difficult to explain, but it is possible that we overlooked a small ventricular septal defect in some cases. It is also possible that the patch closing the atrial septal defect became detached from the atrial septal rim, or more specifically from the valves, where the sutures are placed very superficially to avoid the bundle of His.

The follow-up also shows that late rhythm disturbances are rare and that a complete A-V block can be avoided. Even in older patients the cardio-thoracic index decreases if a good correction can be done.

In conclusion, there has been no deterioration of good primary surgical results and as the operative mortality is low and the late complications few, we consider that this operation is indicated in all patients with significant mitral insufficiency or left-to-right shunt where no special contraindications are present.

Section IV
Surgery of the 4th and 6th aortic canal

21

Results of patent ductus arteriosus ligation in infants and children

R. J. SZARNICKI

Between 1946 and 1974, 1098 children underwent ligation of a patent ductus arteriosus at the Hospital for Sick Children, Great Ormond Street.

We have preferred ligation rather than division of the duct at our institution because we believe it to be a safer and much simpler procedure. With long ducts, up to five ligatures using heavy braided silk have been used to obliterate the lumen throughout its length. Using this method, we believe that the risk of cutting through the friable ductal tissue is reduced. We also believe that the multiple-ligature technique ensures complete closure of the duct while almost eliminating the chance of recurrence, 99% of our children have been managed with this technique. Only six cases of recurrent patency of the ductus arteriosus have been encountered. These were presumably the result of inadequate ligation rather than recanalization. The specific technique and numbers of ligatures used in these cases were not recorded.

Table 1 Indications for ductal division

1. Short wide duct (diameter = aortic diameter)
2. Recurrent duct (i.e., inadequate ligation or recanalization)
3. Recent subacute bacterial endocarditis
4. Aneurysmal dilatation
5. Calcification

There are situations where ductal ligation is unsatisfactory. The risks of haemorrhage, recurrent nerve injury and tedious difficult dissection can be reduced in specific situations by division. Our indications for ductal division are limited (Table 1) and when these situations are present we believe one should be prepared to use a temporary aortic shunt or even left heart bypass if the need for aortic clamping is anticipated for control of bleeding.

AGE DISTRIBUTION

The age distribution of our patients (see Figure 1) ranged from 3 days to 12 years, the majority being between 6 months and 4 years of age. Those patients in the older age groups were more frequently encountered early in the series; 461 patients in this series were less than 1 year of age.

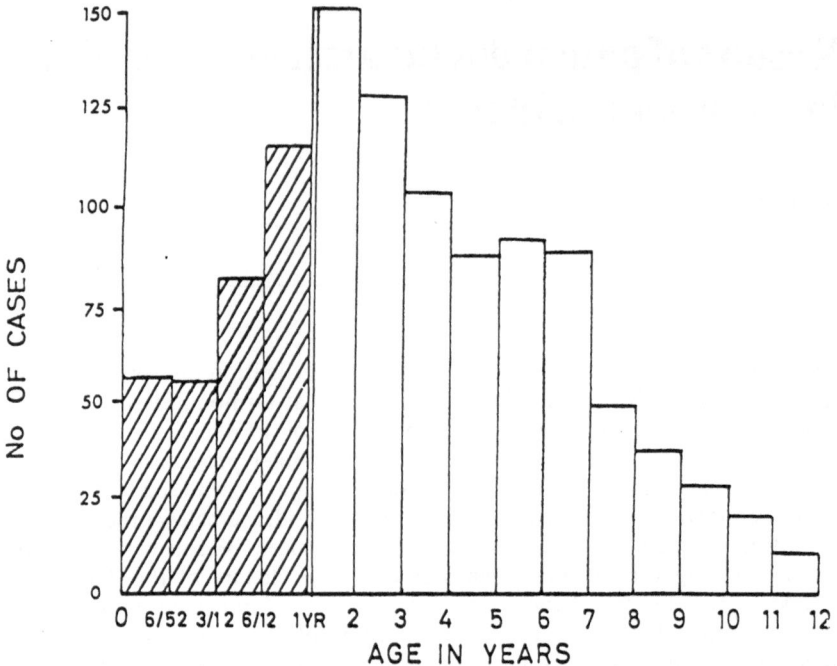

Figure 1   Patent ductus arteriosus in infants and children

Symptoms due to an isolated patent ductus arteriosus were not common; 58% of all patients were asymptomatic and had elective closure of the duct. The remaining 42% had a variety of symptoms related to high pulmonary blood flow (Figure 2). A variety of associated cardiac anomalies was found in 368 patients, or 80%, who presented with symptomatic ducts. Ventricular septal defect was the most common single lesion associated with a patent ductus arteriosus (Table 2). It is interesting to note the relatively high frequency of aortic valve disease in this group of patients; 294 cases, or 80% of these patients with associated cardiac lesions, were noted to be less than 1 year of age. In addition, 167 patients who were symptomatic and were under 1 year of age had an isolated patent ductus arteriosus. These two groups combined represent 85% of all symptomatic patients in the entire series.

There were 637 patients in this group greater than 1 year of age. Amongst these patients, there were 12 deaths, giving a mortality of 1.8%. Ten of the 12 patients died 3–10 years after duct ligation of progressive pulmonary

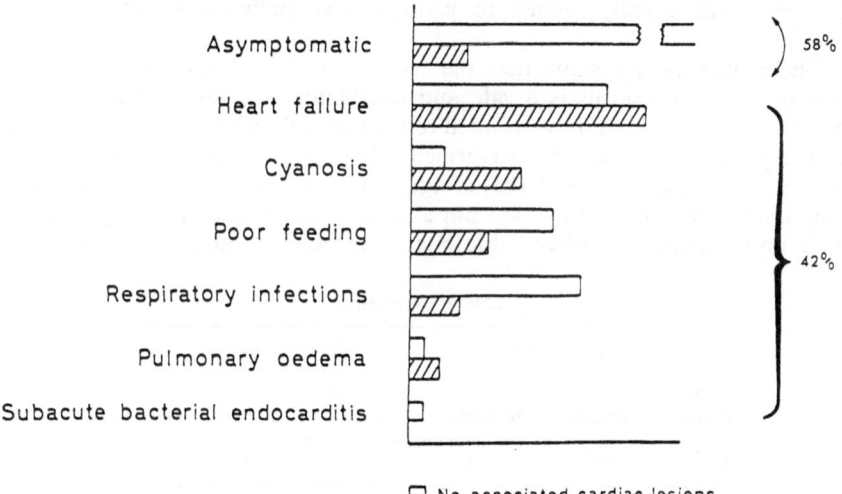

Asymptomatic

Heart failure

Cyanosis

Poor feeding

Respiratory infections

Pulmonary oedema

Subacute bacterial endocarditis

☐ No associated cardiac lesions
▨ With associated cardiac lesions

Figure 2 Patent ductus arteriosus in infants and children

Table 2   Associated cardiac anomalies

VSD	86
VSD + ASD	15
ASD	14
Aortic valve disease	33
Mitral valve disease	14
Pulmonary stenosis	11
TGA	19
Others	49

VSD = ventricular septal defect;
ASD = atrial septal defect;
TGA = transposition of the great arteries

Table 3   Mortality

< 1 year			> 1 year		
No. of patients	deaths	Percentage	No. of patients	deaths	Percentage
461	51	11	637	12*	1.8

* Late deaths due to progressive pulmonary vascular disease

vascular obstructive disease. In the infant group, of less than 1 year of age, there were 461 patients with 51 deaths: a mortality of 11 % (Table 3).

Of the 368 patients who had associated cardiac anomalies, 52 died after ligation of the duct giving a mortality of 14 % in this group of very sick infants; 730 patients had an isolated patent ductus arteriosus and among these, there were 15 deaths: a mortality of 2 %. In this latter group, the cause of death was usually related to postoperative pulmonary complications (Table 4).

These data clearly show that the technique of multiple ligation of the patent ductus arteriosus is a safe and satisfactory technique. None of the deaths in this series can be attributed to the surgical technique used. Ligation of the patent ductus can be performed safely with a very low mortality in that group of patients over 1 year of age and in those in whom the duct is the only lesion present. In the infant population however, the mortality remains high and particularly when additional associated cardiac lesions coexist.

Table 4 Mortality

With associated anomalies			Without associated anomalies		
No. of patients	deaths	Percentage	No. of patients	deaths	Percentage
368	52	14	730	15	2

22

Vascular rings

M. R. DE LEVAL AND L. H. BURR

Vascular rings are congenital anomalies of the aortic arch, causing varying degrees of compression on the trachea and/or the oesophagus.

Most vascular rings result from either a lack of regression, or an abnormal regression of a segment of the aortic arch system. There are six pairs of primitive aortic arches. The first and second pairs disappear. The third pair enters in the formation of the carotid arteries. Both fourth arches persist but their histories differ. On the left side the arch becomes the permanent aortic arch, connecting the aorta distal to the origin of the left carotid to the dorsal thoracic aorta. The right fourth arch forms the proximal portion of the right subclavian artery. The fifth pair of arches disappears. The proximal portion of the six arches form the pulmonary arteries and the distal portion of the left sixth arch remains as the ductus arteriosus.

A double aortic arch results from a failure of regression of the right dorsal aorta distal to the fourth arch.

An obliteration and disappearance of the left dorsal aortic segment situated between the fourth and sixth aortic arches with persistence of the right fourth and right dorsal aorta results in a right aortic arch which may form a vascular ring if a ligamentum connects the descending aorta and the pulmonary artery.

A regression of the fourth right arch and persistence of the right dorsal aorta results in an anomalous origin of the right subclavian artery from the descending aorta.

DOUBLE AORTIC ARCH

This chapter discusses the most common vascular rings: the double aortic arch. In this anomaly, two aortic arches arise from a normally situated ascending aorta and join to form a single descending aorta. One of the aortic arches passes in front of the trachea, whereas the other passes over the right main bronchus and proceeds behind the trachea and the oesophagus. The

167

right common carotid and the right subclavian arteries originate from the posteriorly located right aortic arch, whereas the left carotid artery and the left subclavian artery usually arise from the anterior or left aortic arch. In 80% of the cases, the left aortic arch is smaller than the right. The space bound by the vascular ring is generally not adequate to accommodate the trachea and the oesophagus and compression of the structures is usual.

Most commonly, in this type of vascular ring there is a history of respiratory difficulties and repeated chest infections dating from birth. Stridor is nearly always found. Typically, extension of the head appears to improve the respiratory difficulty, and deflection of the head makes it worse. A persistent brassy cough can also be present, resulting from pressure on the left recurrent laryngeal nerve. Dysphagia is due to the compression on the oesophagus, its degree varying from one patient to another. Sometimes the dysphagia is not observed in an infant while being bottle-fed, but appears only when solid foods are started.

Examination of the oesophagus and the trachea by barium swallow is the most important part of the investigation. On the lateral views, one can see a posterior indentation of the oesophagus and a constriction on both sides of the anteroposterior views. A well-penetrated chest X-ray can also reveal the localized anterior narrowing of the trachea.

Surgical treatment is mandatory in symptomatic infants and is often a life-saving procedure. A left posterolateral incision is used in most cases.

The various major vessels arising from the aortic arch are identified and the smaller arch is divided. If the right arch is smaller, the descending aorta is retracted forward and the right arch is divided as it enters this vessel.

RIGHT AORTIC ARCH WITH LEFT LIGAMENTUM

In this anomaly, there is a right aortic arch which passes to the right of the trachea and continues into the descending aorta. The latter may descend to the right or left of the spinal column. A left ductus arteriosus, which is usually obliterated, may arise from the left subclavian artery, or from the upper descending aorta. In that case, a complete vascular ring exists. If the ligamentum is sufficiently taut, it produces symptoms similar to those with double aortic arch. They are usually less severe and the onset comes later in life than in double aortic arch, usually after 3 years of age. Again, the barium swallow is diagnostic, showing an impression of the oesophagus from both sides and posteriorly. The surgical treatment is simple and consists of dividing the ligamentum arteriosum.

THE ANOMALOUS ORIGIN OF THE RIGHT SUBCLAVIAN ARTERY FROM THE DESCENDING AORTA

It is the most common anomaly of the aortic arch system but rarely produces tracheal or oesophageal compression.

The right subclavian artery originates from the descending aorta, then courses upwards and to the right behind the oesophagus in about 80% of the cases, and between the oesophagus and the trachea in about 20% of them.

Most patients have no symptoms and do not require any treatment. When symptoms do occur they usually present as difficulty in swallowing. The barium shows in these cases a small posterior indentation. The trachea is generally not involved. If surgery is required, it consists of division of the left subclavian artery.

THE ANOMALOUS INNOMINATE ARTERY

This is not really a vascular ring, but a vascular compression of the trachea. It results from an innominate artery which arises further to the left of the arch than normal. If the vessel is short and stretched over the trachea, it may produce dyspnoea. Respiratory difficulties, repeated chest infections and stridor are the main symptoms, but these patients do not have swallowing difficulties. The barium swallow is normal. The air tracheogram shows anterolateral compression on the right side of the trachea, and the diagnosis can be confirmed by an aortogram. For symptomatic patients, Gross suggested relieving the compression by pulling the vessel forward and sewing the adventitia of the innominate artery to the sternum. A reimplantation of the innominate artery on the arch has also been suggested.

PULMONARY ARTERY SLING

In this anomaly, the left pulmonary artery arises from the right pulmonary artery and passes between the trachea and the oesophagus to reach the left lung. The symptoms are mainly respiratory and are present shortly after birth. The diagnosis is based again on the barium swallow which shows an anterior impression and a posterior narrowing of the trachea below the level of the aortic arch. A pulmonary arteriogram may be helpful to confirm the diagnosis.

Surgical treatment consists of reimplanting the left pulmonary artery to the main pulmonary artery.

In Table 1, the anatomic varieties of vascular rings operated on at Great

Table 1   Anatomy of vascular rings (1968–76)

Double aortic arch	18
Right aortic arch and left ligamentum	6
Abnormal subclavian artery	7
Innominate artery compression	2
Anomalous left pulmonary artery	1
Total	34

Ormond Street between 1968 and 1976 are shown. As in most series, the double aortic arches were the most common anomalies. The anomalous left pulmonary artery was seen only in one instance. The preoperative symptoms were mainly related to the compression of the trachea and the bronchial tree (Table 2). Dysphagia was present in only 25% of the cases. The results are quite satisfactory (Table 3). There were two operative deaths.

The first patient went into ventricular fibrillation at the opening of the

Table 2   Vascular rings (1968–76)

Symptoms	No. of patients	(%)
Stridor	26	76
Respiratory tract infections	17	50
Cyanosis	13	38
Dysphagia	12	35
Failure to thrive	3	9

Table 3   Vascular rings (1968–76)

Results	No of patients	%
Operative death (cardiac arrest)	2	5.8
Postoperative stridor	4	11.7
Asymptomatic	28	82.3

chest and the second patient was extubated after division of the vascular ring. He had a persistent stridor which suddenly increased 12 hours postoperatively, and at that time the patient sustained a cardiac arrest. Postoperative stridor was fairly common for several weeks. But only in four cases (11.7%) was the stridor significant requiring prolonged intubation. More than 80% of these patients are now asymptomatic.

CONCLUSIONS

Vascular rings, then, are anomalies of the aortic arch system which are likely to present symptoms in infancy or early in childhood. Respiratory symptoms are the most common. The key to diagnosis is based on the clinical history and on a barium swallow for most cases. The bronchoscopy can be helpful in assessing the degree of tracheal compression. In very few cases is the bronchoscopy helpful in making a diagnosis. This is the case in patients with an abnormal origin of the innominate artery. The pressure of the bronchoscope against the innominate artery is typically accompanied by a loss of the right radial pulse. An aortogram or a pulmonary angiogram are very rarely indicated for making the diagnosis. We think that the surgical treatment should not be delayed in symptomatic patients, because there is always a risk of irreversible damage to the trachea, which can be a disastrous complication.

23

Surgical relief of coarctation of the aorta in infancy using the left subclavian arterial flap technique

D. I. HAMILTON

Coarctation of the aorta presenting with cardiac failure in infancy is usually 'preductal' in type[1]. Approximately two-thirds of the cases fall into the 'complicated' group[2] because they have additional cardiac lesions. Mortality is as high as 80% during the first year of life and medical treatment has little to offer when the stricture is severe and associated intracardiac defects are of haemodynamic significance (Table 1). Such infants frequently present in cardiac failure within the first weeks of life. Some improvement may be obtained following digitalization and diuretic therapy. Early investigation by cardiac catheterization and ciné-angiography is necessary.

Table 1   Royal Liverpool Children's Hospital, 1969–76

36 Infants	Age 4 days to 6½ months
Preductal CoA + PDA	34
Juxtaductal CoA + PDA	2
'Simplex' CoA + PDA	12 in 33%
'Complex' CoA + PDA + associated lesion(s)	24 in 67%

PDA = patent ductus arteriosus; CoA = coarctation

In addition to early digitalization and diuretic therapy, the correction of metabolic acidosis is essential, and occasionally positive pressure ventilation is required during or after cardiac catheterization. Early transfer to a paediatric cardiac centre, with special experience in the neonatal age range, is indicated. This requires transportation in an incubator which provides a controlled environment (temperature and humidity), and the presence of a medically qualified attendant is desirable.

The definitive diagnosis is made at cardiac catheterization and angiography. The frequent association of other significant intracardiac defects (Table 1) necessitate careful and complete assessment of intracardiac haemodynamics and anatomy.

Once the diagnosis has been established, and provided that the infant's condition is reasonably satisfactory and cannot be improved further by medical therapy, then surgical correction is indicated on a semi-emergency basis. It is a mistake to delay surgery for the next planned operating-list unless the baby's condition raises no cause for concern.

SURGICAL PHILOSOPHY

The surgery of this condition in infancy should be directed towards the complete relief of stenosis at the site of coarctation in such a manner that subsequent growth in aortic girth is not restricted significantly. Standard techniques fail because their potential for circumferential growth is limited. It is hardly surprising that the incidence of restenosis is considerable and that hypertension persists above the site of reconstruction in a significant number of cases when resection and end-to-end anastomosis is performed in the first weeks of life. We devised the left subclavian flap aortoplasty in 1969, and have developed its use during the past 9 years, encouraged by the immediate and long-term follow-up of our patients. Waldhausen[3] had previously described this procedure and states: 'I believe it is a basically sound operation and have become more and more convinced that it may be the ideal operation in infants to prevent subsequent stenosis of the suture line as the child grows'.

We now employ the left subclavian flap aortoplasty in virtually all anatomical variations of coarctation of the aorta in infancy because it produces very satisfactory early results and can be expected to continue to do so over an indefinite follow-up period.

SURGICAL TECHNIQUE

The left chest is opened by left lateral thoracotomy through the bed of the fourth rib. The lung is displaced forwards and the mediastinal pleura is opened vertically over the aorta, well below the coarctation, and superiorly over the ductus arteriosus, narrow segment, aortic arch and left subclavian artery. The left superior intercostal vein is ligated and divided.

The coarctation, descending thoracic aorta, patent ductus arteriosus, transverse aortic arch and left subclavian artery are dissected out and are isolated in tape slings. The vertebral artery is ligated at its origin to prevent subsequent 'steal' from the cerebral circulation to the left upper limb. The left subclavian artery is ligated and divided below the first rib after occluding its origin from the aortic arch with a miniature vascular clamp. Additional clamps are placed across the transverse aortic arch, the ductus arteriosus and descending thoracic aorta well beyond the lower level of the coarctation. It may be necessary to ligate one or two pairs of intercostal arteries (in continuity) above the level of this clamp.

An incision is carried along the inferior border of the subclavian artery from its distal open end towards the aorta. This same incision is carried down through the narrow segment of the coarctation, and well beyond, onto the lateral wall of the descending thoracic aorta below. This is an important step in the technique as failure to carry the incision far enough inferiorly will result in residual narrowing just distal to the site of the original coarctation. There is frequently an 'internal shelf' of abnormal tissue at the site of the maximal stricture and this is excised carefully with curved scissors or scalpel. The pedicled flap of subclavian artery is assessed for length and width. A 6/O or 7/O polypropylene suture is passed through the midpoint of the divided end of the arterial flap and this is then passed through the apex of the lowest point of the incision in the descending aorta. When this suture is pulled down the flap is positioned to lie within the margins of the aortic incision. If the flap is wide, the distal corners of the flap are bevelled off with scissors and the 'dog-ears' at the proximal end of the flap are excised. Each 'dog-ear' is cut back with scissors and the two corners of tissue are excised in each case. This provides final architecture of the reconstructed aorta which has a smooth calibre and is of pleasing appearance.

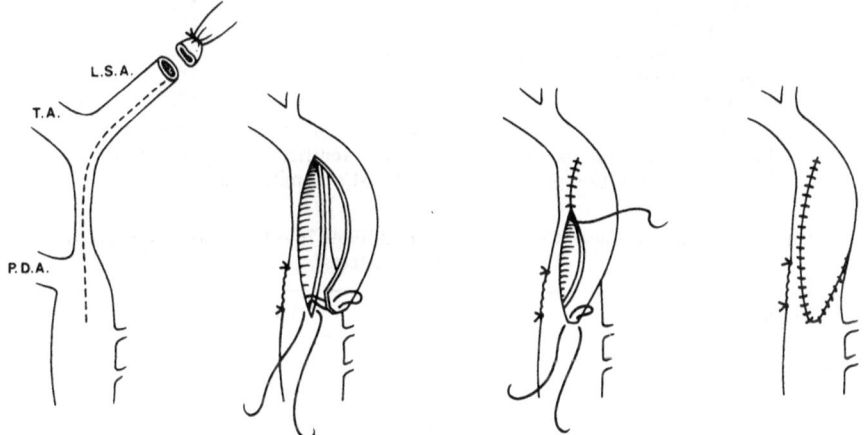

Figure 1 Surgical technique. Steps in the left subclavian flap aortoplasty

The two longitudinal suture lines are inserted using 6/O or 7/O polypropylene material, starting at the proximal end of the flap and proceeding to the apex distally. In this way, a final adjustment in flap length is possible before the suture lines are completed. Clamps are removed and the area is packed. After allowing time for haemostasis the ductus is divided. Division is preferred to ligation in the neonatal period. The surgical technique is summarized in Figure 1. Excellent distal pulsation should be present following reconstruction. If there is an associated ventricular septal defect, which is considered to be large and the right ventricular and pulmonary artery pressures are at systematic level, banding of the main pulmonary artery is performed before the chest is closed.

CLINICAL MATERIAL AND RESULTS

Between late 1969 and September 1976 36 infants aged 4 days to $6\frac{1}{2}$ months at the time of surgery underwent left subclavian flap aortoplasty at the Royal Liverpool Children's Hospital. All had patent ductus arteriosus and two-thirds of the infants had at least one other intracardiac defect. In the great majority this was a ventricular septal defect (Table 2). The patent ductus arteriosus was divided or was ligated in all, and 16 infants underwent banding of the main pulmonary artery also.

Table 2   Royal Liverpool Children's Hospital 1969–76

36 Infants	Coarctation of the aorta	Associated lesions
PDA	36	100%
VSD	22	61%
ASD	3	8%
Hypoplastic aortic arch	1	3%
Hypoplastic left ventricle	1	3%
TGV corrected	1	3%
TGV + VSD	1	3%
TGV + primitive V	1	3%
Aortic V stenosis	2	5%
Parachute MV	1	3%

PDA = patent ductus arteriosus; VSD = ventricular septal defect; TGV = transposition of the great vessels; MV = mitral valve

Table 3   Royal Liverpool Children's Hospital 1969–76—Mortality according to age and associated defects*

36 Infants	Age distribution			
	Under 2 Months	Deaths	2–6½ Months	Deaths
CoA + PDA	7	0 (0%)·	5	0 (0%)
CoA + PDA + additional lesions	17	11 (60%)	7	0 (0%)
	24	11 (46%)	12	0 (0%)

* Hospital mortality overall: 11 cases of 36 = 30%
Abbreviations as in Table 2
CoA = coarctation of the aorta

Two-thirds of the infants (24) were under 8 weeks at the time of surgery and 68% of these had an additional cardiac defect.

The hospital mortality was 30% and was related entirely to the group of infants within the first 8 weeks of life (Table 3). Mortality occurred only in the group who had additional cardiac defects and was not related to the repair of the coarctation itself.

There was no mortality within the group of infants who had coarctation in association with patent ductus arteriosus only, even in the youngest infants.

The 23 survivors have been followed up for at least 1 year and up to 9 years after surgery; two only have femoral pulses that are less than 'good' or 'excellent'. These two children are both normotensive in the upper limbs and one has a gradient of less than 10 mmHg across the reconstructed aortic

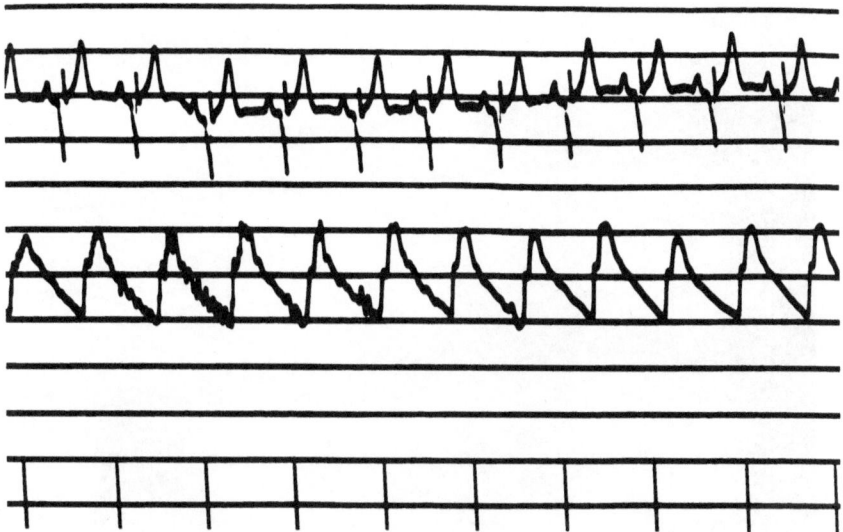

Figure 2 Withdrawal pressure at cardiac catheterization from descending thoracic aorta across the reconstructed site of coarctation of the aorta

segment. Figure 2 demonstrates a withdrawal pressure across the reconstructed area 4½ years after the repair by subclavian aortoplasty was performed. The main feature is the absence of any pressure gradient. Figure 3 is a reproduction of an aortogram 5 years after surgery which was performed on an infant at the age of 6 weeks. The reconstructed area has grown in girth considerably and is of adequate calibre for the present age of the child. Figure 4 charts upper-limb systolic blood pressure, measured at least 1 and up to 7 years postoperatively. All measurements fall within two standard deviations of the normal range for the age of the child at follow-up. This feature, in conjunction with pullback pressure data and the angiographic appearances, suggest that this method of aortic reconstruction is superior to other techniques which are employed in the first months of life. No child has required further surgery to the reconstructed aorta to date – several children have undergone open-heart surgery subsequently, when the ventricular septal defect was closed and the main pulmonary artery was reconstructed at the site of previous banding.

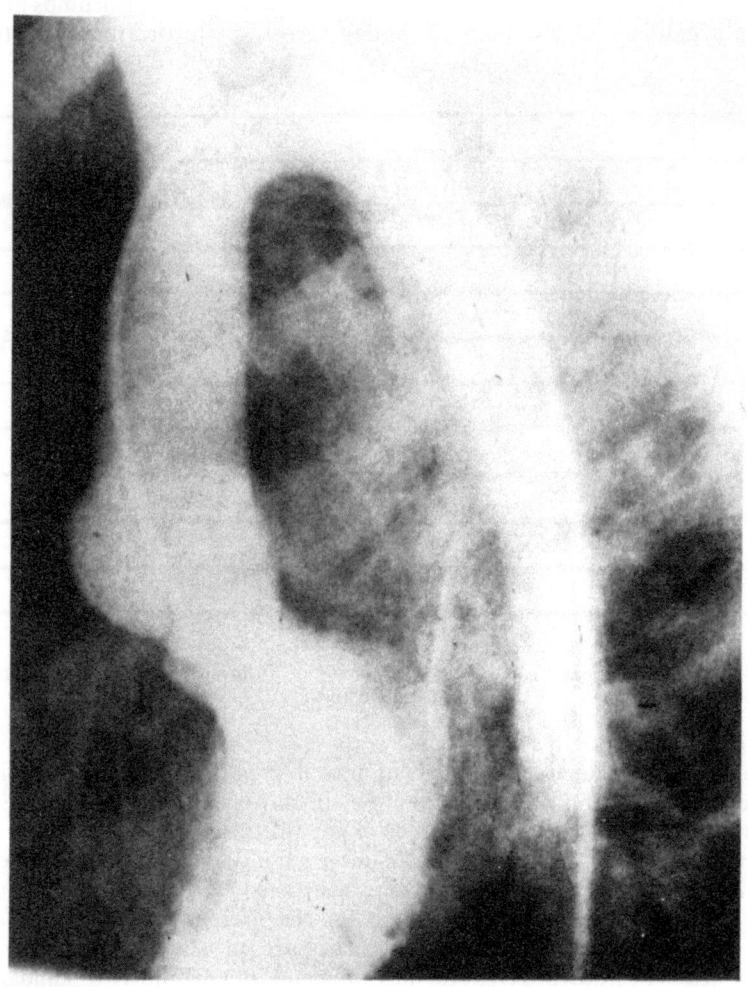

Figure 3 Left ventriculogram and aortogram 5 years after left subclavian flap aortoplasty which was performed at the age of 6 weeks

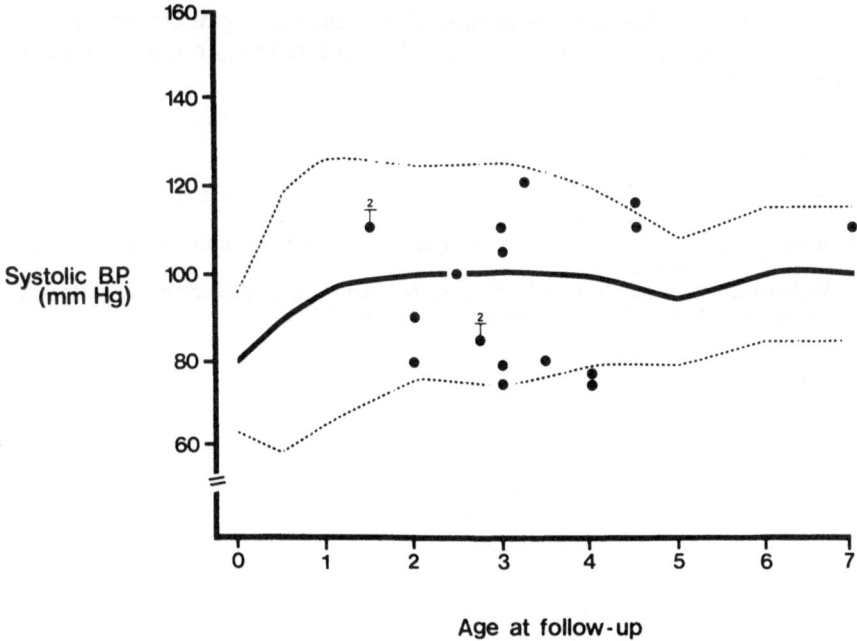

Age at follow-up

Figure 4 Upper-limb systolic blood pressure in 19 infants, measured up to 7 years after left subclavian flap aortoplasty for coarctation of the aorta. The great majority of blood pressures fall within two standard deviations of the mean blood pressure, according to the age of the child

CONCLUSIONS

After 9 years' experience with left subclavian flap aortoplasty for the relief of pre-ductal coarctation in the first months of life, we can draw the following conclusions:

1. The operation is technically straightforward to perform;
2. Hospital mortality and morbidity is no higher than for other procedures used for the correction of this condition;
3. The technique is effective in reducing and possibly in eliminating 're-stenosis' at the site of reconstruction as the repair has excellent growth potential;
4. Normal blood pressure in the upper limbs is maintained in all survivors followed up over a 7-year period.

We are encouraged in the continued use of this procedure and recommend it as the 'operation of choice' for the surgery of coarctation of the aorta in the neonatal and infant periods.

Acknowledgment

I wish to acknowledge the skilled work of my colleagues in the management

177

of these infants. This includes cardiologists, radiologist, pathologist, laboratory, ECG. and theatre technicians, and the ward, recovery room and theatre nursing staff.

References

1. Burford, T. H. (1950). Symposium on clinical surgery: Coarctation of the aorta and its treatment. *Surg. Clin. N. Am.*, **30**, 1249
2. Bahnson, H. T. (1952). Coarctation of the aorta and anomalies of the aortic arch. *Surg. Clin. N. Am.*, **30**, 1313
3. Waldhausen, J. A. and Nahrwold, D. L. (1966). Repair of coarctation of the aorta with a subclavian flap. *J. Thoracic Cardiovasc. Surg.*, **51**, 532

24

Patent ductus arteriosus: indications, operative techniques, and postoperative care in infants

C. LINCOLN

If it is accepted that the incidence of congenital heart disease is six per thousand live births, then the incidence of isolated patent ductus arteriosus is around 7% of all of these with congenital heart disease. In the first year of life the incidence at sea level is 0.04%, and at high altitudes 0.72%.

A recent study by Gittenberger-De Groot[1] at the University of Leiden suggests that a primary anatomical defect of the ductus arteriosus wall is responsible for persistence of the ductus arteriosus, in particular aberrant distribution of elastic material, and the presence of a subendothelial elastic lamina.

Table 1 Patent ductus arteriosus: predisposing causes

1. Maternal rubella (12%)
2. Recessive familial anomaly (3%)
3. Prematurity (20%)

A patent ductus arteriosus must be closed when it persists in prematurity, when there is evidence of a large left-to-right shunt causing congestive cardiac failure with the long-term risk of the development of pulmonary vascular disease, and because of the risk factor of the development of bacterial endocarditis. In addition to these four mentioned medical reasons, a persistent ductus arteriosus must be ligated before the establishment of cardiopulmonary bypass in the treatment of intracardiac congenital or acquired heart lesions. The presence of a persistent ductus arteriosus whilst on cardiopulmonary bypass can cause severe damage to the pulmonary vascular bed and result in a retrograde flow of a large quantity of blood into

179

the pulmonary artery, and then into the right ventricle, obscuring the surgeon's field of operation.

SURGICAL EXPOSURE

A patent ductus arteriosus can be approached through a left posterolateral thoracotomy, through a vertical axillary thoracotomy, or through a median sternotomy, the most common approach being a left posterolateral thoracotomy. The axillary thoracotomy as suggested by Dennis Browne[2] has not gained popular acceptance, but it has the advantage of being an extremely cosmetic incision. Approaching the patent ductus arteriosus from a median sternotomy, as is necessary prior to the institution of cardiopulmonary bypass, is a technique which was first described by Kirklin[3] in 1957 from the Mayo Clinic. In approaching this structure from the front it is helpful to remove both lobes of the thymus gland. This allows a good exposure of the upper ascending aorta and pulmonary artery before bifurcation occurs. Gentle retraction on the adventitia of both great vessels in a caudal direction delivers the upper part of these vessels into the wound. Then the patent ductus arteriosus can be dissected, being sure to dissect around the vessel, not close to the vessel. It is then a relatively simple matter to pass a ligature around for closure (Figures 1 and 2).

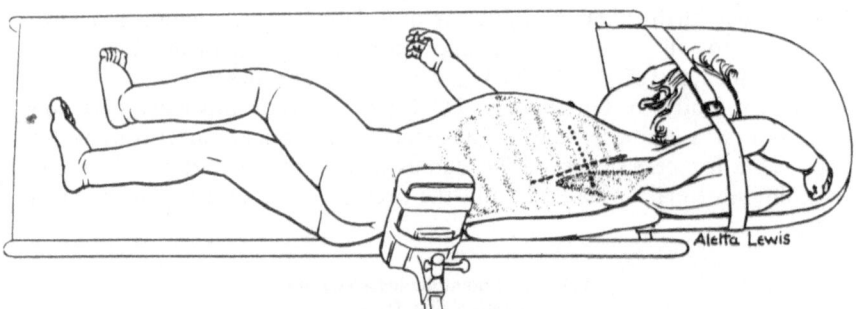

Figure 1 Dennis Browne's axillary incision for transthoracic closure of patent ductus arteriosus

Double ligation in continuity is a safe and effective way of closing a patent ductus arteriosus in infants and young children. However, in adults calcification in the wall of the vessel can occur, and in this instance ligation may be hazardous, since the wall is very friable. In this case division and wide localization of the first part of the descending thoracic aorta is a safe technique. The recurrence rate following the ligation of a patent ductus arteriosus is reported as being 0.5–1 %. When a recurrence occurs closure can be difficult, and in some instances cardiopulmonary bypass (left atrio-femoral bypass) is necessary so that the aorta can be opened opposite the site of entry of the ductus arteriosus into the aortic lumen, and then the orifice of the ductus arteriosus is closed by means of a patch of Dacron cloth (Figure 3). Recent reports of non-surgical closure of patent ductus arteriosus by

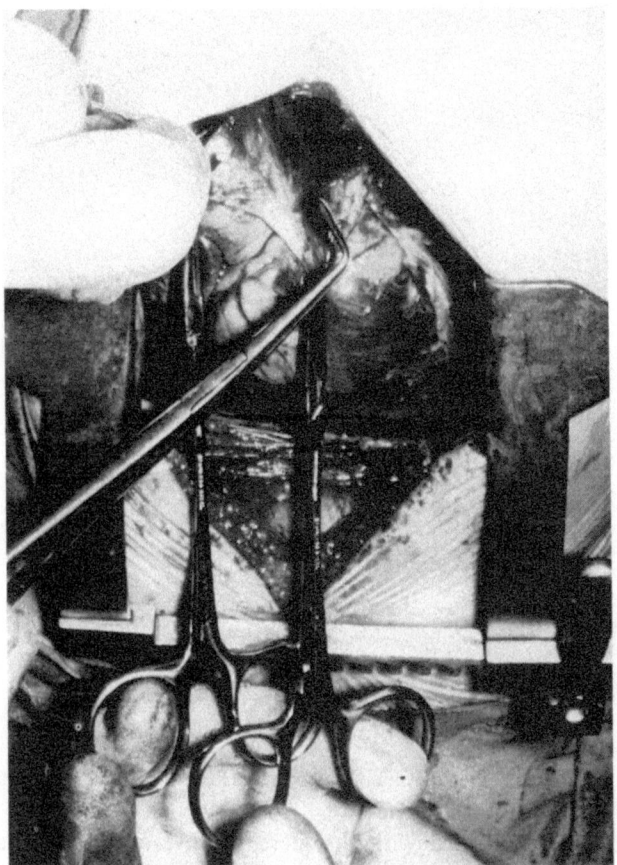

Figure 2 Photograph showing dissection of patent ductus arteriosis through median stenotomy. Note: two artery forceps retracting the great vessels caudally

means of an Ivalon plug[4] passed percutaneously using a cardiac catheter are yet to be proven with long-term follow-up. Closure of complicated ductus arteriosus at cardiopulmonary bypass surgery can also be performed by using profound hypothermia and circulatory arrest, and opening the main pulmonary artery and closing the opening of the ductus arteriosus within the pulmonary artery (Figure 4).

TREATMENT OF PATENT DUCTUS ARTERIOSUS IN INFANCY AND PREMATURITY

In most instances of prematurity the patent ductus arteriosus closes spontaneously. There is, however, a small group of premature infants weighing less than 1500 g in which the presence of a patent ductus arteriosus causes heart failure by left-to-right shunting, which, in the presence of respiratory distress syndrome, can cause difficulty in management. The recent recognition

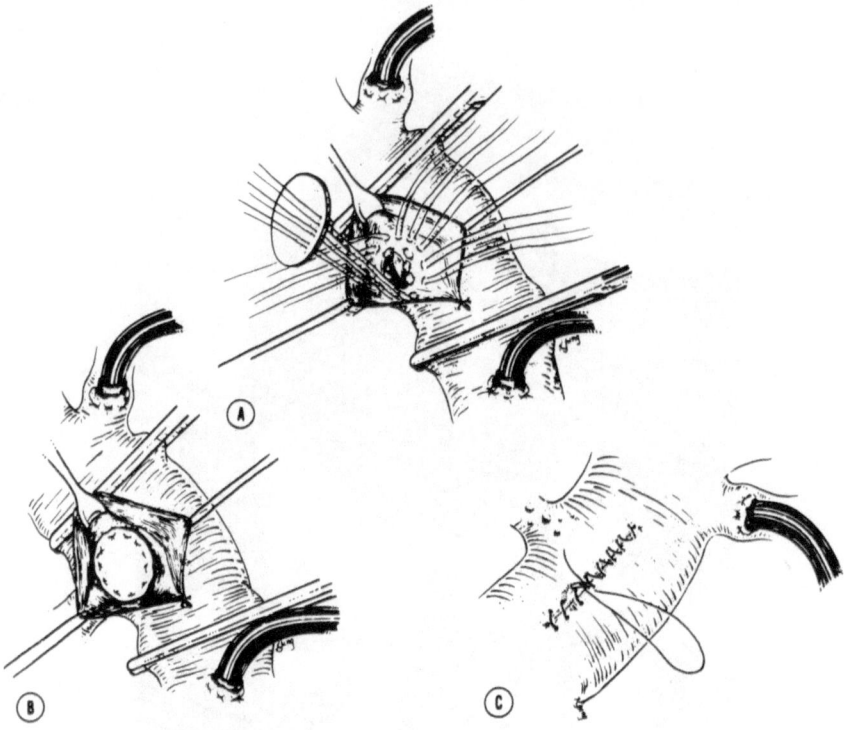

Figure 3 Transaortic patch closure of patent ductus arteriosus using a bypass shunt

of this entity has coincided with the increased use of continuous positive airway pressure breathing, administered by an endotracheal tube or with a close-fitting face-mask. In the respiratory distress syndrome unusually high inspiratory pressures, sometimes greater than 10 cmH$_2$O, are necessary to overcome the primary inability of ventilation; it is probable that the use of such high pressures mitigates against the spontaneous closure of patent ductus arteriosus. The enthusiasm for early closure of patent ductus arteriosus in premature infants must be tempered with the findings of Reynolds and others who note that, in a consecutive series of 300 infants with classical respiratory distress syndrome, the incidence of surgical closure was 0.5%.

POSTOPERATIVE CARE

The postoperative care of children following closure of patent ductus arteriosus is unremarkable. However, in infancy, unless the child is vigorous, great care must be taken to maintain a satisfactory airway, which may necessitate intubation and mechanical ventilation. Since many of these patients have been in congestive cardiac failure and on medical heart failure therapy, continuation of this anti-heart failure therapy into the postoperative period can be useful.

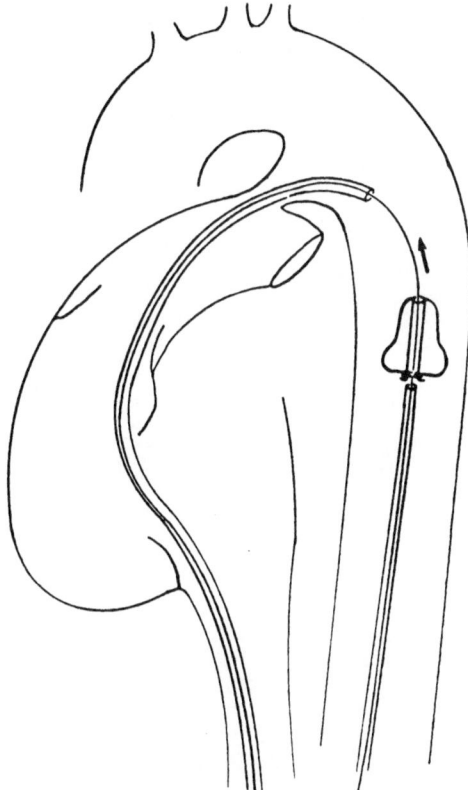

Figure 4   Plug closure of patent ductus arteriosus

References

1. Gittenberger-De Groot, A. C. (1977). Persistent ductus arteriosus: most probably a primary congenital malformation. *Br. Heart J.*, **39**(6), 610
2. Browne, D. (1952). Patent ductus arteriosus. *Proc. Roy. Soc. Med.*, **45**, 719
3. Kirklin, J. W. and Silva, A. W. (1958). Technique of exposing the ductus arteriosus prior to establishing extracorporeal circulation. *Proc. Staff Meet., Mayo Clin.*, **33**, 432
4. Patto, K. Fugino, M. *et al.* (1975). Transfemoral plug closure of patent ductus arteriosus. *Circulation*, **51**, 337
5. Kiterman, J. A., Edmunds, L. H. *et al.* (1972). Patent ductus arteriosus in premature infants. *N. Engl. J. Med.*, **287**, 473
6. Murphy, D. A. and Outerbridge, E. (1974). The management of premature infants with patent ductus arteriosus. *J. Thorac. Cardiovasc. Surg.*, **67**(2), 221
7. Kilman, J. W. and Sirac, H. D. (1970). The case for the early closure of a patent ductus arteriosus. *Surgery*, **67**(1), 197
8. Zachman, S. (1970). The incidence and treatment of the patent ductus arteriosus in the ill, premature neonate. *Am. Heart J.*, **87**(6), 697

25

Recoarctation of the aorta

J P. BYRNE AND L. H. BURR

A satisfactory result is usually obtained in patients who have survived resection of coarctation of the aorta. However, in some patients, obstruction may recur and require reoperation. We will examine this problem utilizing the experience of the Thoracic Unit, The Hospital for Sick Children, Great Ormond Street, during the years 1953–1975.

During this period 33 patients with recurrent coarctation were seen, of which 32 had the initial operation in our institution. The incidence of recoarctation based on age is shown in Table 1. The incidence is highest in those who underwent initial operation in the first 6 months of life.

Table 1   Recoarctation 1953–75

Age at first operation	No. at risk	No. of recoarctations	Percentage
< 6 weeks	66	13	20
6 weeks–3 months	43	10	23
3–6 months	44	5	11
6–12 months	34	0	0
> 1 year	257	4	1.6
TOTAL	444	32	7.5

One patient had initial operation elsewhere

The signs and symptoms of recoarctation are similar to those of the initial presentation. Upper extremity hypertension was present in 12 patients, congestive heart failure in nine and claudication in one. Evidence of cardiac enlargement or ventricular hypertrophy by chest roentgenogram or electrocardiogram was present in 31 patients. In general, these findings have also been our indications for reoperation.

The age at reoperation and the interoperative time interval are shown in Tables 2 and 3. The majority of patients were operated upon 5 or more years following the initial operation, emphasizing the need for prolonged follow-up. The occurrence of recoarctation is not necessarily related to an increase in postoperative interval, however, as evidenced by six patients who required reoperation in the first 6 months following the initial operation.

Table 2   Recoarctation 1953–75

Age at reoperation	Number
< 6 months	3
6–12 months	2
1–5 years	7
5–10 years	15
> 10 years	6
TOTAL	33

Table 3   Recoarctation 1953–75

Interoperative interval	Number
< 6 months	6
6–12 months	0
1–5 years	9
5–10 years	12
> 10 years	6
TOTAL	33

Seventeen patients had an end-to-end anastomosis with one continuous suture at the initial operation, whilst in 14, an end-to-end anastomosis with interruption of the anterior row was done. One patient had a Blalock-Park operation and the type in one patient is unknown. At reoperation, the majority of patients again had an end-to-end anastomosis (Table 4). An onlay patch or Dacron conduit were other techniques utilized. Two patients underwent reoperation with the aid of left heart bypass.

Table 4   Recoarctation 1953–75

Technique at second operation	No.
End-to-end anastomosis	28
Onlay patch	4
Dacron conduit	1
TOTAL	33
Left heart bypass	2

There were two hospital deaths and no late deaths. There were no serious complications. All surviving patients have had satisfactory relief of the signs of recoarctation.

Certain technical points merit emphasis. Some of these patients may have inadequate collateral circulation. We therefore measure proximal and distal pressures with the aorta occluded at the site of recoarctation to assess the need for a temporary shunt or left heart bypass. Proximal as well as distal pressures should be considered. However, firm criteria for the determination of safety during temporary aortic occlusion have not been established.

The use of a bypass graft, as described by Edie *et al.*[1] may avoid aortic occlusion, a difficult dissection with possible haemorrhage or recurrent laryngeal nerve damage.

Our study has not elucidated the causes of recoarctation. Failure of the anastomosis to grow is probably the basic cause but the factors which lead to this are not completely understood. The technique of anastomosis is undoubtedly of importance. Experimentally, one interruption of the suture line has resulted in normal growth of an aortic anastomosis[2]. However, in our patients with recoarctation, those who had continuous suture technique and those in whom interruption of the anterior row was done were almost equal in number. Other factors such as inadequate resection, inclusion of ductal tissue in the anastomosis and inadequate mobilization of the aorta with tension on the anastomosis may also prevent growth.

Although reoperation may be carried out with acceptable morbidity and mortality, there is need for new techiques of coarctation repair which will prevent this complication.

References

1. Edie, R. N., Janini, J., Attati, L. A., Malm, J. R. and Robinson, B. (1975). Bypass grafts for recoarctation or complex coarctation of the aorta. *Ann Thoracic Surg.*, **20**, 558
2. Tawes, R. L., Aberdeen, E. and Berry, C. L. (1968). The growth of an aortic anastomosis: an experimental study in piglets. *Surgery*, **64**, 1122

26

Coarctation of the aorta in the adult

W. P. CLELAND

The special features relating to the adolescent or adult patient with coarctation are due to a considerable increase in variety and incidence of complicating lesions, the presence of substantially higher levels of hypertension, and the fact that no allowance has to be made for future growth of the anastomostic site. These various factors will be discussed in some detail.

Table 1 gives the age distribution of 203 patients on whom I have operated over a 20-year period together with the incidence of complicating factors; the Table shows the increasing incidence of berry aneurysms and of atheroma with age, whereas vegetations and mycotic aneurysms are found at all ages; it shows also that apart from the infant group there is little variation in operative mortality in the various decades and even in those patients over the age of 50.

Table 2 lists the causes of early death in 12 of the patients. It is important to note that in eight of these death was due wholly or partially to haemorrhage. One patient with severe coronary atheroma developed cardiac arrest after a sudden but not severe loss of blood on the operating table. Two deaths were in infants with complicated congenital heart disease, and one was related to an unusual drug reaction.

Table 1 Coarctation of aorta

Age (years)	Total	Early death	Late death	Berry aneurysms	Vegetations	Atheroma	Aortic aneurysms
0–2	10	3	0	0	0	0	0
2–9	40	1	1	0	2	0	1
10–19	56	4	3	5	3	0	1
20–29	41	1	2	13	1	1	1
30–39	33	1	3	14	3	5	2
40–	23	2	3	12	2	6	2
TOTALS	203	12	12	44	11	12	7

189

Table 2 Coarctation of aorta (early deaths)

Haemorrhage	8
Neurological	1
Complex infants	2
Coronary atheroma	1

Table 3 gives a list of later deaths. It is important to note that in five of the twelve patients death was related to coronary artery disease and was probably related to coronary artery disease in two others who died suddenly, although no autopsy had been carried out. In two patients with dissecting aneurysms, later death was related to extension of the dissections. One patient died following a subarachnoid haemorrhage, emphasizing the increased prevalence of berry aneurysms on the cerebral vessels amongst patients with a co-arctation.

Table 3 Coarctation of aorta (late deaths)

Coronary artery disease	5
Dissecting aneurysm	2
Subarachnoid haemorrhage	1
Left ventricular failure (after arteriovenous resection)	1
Perforation infected suture line (9 years)	1
Sudden; no autopsy	2

OPERATIVE SURGERY

At the time of the operation I believe it is essential to excise all the abnormal fibrous or muscle tissue in or around the area of the coarctation (see Figure 1) and the ligamentum arteriosum with the restoration of a good-sized lumen and preservation of the curve of the aortic arch. If this cannot be achieved by direct anastomosis one should not hesitate to use a graft. It is important

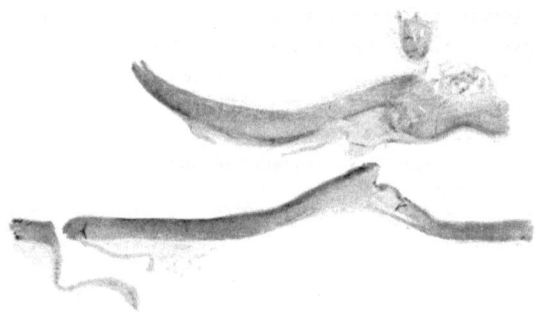

Figure 1 Longitudinal section across coarctation showing abnormal fibrous and muscle tissue

that there should be no gradient across the suture line, and if one is recorded of 15 mm or more under the conditions on the operating table, it is likely that this will be considerably higher during active life and the relief of hypertension will be less than optimal. If a gradient persists the surgeon must seriously consider redoing the anastomosis or employing a prosthetic graft.

Table 4   Coarctation of aorta (artificial graft replacement)

Ivalon (3)	
Died early leak	2
Satisfactory	1
Terylene (1)	
Replaced 3 years (obstruction)	1
Crimped Teflon (15)	
Replaced 1 year (obstruction)	1
Satisfactory	14
Crimped Dacron (12)	
Satisfactory	12

PROSTHETIC GRAFTS

In all, 42 grafts have been used in the 206 patients, an incidence of about 20%. Initially, freeze-dried homografts were inserted in 11 patients, but in only five are these grafts still *in situ*. Of the remainder two were successfully resected and replaced, but one of these died after a subsequent aortic valve replacement. The third patient died at the time of the second operation. Satisfactory results followed the use of crimped Teflon (15 patients) and, more recently, crimped Dacron (12 patients). Only one of the former became obstructed 1 year after insertion (see Figure 2) and all the remainder of both Teflon and Dacron are working satisfactorily.

Finally, I would like to mention the problem of associated aortic valve disease, as this appears to be particularly relevant to the adult patient.

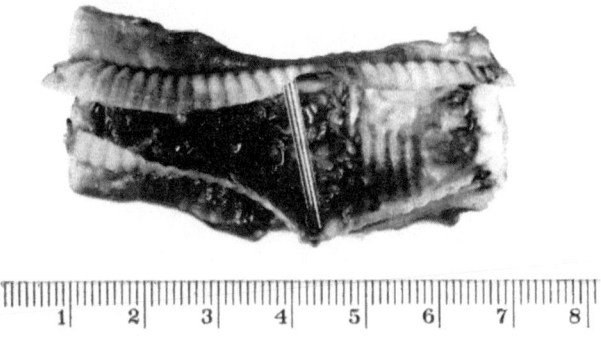

Figure 2   Crimped Teflon graft which became obstructed

Between 15 and 20% of all patients with coarctation have signs suggesting either a bicuspid aortic valve or mild aortic stenosis. In no instance in my experience has there been significant or severe aortic valve obstruction, and there has been no occasion to consider aortic valvotomy in this group. However, over the years we have had nine patients with severe aortic regurgitation. Our initial attitude to this combination was to resect the coarctation with atriofemoral bypass standing by; in practice it was never required. Having successfully survived resection of the coarctation, all patients appeared to be benefited for a time, with evidence of decreased aortic regurgitation, and no further action was taken. But as time went on the aortic leak became worse and eventually valve replacement became necessary. Table 5 summarizes the subsequent events, and shows that four of the patients have died

Table 5   Coarctation of aorta (homograft replacement)

Late stenosis with replacement	1
Late stenosis and calcification. Died after arteriovenous resection	1
Died at operation	1
Died at 2 weeks; perforated intercostal	1
Died at 1 month; Rup. Diss. Ann.	1
Died at 4 years; I.H.D.	1
Still functioning	5

and only three can be regarded as reasonably satisfactory. Two are awaiting valve replacement but both have poor left ventricular function. The combination of coarctation with aortic regurgitation is a sinister one. The ventricle is frequently found to be dilated and functioning poorly; more so than one would expect from the degree of aortic regurgitation. We are not certain whether this is mere coincidence or whether these two lesions are linked in some special way. But as a result of our experience we believe that early correction of both the coarctation and the aortic lesion is advisable.

Section V
Pulmonary atresia

27

The development of the pulmonary circulation in pulmonary atresia

SHEILA G. HAWORTH

In pulmonary atresia the intrapulmonary arterial circulation fails to grow and develop normally. When the ductus arteriosus is the only source of blood supply, the reduction in blood flow before birth impairs fetal development and such children die at birth, if untreated, with abnormally small pre- and intra-acinar arteries and a reduction in intra-acinar arterial number. The muscle coat is abnormally thin although the distribution of muscle along the arterial pathway is normal. An aortopulmonary anastomosis increases arterial size and if too large arterial medial hypertrophy develops rapidly in the first days of life, but peripheral arterial number remains low.

Large collateral arteries which arise from the aorta to supply the lung in pulmonary atresia originate *in utero* as segmental arteries. They normally perfuse the pulmonary vascular bed, at about the fifth week of gestation, before the sixth branchial arteries appear, and then regress. In pulmonary atresia, with or without development of the sixth arch they frequently persist, capturing a portion of lung in early fetal development before the bronchial arteries appear. One or more may anastomose with the sixth arch at the hilum of the lung and empty into a normal intrapulmonary arterial branching system, or they may enter the lung and anastomose with the lobar branches of the pulmonary arteries, or they may distribute blood to various lobes or segments of lung directly, either running alongside arteries seen to communicate with the sixth arch or as the only arterial supply to a segment or lobe (Figure 1). At the lung periphery, within the respiratory unit, all arteries, irrespective of their origin, run normally with the peripheral airways, suggesting early fetal capture of a part of the intrapulmonary plexus by persisting segmental arteries. Variation in arterial wall thickness between intrapulmonary arteries having a different source of blood supply indicates that there is little territorial overlap between them. Collateral arteries should not be ligated before their peripheral distribution has been clearly demonstrated by pulmonary angiography. Peripheral arterial wall structure is determined mainly by the presence or absence of a proximal stenosis. Stenoses occur at the junction of a systemic artery with the sixth arch at the hilum, or within the lung at the origin of the segmental branches of the pulmonary artery, or where vessels of systemic origin branch. An artery arising from the aorta and branching within the lung without a stenosis can finally give rise, at the level of the respiratory bronchioli, to thick-walled arteries with intimal occlusion.

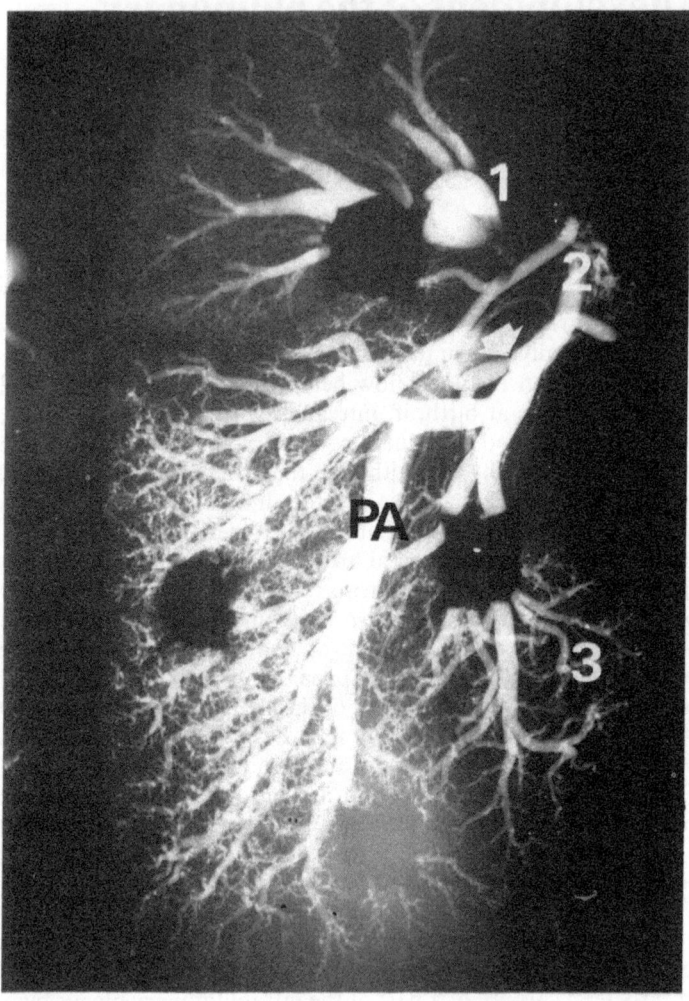

Figure 1 Pulmonary atresia with large collateral arteries to the lung. Arteriogram of a slice of right lung ($\times$ 0.9). (1) Artery arising from the aorta and anastomosing at the hilum with the pulmonary artery to the right upper lobe. (2) Arteries arising from the aorta and branching within the lung. Note stenoses ($\rightarrow$). (3) Segment of lung perfused only by an artery originating from the aorta

196

Nearby vessels supplied by a different vessel may appear relatively normal (Figure 2).

Thus in pulmonary atresia where the lungs are perfused only by a ductus arteriosus, the lung fails to grow and develop normally *in utero*. In the presence of large collateral arteries arising from the aorta to supply the lung the intra-pulmonary branching pattern can be abnormal and the systemic arterial supply may be the only blood supply to certain segments of lung. Lung structure, and therefore pulmonary vascular resistance, can vary considerably within one lung; even within one lobe or segment of lung.

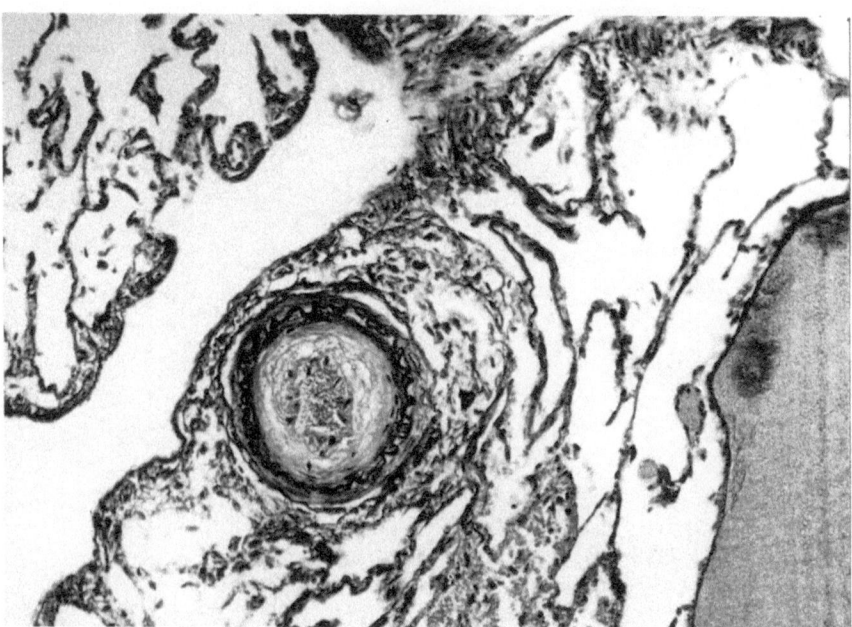

Figure 2 Photomicrograph of a section from lung in Figure 1. Arteries accompany the respiratory bronchioli; one is thick-walled with an obliterated lumen; the other has the appearance of a normal pulmonary artery in this position. ($\times$ 180)

28

Surgical management of pulmonary atresia with confluent pulmonary arteries

J. P. BYRNE

In order to clarify the group which we are discussing, this condition may be defined as follows:

1. there is hypoplasia or atresia of the right ventricular outflow, pulmonary valve or main pulmonary artery;
2. there are confluent left and right pulmonary arteries; they may be hypoplastic or adequately developed;
3. pulmonary blood supply is from large collateral arteries, patent ductus arteriosus or surgically created systemic to pulmonary artery shunts; and
4. there is a large ventricular septal defect.

The surgical management of this entity is concerned with three factors:

1. the exact anatomy of the pulmonary arteries;
2. the sources of pulmonary blood flow; and
3. the anatomy of the right ventricular–pulmonary artery discontinuity.

The major factor in the surgical repair is management of the large collateral arteries. Their characteristics may be listed as follows:

1. they are one to six in number;
2. their origin most commonly is from the anterior aspect of the proximal descending aorta;
3. they may also originate from the brachiocephalic vessels or the abdominal aorta;
4. they may emerge from common or separate aortic ostia;
5. they may be stenotic at their origin from the aorta, or at their junction with the pulmonary arteries.

Several points in the preoperative evaluation deserve emphasis. Accurate mapping of the number, course, origin and size of each collateral vessel is necessary. This means that aortography and preferably selective opacification of the collateral vessels should be done. A determination of the adequacy of the central and peripheral pulmonary arteries is necessary. In those patients with hypoplastic pulmonary arteries, it may be necessary to do a preliminary palliative procedure with the intention of inducing growth and development of the pulmonary arteries. An assessment of pulmonary blood flow and pulmonary vascular resistance is necessary, as some of these patients may have pulmonary vascular obstructive disease.

The operative management of these patients consists of three phases. The first is the control of the collateral vessels (or shunts). This is necessary in order to prevent excessive return with cardiac distension and flooding of the operative field once cardiopulmonary bypass is established. Also, if collateral vessels are not ligated, and intraoperative difficulties do not occur, there may be a large left-to-right shunt postoperatively, and congestive heart failure. The control of the collaterals must be gained prior to initiating bypass so that they may be ligated immediately after bypass is begun. As most of the collaterals originate from the descending aorta it may be necessary to do a separate left thoracotomy as described by Doty et al.[1] However, in some patients, the collaterals may be ligated through the sternotomy incision (McGoon et al.)[2]

The second phase is closure of the ventricular septal defect. Two types of ventricular septal defects have been described in these patients; one is the typical defect seen in tetralogy of Fallot in which the septal leaflet of the tricuspid valve forms the inferior margin. The other type is that seen in truncus arteriosus in which a muscular rim is present around the entire circumference of the defect.

The third phase of the operation consists of restoration of right ventricular pulmonary artery continuity. This may be done by using either a patch or a conduit, depending on the anatomy. If there is a possibility of residual right ventricular hypertension postoperatively due either to small pulmonary arteries or pulmonary vascular obstructive disease, we prefer to employ a valved conduit, in order to prevent pulmonary insufficiency.

Five patients have undergone repair of this defect at the Hospital for Sick Children, Great Ormond Street. Three of them had large collaterals which required separate ligation. In two of these, the collaterals originated from the descending aorta and required closure through a separate left thoracotomy. In the third patient, the collaterals originated from the ascending aorta and the brachiocephalic vessels, and these were ligated through the sternotomy incision. The other two patients had pulmonary blood supply from previous surgically created shunts and patent ductus arteriosus. All five patients underwent reconstruction of the right ventricular outflow utilizing a valved conduit. All patients survived .the operation and have had satisfactory postoperative results.

References

1. Doty, D. B., Kouchoukos, N. T. and Kirklin, J. W. (1972). Surgery for pseudotruncus arteriosus with pulmonary blood flow originating from upper descending thoracic aorta. *Circulation*, **45, 46**: (Suppl. I)
2. McGoon, D. C., Baird, D. K. and Davis, G. D. (1975). Surgical management of large bronchial collateral arteries with pulmonary stenosis or atresia. *Circulation*, **52**, 109

29

Pulmonary atresia with non-confluent pulmonary arteries

R. J. SZARNICKI AND M. R. DE LEVAL

The role of surgical treatment of patients with severe pulmonary atresia with non-confluent pulmonary arteries remains highly controversial. Many of these children are considered inoperable by most standards.

These children usually have a multifocal source of pulmonary blood flow as has been described by Professor Macartney in Chapter 31 of this volume. Because of frequent stenoses at the junction of the aortopulmonary collaterals and the pulmonary artery, and the small size of the vessels, pulmonary blood flow is often inadequate. The ultimate goal in these patients is to convert this situation to one in which adequate pulmonary blood flow arises from a unifocal source. In order to achieve this, and to make surgical correction feasible, it is necessary to increase blood flow in the pulmonary arteries themselves to ensure eventual growth.

We have recently embarked upon a staged approach to this difficult problem. Before any palliative intervention can be contemplated, meticulous detailed angiocardiography with selective injection of all aortopulmonary collaterals is essential. This enables precise determination of hilar anatomy of the pulmonary arteries and localization of all collateral vessels. The origins of aortopulmonary collaterals may be found almost anywhere along the aorta, and its branches distal to the origin of the innominate artery. In spite of detailed investigations, identification of a distinct pulmonary artery is not always possible.

In these children, we currently perform an exploratory thoracotomy and carry out a meticulous, and sometimes tedious, dissection to identify a pulmonary artery deep in the hilum of the lung. At times it has been possible, by opening the pericardium, to identify a minuscule vessel lying posterior to the aorta and to follow it to the hilum. In our limited experience so far, we have always been able to find a pulmonary artery. When this is done, an aortopulmonary shunt is created. It has been quite surprising to find a vessel measuring up to 4–5 mm in diameter in these patients, even though none was visualized on preoperative angiography. Upon completion of the aorto-pulmonary shunt, aortopulmonary collateral arteries can sometimes be ligated, if flow through the shunt is believed to be satisfactory based on frequent intraoperative monitoring of arterial blood gases during temporary occlusion of the collateral vessel. This was of particular benefit to one of our patients who had chronic congestive heart failure and failure to thrive.

TECHNIQUE

A standard thoracotomy in the fourth intercostal space is performed (see Figure 1). If the location of the aortic arch is contralateral to the side being explored, a Blalock–Taussig anastomosis may be possible. If it is felt that

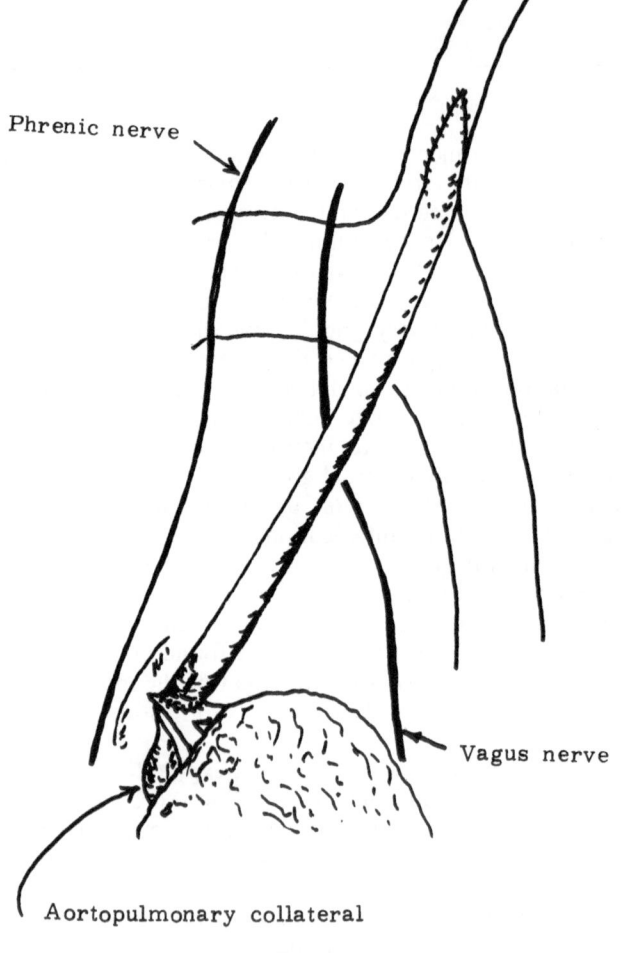

Phrenic nerve

Vagus nerve

Aortopulmonary collateral

Figure 1

even slight tension would be created on the anastomosis, a prosthetic conduit* (4–6 mm in diameter) is used. The proximal anastomosis of the conduit is placed on the subclavian artery just distal to its origin. An end-to-side anastomosis is then made with the pulmonary artery proximal to any lobar branches.

Fine monofilament suture material is used on the anastomosis. We currently prefer to use the Gore-tex graft in these cases, because of the easy handling and suturing during creation of very small anastomoses.

To date, we have used this approach in ten patients with one mortality and one shunt failure (Table 1). Seven of our patients had pulmonary atresia and ventricular septal defect. Two patients had tetralogy of Fallot with an absent pulmonary artery. In one of these patients, the left pulmonary artery was noted to be supplied by a duct arising from the left subclavian artery at the initial catheter study. On a repeat angiogram only a duct remnant còuld be identified, and there was no communication with the left pulmonary artery. Having demonstrated a pulmonary artery to the left lung earlier, it was felt reasonable to explore the left chest and create a shunt to allow growth of this vessel prior to contemplating corrective surgery. At operation, a small pulmonary artery was found and a shunt created without difficulty.

Table 1   Results of surgery for 10 patients with pulmonary atresia

Patient	Age	Condition	Result
J.H.	1 year 9 months	Pulmonary atresia + VSD	Improved
J.B.	14 years 2 months	TGA + pulmonary atresia + VSD	Shunt failure
E.S.	3 years 6 months	Pulmonary atresia + VSD	Improved
O.P.	5 months	Pulmonary atresia + VSD	Died
C.H.	1 year 4 months	Pulmonary atresia + VSD	Improved
L.S.	9 years	Pulmonary atresia + VSD	Improved
K.H.	5 months	Pulmonary atresia + VSD	Improved
D.S.	9 years	Tet + absent LPA	Improved
K.E.	6 months	Tet + absent LPA	Improved
M.D.	14 years	Pulmonary atresia + VSD	Improved

VSD = ventricular septal defect; Tet. = tetralogy of Fallot; LPA = left pulmonary artery; TGA = transposition of the great arteries

The patient with pulmonary atresia, transposition of the great arteries and ventricular septal defect was the only one in the series in whom shunt failure has been documented. She has subsequently undergone reoperation and a central shunt was created from the ascending aorta to the right pulmonary artery under cardiopulmonary bypass.

Our present policy is to recatheterize all of these patients 6–12 months after creation of the shunt, to determine patency and to evaluate growth of the pulmonary arteries. If, as we believe, the pulmonary arteries do in fact grow sufficiently, corrective surgery with creation of a unifocal source of pulmonary blood flow should be possible.

* We have found the Gore-tex prosthesis very useful in performing this anastomosis.

Section VI

Palliative surgery for cyanotic heart disease in infancy

30

The development of palliative operations for the tetralogy of Fallot

LORD BROCK

I was recently approached by a registrar who was interested in the early development of operations for congenital heart disease. I was rather taken aback by the absence of knowledge shown until I realized that we were concerned with happenings fully 30 years ago and that my questioner was not even born then. I began to realize how much things have altered. I suppose the really difficult thing to grasp is the complete change that occurred as a result of the Blalock–Taussig contribution when we were at last able to achieve something with the relief of congenital heart disease whereas previously nothing could be done. From the initial palliation has sprung a progressive improvement in understanding, in high standards of diagnosis and in treatment that can now achieve complete cure in many cases. This brilliant evolution towards successful treatment owes its origin to the palliative methods that began the saga and that are still of great value.

Blalock's first epoch-making operations were done in 1945, and it was in 1947 that his visit as exchange professor to Guy's Hospital caused such intense interest. His visit was a total and brilliant success. He operated on nine patients at Guy's and although the immediate results were so successful four of the nine have since died, four have had a secondary direct operation for relief of pulmonary stenosis because of failure or regression of the original anastomosis, and one has proceeded to total correction.

Even in the presence of Blalock's success objections were soon being advanced against his operation and the various alternatives such as Potts' operation. It was pointed out that nothing direct was being done to relieve the obstruction to the flow of blood to the lungs. A fundamental surgical step in such cases should be to relieve the obstruction, and not to rely on a short-circuiting procedure that in fact adds yet a new lesion, another burden, to the existing one. Hence the next step in palliation lay in attempts to relieve the pulmonary stenosis and so increase the blood flow to the lungs directly, thus also lessening or correcting the shunt through the ventricular septal defect. A frequent cause of disability or of death even in the most successful cases after a Blalock's or a Potts' operation was paradoxical cerebral embolism or abscess, whereas after a direct operation on the pulmonary outflow this was rare. The persistence of the ventricular septal defect meant that an important lesion remained and that until this could be closed total correction could not be achieved. Moreover if the stenosis was overcorrected the lung circulation might be flooded or nearly so.

Direct relief of the outflow tract obstruction was by no means generally accepted. In fact many denied that it was possible to achieve. Valvotomy was accepted, but the infundibular element that could accompany and often dominated the obstruction was said to be an inoperable condition. This was shown to be just not so and in fact it could easily give excellent results. Today we do not hear of the infundibular stenosis being inoperable. It is an essential routine step as part of the operation for total correction and is fully accepted.

It was still not possible in the absence of heart–lung bypass to close the ventricular septal defect and thus obtain total correction. Although relief of the outflow obstruction was a palliative procedure it was suggested, indeed stated, that these lesser procedures could be permanently satisfactory and that nothing more need be done in many cases if a nice circulatory balance was achieved. Later experience, however, showed that this was not so. Although many patients did continue with a good result and have continued for as long as 20 years or more, there was always the possibility of deterioration. Consequently it soon became apparent that total correction should be aimed at in all cases as a secondary operation and certainly before the late teens. Time does not allow a full statistical presentation of results after these direct palliative procedures, but I am convinced that total correction should be aimed at in all cases and this is indeed the commonly accepted practice today.

This brings the problem of the total objection to all palliative procedures and the insistence of aiming always at total correction as the sole step for all patients however young and however ill. Again time does not permit a statistical presentation of results of such a policy but I can comment that excellent results have been obtained in many patients and it gives operative figures that would scarcely have been thought possible 10 or 20 years ago.

Although I accept unreservedly that total correction is to be aimed at whenever possible I am still not convinced that this can be done at once in all cases especially those who are severely ill and in infants and small children. Indeed the patient may be so ill that some form of palliation is unavoidable. It may well be asking too much to expect a fully satisfactory result in one stage. It is, for example, common for a substantial degree of pulmonary stenosis to remain uncorrected even though an outflow tract patch is used. This residual pulmonary stenosis element cannot be desirable and to describe such a case as having been totally corrected is quite wrong. It is in these patients that a place still exists for a preliminary procedure that will allow adequate changes to occur in the right outflow tract and ventricle so that total correction can be done later with much greater safety. This is especially so in infants and young children.

As a first-stage operation many surgeons, especially those in the United States where most of the anastomotic operations originated, still prefer an anastomosis. I maintain that an operation for direct relief of the right outflow tract obstruction is far better, can give excellent results and is the logical first step to a secondary total correction. It has been shown by many surgeons, both in Great Britain and abroad, that these operations are well tolerated even by very small infants and the excellent results have well justified their use as a palliation. I suggest that we should recognize and accept the feasibility and desirability of a preliminary direct operation on the outflow tract stenosis as a proper palliative procedure to allow readjustment before proceeding to secondary total correction and not accept one-stage total correction in all cases. We should retain a proper sense of proportion and recognize that there are limits to our ability to achieve routine one-stage total correction and not be paranoic in this matter in regard to the triumphant success of modern open heart surgery however much we have advanced in the treatment of Fallot's tetralogy.

31

Tetralogy of Fallot: haemodynamic and angiocardiographic considerations

F. J. MACARTNEY

How is one to define tetralogy of Fallot? One can attempt to do this haemo-dynamically, as in fact many other people have done in the past. The haemo-dynamic criteria would include first, equalization of the ventricular pressures, second, subvalvular and possibly valvular pulmonary stenosis, and third, favourable streaming, that is to say, aortic oxygen saturation higher than pulmonary artery oxygen saturation. But that definition includes such entities as double outlet right ventricle with pulmonary stenosis, and primitive ventricle, with or without transposition and pulmonary stenosis.

So I would suggest that tetralogy of Fallot must be defined morpho-logically as a condition characterized by anterior deviation and/or rotation of the infundibular septum. This has two consequences, first, right ventricular outflow tract obstruction, and second, a ventricular septal defect over-ridden by the aorta. In addition, one has to specify mitral—aortic fibrous continuity.

Figure 1 shows an angiocardiogram from such a patient, which was

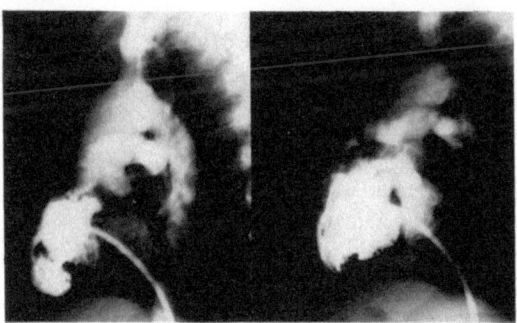

Figure 1 (Left) lateral view, selective right ventricular angiocardiogram in tetralogy of Fallot with accessory tricuspid valve tissue blocking the ventricular septal defect. (Right) the same patient, demonstrating that when the left ventricle opacifies, there is a crescent shaped filling defect between the two ventricles

proven at surgery to fulfil the morphological criteria of tetralogy of Fallot just proposed, but which has an associated abnormality. On the right, during ventricular systole, but prior to opacification of the left ventricle, the contrast medium, instead of mingling with unopacified blood as it traverses the ventricular septal defect, is sharply outlined, at least over part of its diameter. Later on, as can be seen on the left, there can be seen a crescentic filling defect of the same shape within the ventricular septal defect. This is in fact a pouch of accessory tricuspid valve tissue prolapsing through the ventricular septal defect and partially occluding it. As a result, the right ventricular pressure was twice that in the left ventricle. By the usual haemodynamic criteria, this is not a tetralogy of Fallot. However, common sense dictates that it should be included in that category. This is another argument against use of a haemodynamic definition.

Let us for the moment forget the question of obstruction of the ventricular septal defect, and instead consider the haemodynamics of straightforward tetralogy of Fallot. There is a large ventricular septal defect. The simple haemodynamic story is that when the ventricular septal defect is large, since it is easier for the left ventricle to eject blood into the pulmonary circulation than into the aorta, there is a left-to-right shunt through the ventricular septal defect. If there is pulmonary stenosis, however, this makes it easier for the left ventricle to eject into the aorta than into the pulmonary artery and indeed it is easier for the right ventricle to eject into the aorta than into the pulmonary artery. Hence, a right-to-left shunt. The next two figures, taken from Levin's work in 1966, demonstrate that this is an over simplification.

Figure 2 refers to moderately severe tetralogy of Fallot. In the centre are simultaneous, closely matched pressures from the right ventricle, the left ventricle, and the ascending aorta. At the top of the illustration, the right ventricular pressure is subtracted throughout the cardiac cycle from the aortic pressure. Since the aortic pressure is usually higher, the result is usually positive, but you will see that at the onset of ejection into the aorta there is a

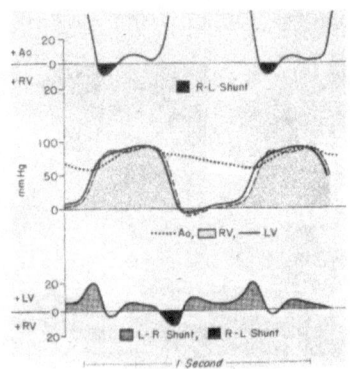

Figure 2 Relationship between simultaneous pressures in the aorta, right ventricle, and left ventricle of moderate tetralogy of Fallot (middle curve). The upper curve shows the difference between the simultaneous aortic and right ventricular pressures, while the lower curve shows the difference between simultaneous ventricular pressures. From Levin *et al.*, *Circulation*, **34**, 4, 1966, reproduced by kind permission of the Editors

pressure gradient in favour of the right ventricle, which is associated with an angiocardiographic right-to-left shunt from the right ventricle to the aorta. Simultaneously with this, there is a pressure gradient in favour of the right ventricle as opposed to the left ventricle, but a shunt into the body of the left ventricle is not seen. However, during the phase of so-called isovolumic relaxation, between closure of the aortic valve and opening of the mitral valve, because of the delay in right ventricular relaxation, there is a pressure gradient in favour of the right ventricle during this period. In Figure 3, where

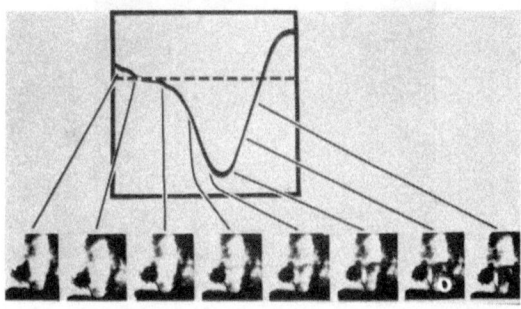

Figure 3 Comparison of difference between right and left ventricular pressures with simultaneous cine angiography. The upper square contains a dotted line representing equality between the ventricular pressures. Values above this line represent a pressure gradient in favour of the left ventricle, whereas pressures below this line represent a pressure gradient in favour of the right ventricle. From Levin *et al.*, *Circulation*, **34**, 4, 1966

the differential pressure trace begins at the onset of isovolumic relaxation, and ends at the beginning of diastole, it can be seen that if we correlate the angiocardiogram with the difference between left and right ventricular pressure, there is no right-to-left shunt during early isovolumic relaxation. Instead, as so-called isovolumic relaxation continues, a right-to-left shunt appears and this is only terminated, as far as the pressure is concerned, at the beginning of diastole.

Returning to Figure 2, it can be seen that in moderate tetralogy of Fallot, far from there being a pure right-to-left shunt, in fact, during the majority of the cardiac cycle, there is a pressure gradient in favour of the left ventricle over the right. This begins at the beginning of diastole and continues right through up to the end of so-called isovolumic systole, after which ejection into the aorta is associated with pressure gradient reversal, as already stated.

Analysis of left ventricular ciné angiography during this phase of a pressure difference in favour of the left ventricle reveals a left-to-right shunt, increasing in intensity toward the end of the phase, during so-called isovolumic systole. This left-to-right shunt is terminated with the reversal of pressure differences which occurs during ejection into the aorta. So shunting in tetralogy of Fallot is a far more complex subject than most people think, and indeed there is some evidence that in severe tetralogy of Fallot, the timing of the right-to-left shunt is different from that which I have outlined in moderate tetralogy. However, rather than continued on that theme I would rather talk now about complexities of pulmonary arterial supply in tetralogy.

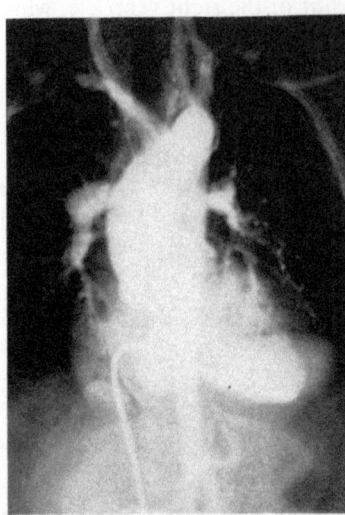

Figure 4 Frontal view, selective right ventricular angiocardiogram, in a patient with tetralogy of Fallot and additional supply to the lungs from a major aortopulmonary collateral artery

Figure 4 shows an apparently straight forward frontal right ventricular angiocardiogram in tetralogy. The observant might comment on the curious appearance of the right pulmonary artery, and indeed on close inspection, there seem to be two parallel arteries supplying the lungs in the region of the right hilum.

Selective injection of contrast medium into the right ventricular outflow tract (Figure 5) demonstrates that the lower of these two arteries is the true main right pulmonary artery, and also demonstrates rather a lack of opacification to the right upper zone of the lung fields.

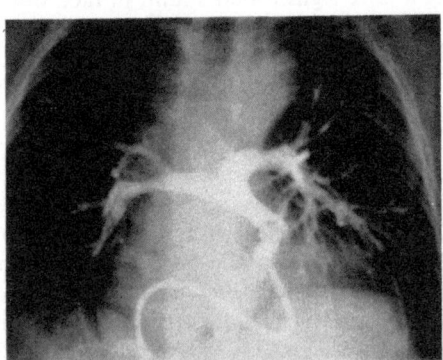

Figure 5 Same patient as in Figure 4. Selective injection into right ventricular outflow tract in the frontal projection, with 45° head-up tilt

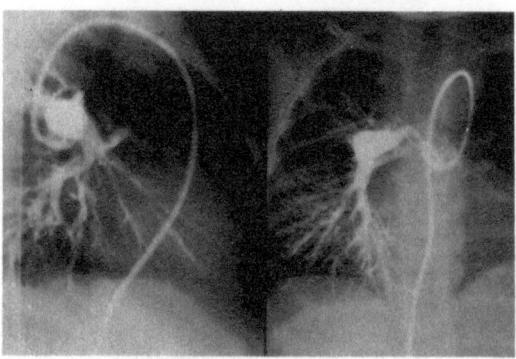

Figure 6 Same patient as in Figures 4 and 5. Lateral and frontal projections of selective injection into major aorto-pulmonary collateral arteries

The upper of the two arteries at the right hilum was in fact a major aorto-pulmonary collateral artery (Figure 6), just as one sees in pulmonary atresia with ventricular septal defect. Retrograde filling of the main right pulmonary artery is seen, and the anastomosis between the collateral artery and the main right pulmonary artery is clearly identified within the hilum of the right pulmonary artery, but somewhat distal. There is a dual pulmonary blood supply here, which will cause problems on cardiopulmonary bypass if it is not recognized, because of excessive return to the left side of the heart even when the aorta is cross clamped. On the other hand, pulmonary blood supply is unifocal, since the pressure head in all these arteries supplying both lungs is the same, and both systems are in free communication with each other.

This situation is to be contrasted with that depicted in Figure 7. I doubt if anyone would argue against a diagnosis of straight-forward tetralogy of Fallot with a right aortic arch on this picture.

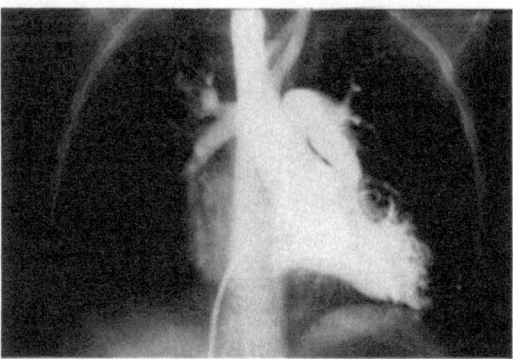

Figure 7 Tetralogy of Fallot with anomalous origin of right pulmonary artery. Frontal view of selective right ventricular angiocardiogram

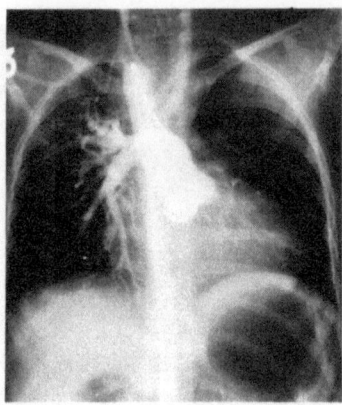

Figure 8 Same patient as in Figure 7. Aortogram to display anomalous origin of right pulmonary artery

However, on injection into the aortic root (Figure 8), it can be seen that the right pulmonary artery originates anomalously from the ascending aorta. Here there is dual pulmonary blood supply, which will certainly cause problems with flow on bypass if not recognized. However, it also causes problems in calculation of pulmonary resistance, since both lungs are perfused at different pressures and at different oxygen saturations. Here the pulmonary blood supply is multifocal.

Finally another example of multifocal pulmonary blood supply with tetralogy is shown. Figure 9 was taken in infancy'and might be regarded as straight forward tetralogy except that there appears to be a persistent ductus arteriosus, which is unusual in tetralogy.

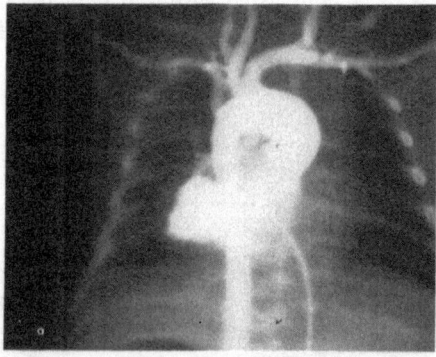

Figure 9 Tetralogy of Fallot with interruption of pulmonary artery. Frontal view of selective right ventricular angiocardiogram in infancy, demonstrating ductus arteriosus

This patient had a right Blalock–Taussig anastomosis and here is the reinvestigation 5 years later (Figure 10). An injection has been made into the right ventricular outflow tract to demonstrate that there is no filling of the left main pulmonary artery from the pulmonary trunk. However, contrast

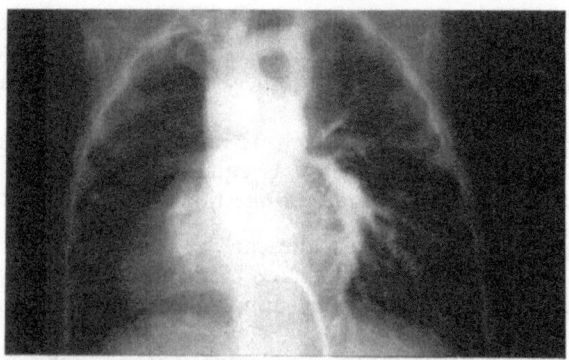

Figure 10 Same patient as in Figure 9, following right Blalock–Taussig anastomosis and spontaneous closure of persistent ductus arteriosus. There is now no apparent blood supply to the left lung

medium has also passed into the left ventricle and the aorta, and you will see that there is no filling of the left main pulmonary artery from the aorta either.

The explanation for this is that the left pulmonary artery was in fact interrupted, and derived its sole blood supply from the persistent ductus arteriosus. When the child was palliated by a Blalock–Taussig anastomosis, the ductus arteriosus was free to close without any adverse effect being noted. The patient would probably have been diagnosed as having absence of the left pulmonary artery, had not the angiocardiogram in infancy been available. Distinction of these two conditions is important, because postoperative pulmonary hypertension in the presence of major obstruction of one pulmonary artery is a major cause of increased operative mortality for tetralogy of Fallot. Figure 11 shows that the anatomy of the left pulmonary artery was restored by a synthetic conduit from left subclavian to left pulmonary artery. It seems to us, though the evidence is not yet to hand, that preservation of the function of the interrupted pulmonary artery is an important part of the

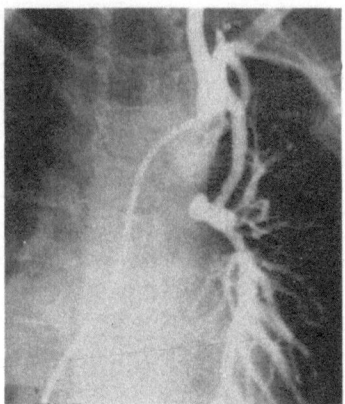

Figure 11 Same patient as in Figures 9 and 10, following conduit from left subclavian artery to left pulmonary artery. The anatomy of the left pulmonary artery has been restored

217

management of interruption of the pulmonary artery in infancy. Since the blood supply to the two lungs in the case of interruption of the pulmonary artery is quite independent we have another example of multifocal pulmonary artery blood supply.

For this reason, the check list which we originally devised for pulmonary atresia with ventricular septal defect is equally applicable to any case of tetralogy of Fallot. The following four questions are well worth asking.

1. Is either main pulmonary artery present?
2. What are the sources of pulmonary blood supply, the right ventricle alone, or is there pulmonary blood supply derived from the aorta by one means or another?
3. How and where do the sources of pulmonary blood supply interconnect?
4. (The most difficult to answer) What is the resistance to blood flow relative to the focus or foci which are to be connected to the right ventricle?

32

Late results of aortopulmonary shunts

S. C. LENNOX

Between 1968 and 1975 I performed 86 shunt operations for a variety of conditions. There were 13 deaths in this series giving a mortality of 15% (Table 1). However when one looks at the results for tetralogy of Fallot one sees that there were 37 operations with only one death, a mortality of 2.7%. Therefore the first point I would like to make is that the mortality for shunting tetralogy of Fallot is quite different to that for shunting other conditions, especially lesions such as pulmonary atresia with intact septum.

Table 1   Shunt operations 1968–75

	No.	Deaths	
Tetralogy of Fallot	37	1	2.7%
Tricuspid atresia	13	2	15%
Pulmonary atresia with VSD	7	2	28%
Pulmonary atresia with intact septum	7	5	70%
DORV and PS	4	1	25%
DOLV and PS	1	0	0%
Truncus arteriosus	1	0	0%
TGA VSD PS	5	0	0%
Complex	11	2	18%
TOTALS	86	13	15%

VSD = ventricular septal defect; DORV = double outflow right ventricle; PS = pulmonary stenosis; TGA = transposition of the great arteries

Of the 37 patients the youngest was 2 days old, five were under 1 month of age, 16 under 1 year and 27 under 2 years (Table 2). Four patients required a further operation and in each of these a Blalock operation was performed. One death occurred in a child whose Waterston shunt was made too large and who developed pulmonary oedema during the evening following surgery.

219

In view of this he was treated by intubation and positive pressure respiration. However, due to a technical mishap during intubation the patient had a period of hypoxia. Although the shunt was easily controlled the next day and his pulmonary oedema relieved, the patient had sustained irreversible cerebral damage and eventually died from that cause.

Table 2   Tetralogy of Fallot—Shunt operations

Total	37
Youngest	2 days
Under 1 month	5
Under 1 year	16
Under 2 years	27

In the last 2 years we have been using the Shumway technique of topical hypothermia while doing total correction. In that time, between October 1975 and April 1977, 18 patients have undergone total correction (Table 3). Of these 13 have had a previous shunt and five had had no previous shunt. Their ages, as will be seen from Table 3, range from 4 to 8 years for those with a shunt, while those without a shunt were slightly younger, ranging from 2 to 6 years. In the 12 patients who had had previous shunts eight required reconstruction of the outflow tract and this was performed with an aortic

Table 3   Tetralogy of Fallot—Total correction
October 1975–February 1977

Previous shunt	No.	Age	Homograft
Waterston	9	4–8 years	5
Right Blalock	2	4–8 years	2
Waterston–Blalock	2	4–5 years	1
No Shunt	5	2–6 years	3

homograft using a monocusp valve. There have been no deaths in this group. In the five who had no previous shunt three had reconstruction of the outflow tract with homograft patches and there was one death from low output syndrome 3 days following operation. In three of these patients there was one other significant lesion. One patient had a complete absence of the left pulmonary artery, another had stenosis of both pulmonary artery branches and these had to be repaired, while the third patient had an interrupted inferior vena cava and this lower body venous drainage was to a left azygos system (Table 4).

Table 4   Tetralogy of Fallot—additional problems

1. Absent left pulmonary artery
2. Bilateral pulmonary artery stenoses
3. Interrupted inferior vena cava
   Lower body venous drainage to left azygos system

The results of this small personal series suggest that, in common with many other centres, tetralogy of Fallot can be palliated with extremely low operative mortality, and that these children can then subsequently be corrected from the age of 4 onwards, with again a very low operative mortality.

33

Palliative surgery for cyanotic heart disease in infancy

The Blalock-Taussig anastomosis for the palliation of tetralogy of Fallot in children under the age of one year. (A co-operative study – The Brompton Hospital and The Hospital for Sick Children, London)

C. LINCOLN

In November 1944 Dr Alfred Blalock performed his first systemic artery/ pulmonary artery anastomosis (Blalock–Taussig shunt), thereby instigating the palliation of patients with cyanotic congenital heart disease. Since that date, other palliative operations have been suggested and performed for cyanotic congenital heart disease, and more recently there has been a trend towards one-stage total corrective surgery for patients, rather than a two-stage palliative/corrective surgical approach.

This is a cooperative review of 31 patients under the age of 1 year, with a diagnosis of tetralogy of Fallot, who were palliated by Blalock–Taussig anastomosis, at the Brompton Hospital and the Hospital for Sick Children, London.

When using an eponymous operation it is pertinent that the operation is performed according to the description by its originator. Only when a classical operation is performed can a realistic appraisal of its value be formulated.

'The performance of the anastomosis is not very difficult when the left pulmonary artery can be used. The anastomosis of the innominate artery to the left pulmonary artery is possible only in patients with a right aortic arch and hence an innominate artery on the left. With the innominate artery in its normal position the anastomosis of this vessel to the right pulmonary artery is more difficult because so much of the latter artery lies behind the aorta and the superior vena cava.'

Alfred Blalock[1]

Since this classical description, this anastomosis has been the subject of many reports for the treatment of cyanotic congenital heart disease[2-4] (See Table 1).

Table 1   Blalock-Taussig shunt – tetralogy of Fallot

	< 1 year	Percentage mortality	< 6 months	Percentage mortality	< 1 month	Percentage mortality
Neches[2]	32	6			1	100
Laks[3]			18	33	2	100
Truccone[4]	26	19	10	26		

RESULTS

Thirty-one patients under the age of 1 year (mean age 4.7 months, age range 1 day to 12 months) and whose mean weight was 5 kg (weight range 1.9–9.9 kg.) underwent palliation of their tetralogy of Fallot cardiac anomaly by the Blalock–Taussig anastomosis. Twenty-three were performed on the right, and eight on the left.

The duration of palliation ranged from 1 month to 6 years, and there were three early failures related to thrombosis or technical error, with one late failure of which the cause was unknown. The 30-day hospital mortality was two (6.4%). Five of the 31 patients proceeded to corrective surgery, with one hospital death.

Review of the recent literature for palliation of tetralogy of Fallot using the Blalock-Taussig shunt shows a wide variation in the mortality for this operation. It is evident that when performed between birth and 6 months of age the mortality is higher than when performed between 6 months and 12 months of age. This reflects the severity of the condition when presenting in early infancy.

The use and efficacy of the Blalock–Taussig anastomosis in the treatment of tetralogy of Fallot is not in dispute. However, the recent concept of one-stage totally corrective surgery for such patients causes the clinician to review again the use and results of this palliative operation. It is evident that there is wide variation from centre to centre in the operative and long-term results. However, with improved microsurgical techniques, it is still possible that the Blalock–Taussig anastomosis may, in most instances, be a preferable palliative operation in relation to corrective surgery, particularly in those infants under the age of 6 months.

References

1. Blalock, A. and Taussig H. B. (1945). The surgical treatment of malformations of the heart in which there is pulmonary stenosis or pulmonary atresia. *J. Am. Med. Assoc.*, **128**, (3), 189
2. Neches, W. H., Naifeh, J. G., *et al.* (1975). Systemic pulmonary artery anastomoses in infancy. *J. Thorac. Cardiovasc. Surg.*, **70** (5), 921
3. Laks, H., Marco, J. D. and Willman, V. L. (1975). The Blalock–Taussig shunt in the first six months of life. *J. Thorac. Cardiovasc. Surg.*, **70** (4), 687
4. Truccone, N. J., Bowman, F. O., *et al.* (1973). Systemic pulmonary arterial shunts in the first year of life. *Circulation* **49**, 508

34

Open infundibulectomy in Fallot's tetralogy and hypoplastic pulmonary arteries

H. OELERT

For surgical treatment of Fallot's tetralogy various palliative and corrective operations are available. Palliative measures consist mainly of the creation of aortopulmonary shunts which, inherently, carry certain disadvantages:

1. Complete intracardiac correction remains to be done at a later date.
2. The shunt operation has a high mortality rate when performed in patients under 1 year of age with hypoplastic pulmonary arteries. Even if infants survive operation, because of the limited size of the pulmonary arteries their shunts often do not remain open.
3. A well-functioning Blalock–Taussig anastomosis lasts no longer than 4.6 years on the average.
4. Following the Waterston anastomosis, congestive heart failure and pulmonary oedema can occur early after operation or pulmonary vascular disease may develop late. Also, obstruction of the right pulmonary artery sometimes occurs, requiring extensive reconstructive measures at the time of intracardiac repair.
5. After shunt operation to one of the pulmonary artery branches a hypoplastic pulmonary artery trunk will usually remain small.
6. Finally, the corrective operation has proved to carry a higher surgical risk when the patient has undergone a shunt procedure before the age of 6 months, mainly because of late-developing pulmonary vascular disease.

The alternative for any palliative operation is primary intracardiac repair. This has become an accepted form of management in Fallot's tetralogy with well-developed pulmonary arteries, but not in cases with pulmonary artery hypoplasia. Most children with this additional defect had died during attempts at early correction.

In Fallot's tetralogy not suitable for one-stage repair, surgical enlargement of the right ventricular outflow tract without closure of the ventricular septal

225

defect (VSD) seems superior to the shunt operation. This direct attack on the outflow tract relieves some of the afterload on the right ventricle and achieves part of the ultimately desired result. Closed pulmonary valvotomy and blind infundibular resection with the infundibular punch have led to good results in some hands; however, these procedures may be dangerous and even unsuitable in the presence either of a hypoplastic main pulmonary artery or a narrow or atretic pulmonary valve ring.

In our own series, three children with small pulmonary arteries underwent open enlargement of the right ventricular outflow tract without VSD closure and with limited or no infundibulectomy. Details of the operative procedure are outlined in Figure 1. Extensive muscular resection appeared inadvisable

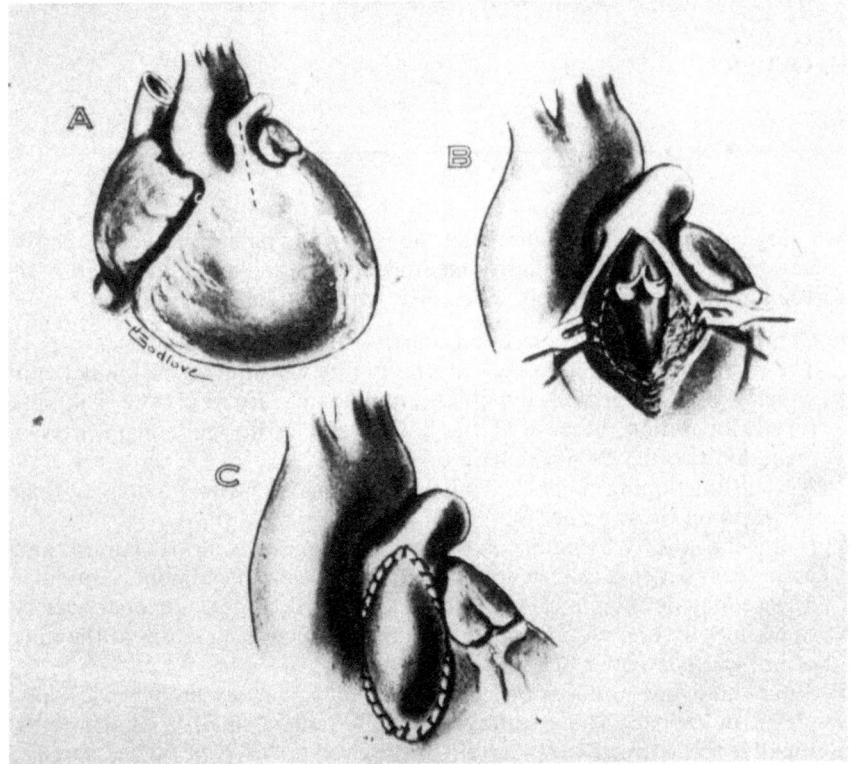

Figure 1 Patch enlargement of the right ventricular outflow tract (from Davidson with permission)

in one instance because the infundibulum was primarily hypoplastic; that is, narrow but not hypertrophied. In the other two it was thought that, after enlargement of the right ventricular outflow tract with a pericardial or Teflon gusset, an excessively large akinetic area would have been created.

The indications for surgical intervention in all three children with primarily uncorrectable Fallot's tetralogy were severe cyanosis and disability. Two were infants, the other a 4-year-old child. One infant had pulmonary valve atresia

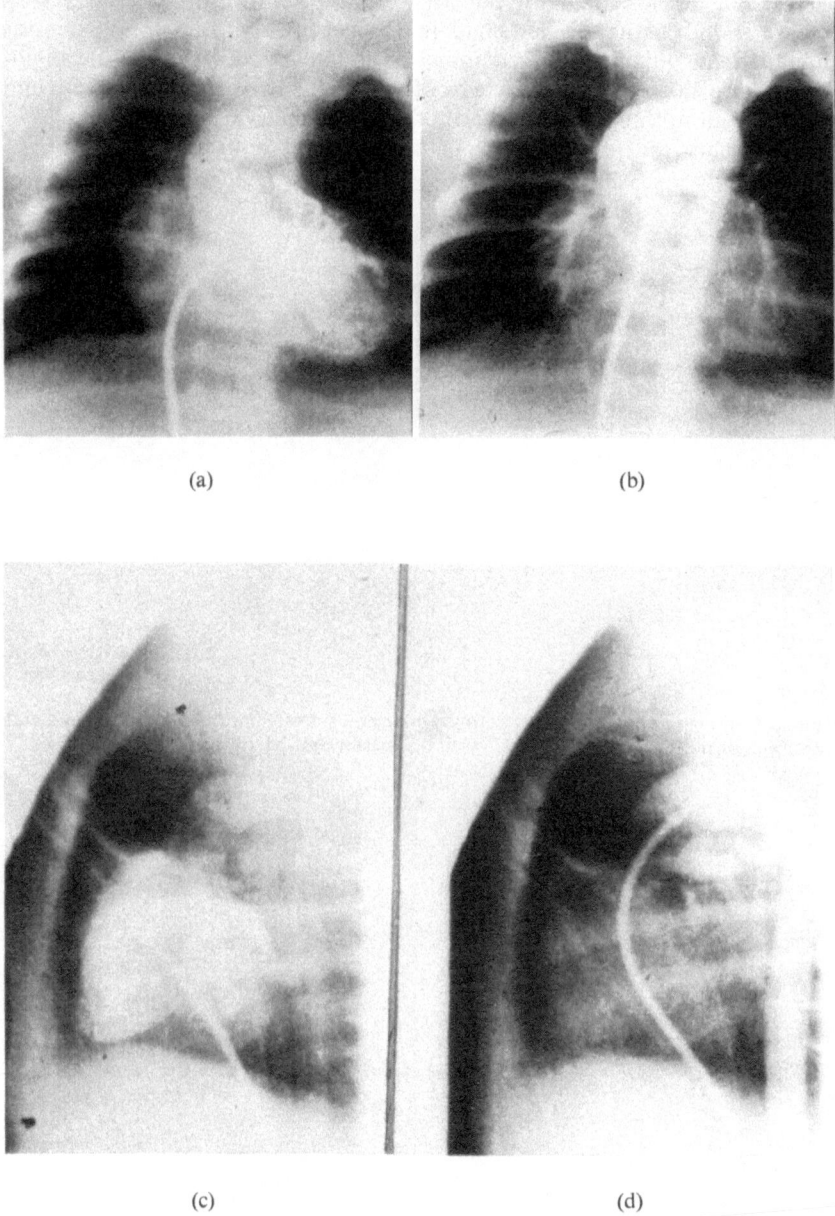

(a)   (b)

(c)   (d)

Figure 2　Fallot's tetralogy with pulmonary (valve) atresia: a and b: anteroposterior view after right ventricular and aortic injection; c and d: lateral view after right ventricular and aortic injection

with a closing duct (Figure 2a–d), the other showed valvular and infundibular obstruction with extreme hypoplasia of the central pulmonary vessels (Figure 3a and b). In the oldest child, in whom a Blalock–Taussig anastomosis had failed, the pulmonary vasculature was equally hypoplastic. On the angiofilm (Figure 4) only the obstructed outflow tract of the right ventricle could be seen, with no further appearance of the pulmonary artery branches.

All patients underwent enlargement of the right ventricular outflow tract

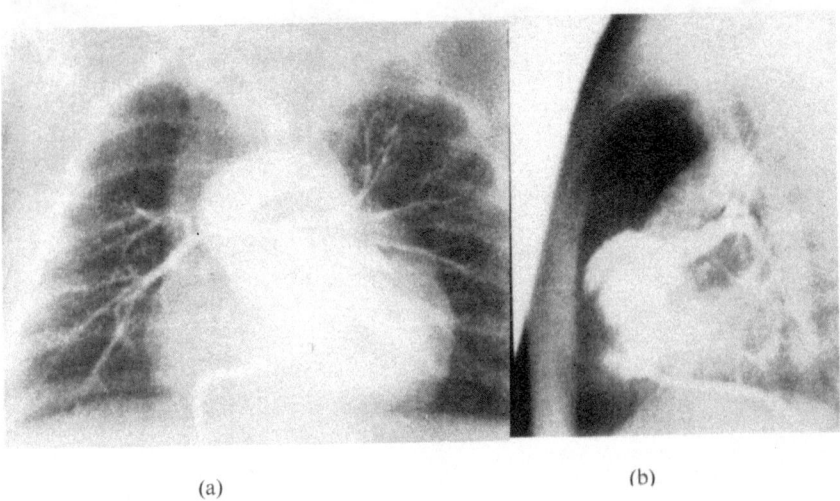

(a)   (b)

Figure 3 a and b Fallot's tetralogy with valvular and subvalvular pulmonary stenosis and hypoplasia of the pulmonary arteries—anteroposterior and lateral view

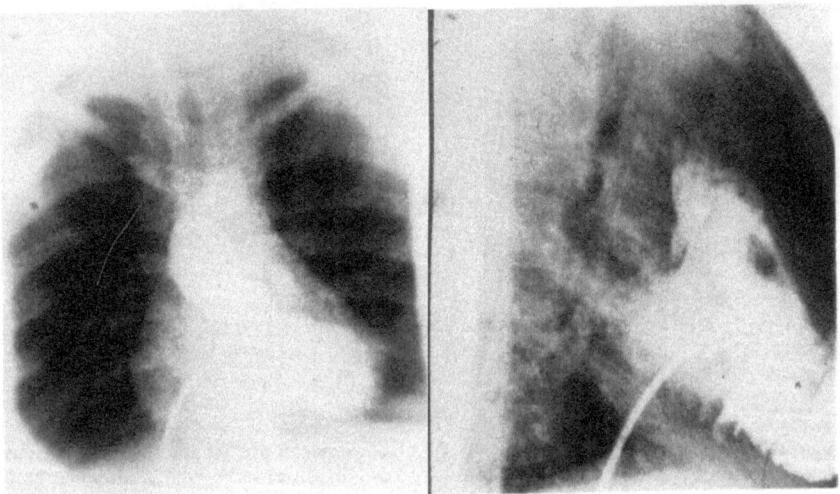

Figure 4 Fallot's tetralogy with right ventricular outflow-tract obstruction and no further appearance of the pulmonary arteries. A previous Blalock–Taussig anastomosis had failed

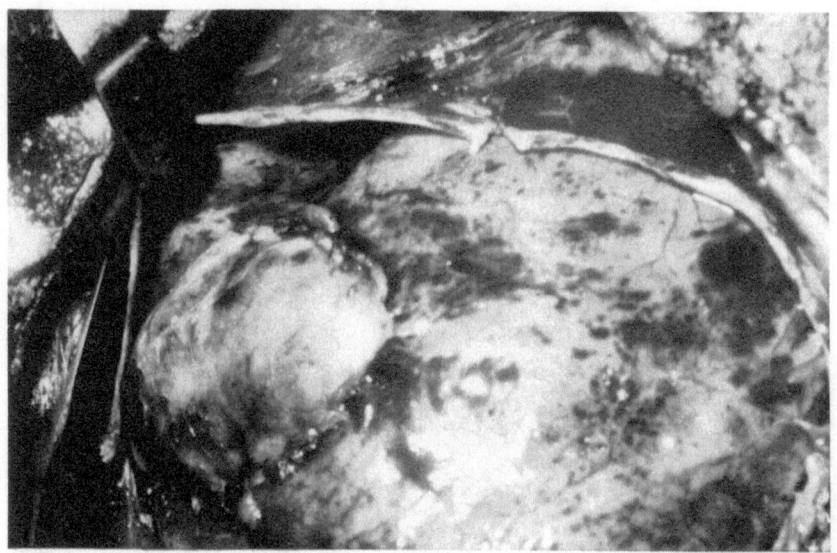

Figure 5 Patch enlargement of the right ventricular outflow-tract, operative view

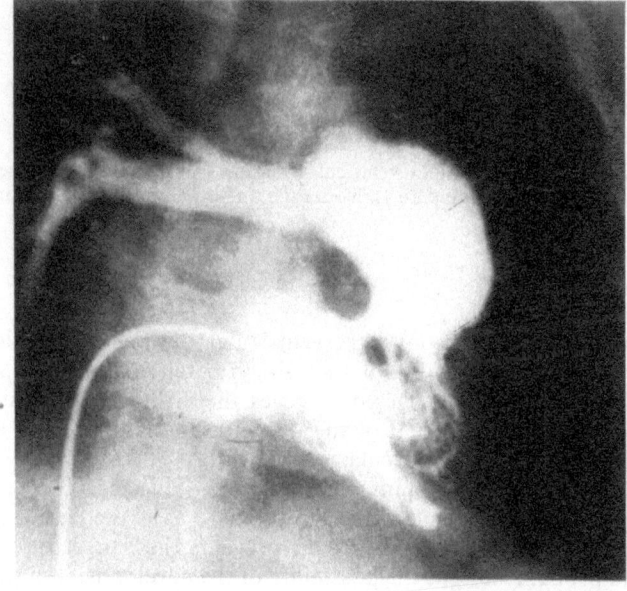

Figure 6 Angiogram of the right ventricular outflow tract 6 months after infundibuloplasty (same patient as in Figure 3). Notice the well-developed right pulmonary artery with no major right-to-left shunt

by insertion of a pericardial or Gore–Tex gusset (Figure 5). The postoperative course was uneventful and half a year after operation patients had all become 'pink' with a balanced or only minor left-to-right shunt. On re-study, a residual gradient at the ventricular or distal pulmonary artery level was found with no significant overcirculation of the lungs. Nevertheless, the pulmonary vasculature had developed well (Figure 6). The 4-year-old child whose postoperative findings are shown in Figure 7 has subsequently undergone closure of the VSD with only minor resection of residual infundibular obstruction being required. Both infants are awaiting intracardiac repair.

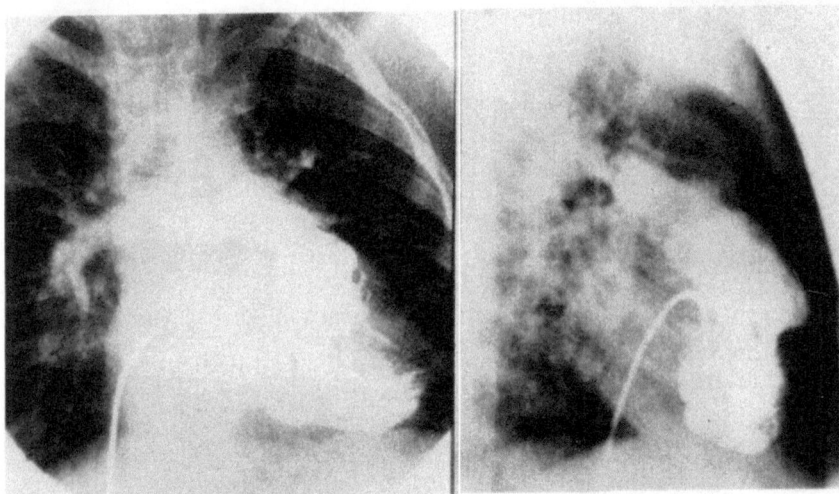

Figure 7 Angiogram of the right ventricular outflow-tract 1 year after open infundibulectomy (same patient as in Figure 4). Notice the well-developed pulmonary arteries with no major right-to-left shunt

DISCUSSION

In severe proximal or distal right ventricular outflow obstruction which precludes primary repair of Fallot's tetralogy, patch enlargement across the pulmonary valve ring diminishes or relieves the right-to-left shunt, thereby leading to a better development of the whole pulmonary vascular system as well as the left atrial and ventricular cavities.

After this operation, the pulmonary artery is subjected only to a higher systemic systolic, not systemic diastolic, pressure as is the case after a too-large aortopulmonary anastomosis. This prevents the danger of pulmonary oedema and probably lessens the possibility of the development of pulmonary vascular disease. Additionally, the capacity of the pulmonary vascular system increases and enables the surgeon to proceed with intracardiac correction in the relatively short interval of 1–2 years.

Patch infundibuloplasty as a preliminary part of total correction in Fallot's tetralogy with severe pulmonary artery hypoplasia differs from the Brock procedure in that a hypoplastic pulmonary valve ring is also enlarged. This ring necessarily remains narrow after a shunt or Brock operation and requires major reconstructive measures at the time of definitive repair. On the other hand, the open procedure results in at least partial total correction, for in the second operation there remains basically only closure of the ventricular septal defect. When insertion of a biological valve into the pulmonary valve ring position or the implantation of a valved conduit also becomes feasible, nearly normal haemodynamics can be achieved.

35

Anatomical correction of complete transposition of the great arteries in infancy

M. YACOUB

Until lately the only treatment for complete transposition of the great arteries (TGA) was early atrial septostomy[1,2] followed by inflow correction by the Mustard[3] or Senning[4] operation at a later age. These procedures, however, are not totally corrective since the right ventricle continues to serve the systemic circulation and tricuspid regurgitation[5], obstruction of systemic or pulmonary venous drainage[6] and late arrhythmias[7] may constitute late serious complications.

Total correction of transposition of the great arteries can be accomplished by transecting the aorta and pulmonary arteries and reattaching them to the appropriate ventricles[8–10]. This should include transferring the coronary ostia to the posterior vessel.

TECHNICAL CONSIDERATIONS

In transferring the coronary ostia it is essential to avoid undue tension, tortion or kinking of the main coronary arteries and their early branches. To achieve this, the coronary anatomy in TGA was studied and four main types or coronary anatomy were identified[11]. In Type A (the commonest) the right and left coronary arteries arise from the middle of the right and left posterior aortic sinuses (Figure 1) and run for several millimetres in the atrioventricular groove before branching, thus allowing mobilization of the coronary ostia, a disc of surrounding aortic wall and the proximal part of each main coronary artery. The discs are then anastomosed to the posterior vessel at preselected sites (Figure 2). In the other three types this technique cannot be applied because of common, or close, origin of the coronary arteries from the back of the aorta, Type B and C (Figure 1) or origin of the circumflex from the right coronary Type D (Figure 1). In Type D the circumflex reaches the left side of the heart by passing around the right and posterior aspect of the

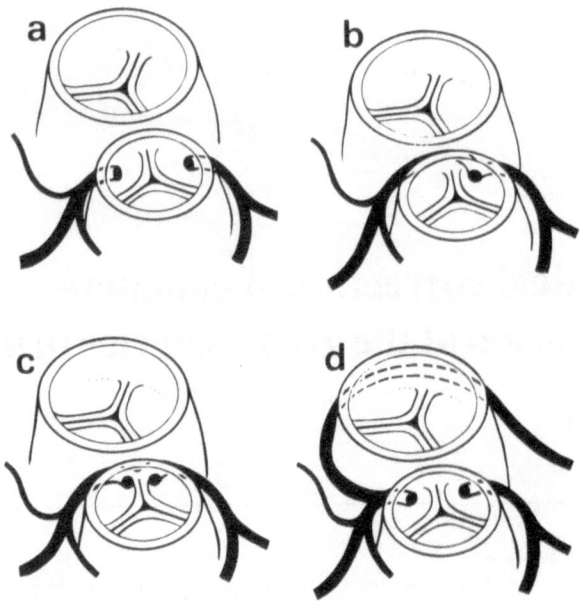

Figure 1 Showing the various sites of origin of the coronary arteries. They usually do not branch immediately, and can be mobilized and transplanted

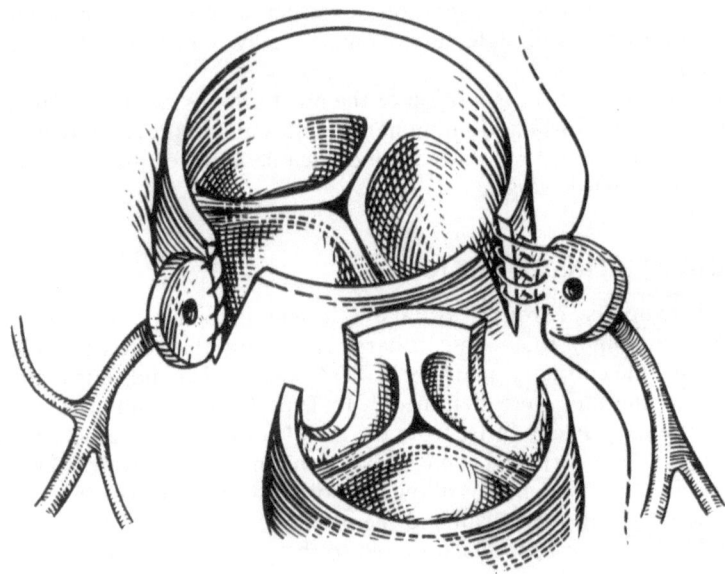

Figure 2 Showing the mobilized coronary arteries transplanted to a new site on the new aortic root

posterior vessel. Direct transfer, as in the technique described for Type A, would result in serious kinking of one of the main coronary arteries or their branches. For this reason an alternate technique has been developed which allows the coronary ostium and proximal parts of the coronary arteries to remain in the same position without tension, torsion or kinking (Figure 3). It is, therefore, possible to effectively transpose the coronary ostia to the posterior vessel in all types of coronary anatomy in TGA.

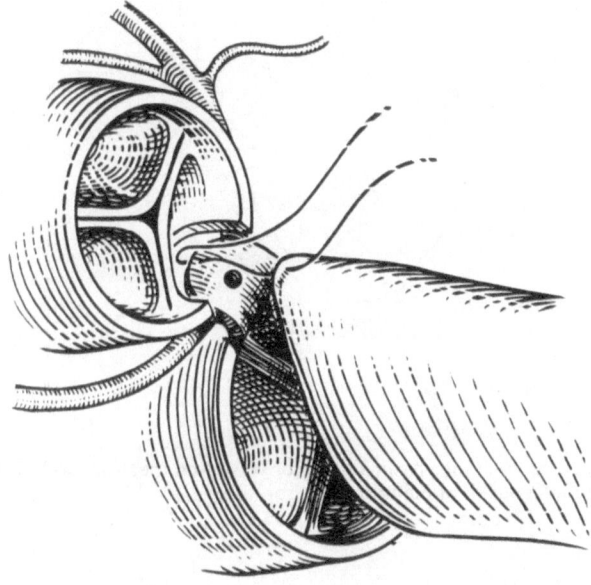

Figure 3 A technique for transferring the coronary arteries without torsion or tension

Following transection of the vessels and restoration of continuity between the proximal posterior vessel and distal aorta, a gap between the proximal anterior vessel and distal main pulmonary artery results which can be bridged by either a dacron graft (Figure 4) or a large tube made of a homologous dura, which we have used in our later cases.

THE STATE OF THE POSTERIOR VENTRICLE

The posterior ventricle in TGA is well developed only in patients with additional defects which maintain a high pressure within the ventricle, such as large ventricular septal defects, persistent ductus arteriosus and subpulmonary stenosis. In the absence of one of these defects regression of fetal pulmonary vascular resistance leads to a fall in systolic posterior ventricular pressure with rapid diminution in left ventricular mass[12,13]. It is estimated that after the first 2 weeks of life, approximately half the infants with transposition will have left ventricles incapable of supporting the systemic circulation[14]. The percentage increases rapidly with age, rendering most patients with TGA and intact interventricular septum unsuitable for anatomical correction. In an

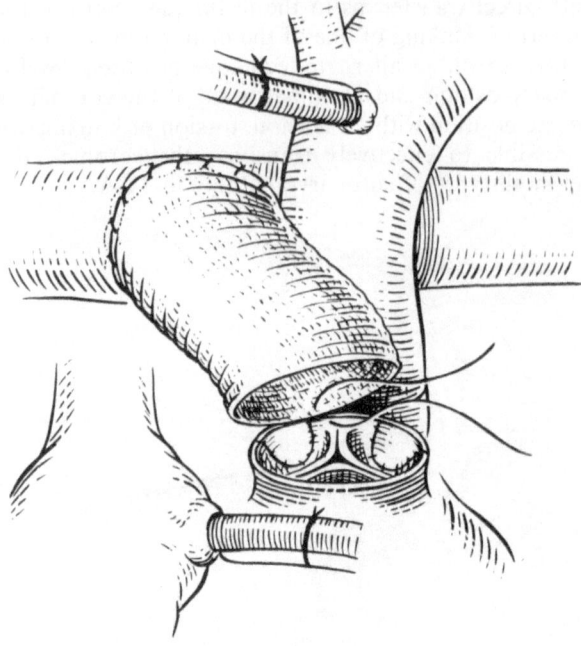

Figure 4 The gap between the proximal anterior vessel and the distal aorta bridged with a large tube of homologous dura mater or a dacron tube

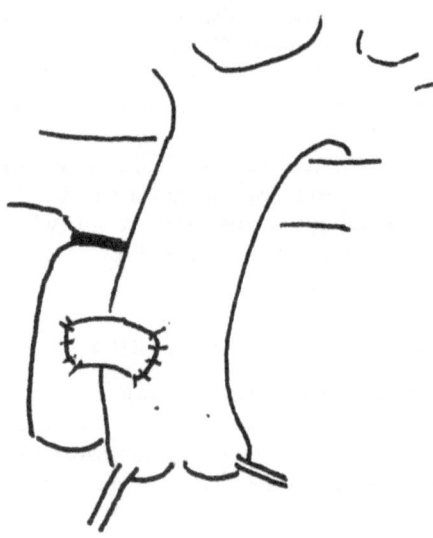

Figure 5 Technique for banding and creation of aortopulmonary shunt as a first stage operation to redevelop the posterior ventricle

attempt to overcome this difficulty a first stage operation to redevelop the posterior ventricle in these patients has been developed[15]. This consists of banding of the pulmonary artery and creation of an aortopulmonary shunt proximal to the band (Figure 5). This procedure is combined with atrial septectomy, if a sufficiently large interatrial communication is not already present. Apart from its beneficial effect in favouring mixing we believe that the interatrial communication acts as a safety mechanism in case of temporary posterior ventricular failure after banding. The addition of an aorto-pulmonary shunt proximal to the band renders pulmonary blood flow less dependent on posterior ventricular function and acts as a safeguard against excessive rise of peak posterior ventricular pressure above systemic level, particularly during exercise which can lead to severe hypertrophy and possibly fibrosis of the posterior ventricular myocardium.

PATIENTS AND RESULTS

Our early experience consisted of three patients operated on between 1972 and 1975, who had intact interventricular septums with low left ventricular pressure. The operations were performed very early in life in an attempt to prevent excessive diminution in left ventricular mass (Table 1). All three

Table 1   Early experience with TGA and intact ventricular septum 1972–1975

Date	Age at operation	LV/RV	Outcome
November 1972	6 months	25/90	Died soon after bypass
July 1974	17 days	30/70	Survived 5 hours
February 1975	24 days	55/70 (PA 30)	Survived 4 hours

patients developed acute left ventricular failure in the immediate postoperative period in spite of satisfactory technical repair (Figure 6). Since then four patients, varying in age between 8 weeks and 6 years, have undergone anatomical correction. There was one early death. In three of the patients there were large ventricular septal defects present and in two a previous banding had been performed. The fourth patient had an intact interventricular septum and for that reason a first stage operation to redevelop the posterior ventricle was performed (Figure 7). Following the anatomical correction the left ventricle took the load of the circulation quite readily and postoperative tests showed normal movement of the left ventricular wall, as shown by echocardiography (Figure 8). Computer analysis, by the method of Gibson and Brown[16], showed normal left ventricular function (Figure 9).

Postoperative angiography showed normal appearances of the anterior ventricular outflow to the lung (Figures 10a and b). In one of the patients who had previous banding there was marked discrepancy between the ascending aorta and its new 'root' as shown in Figure 11, however, the new aortic valve was completely competent. Late repeat angiography showed that both the aortic and coronary anastomoses are capable of growth following correction in early infancy.

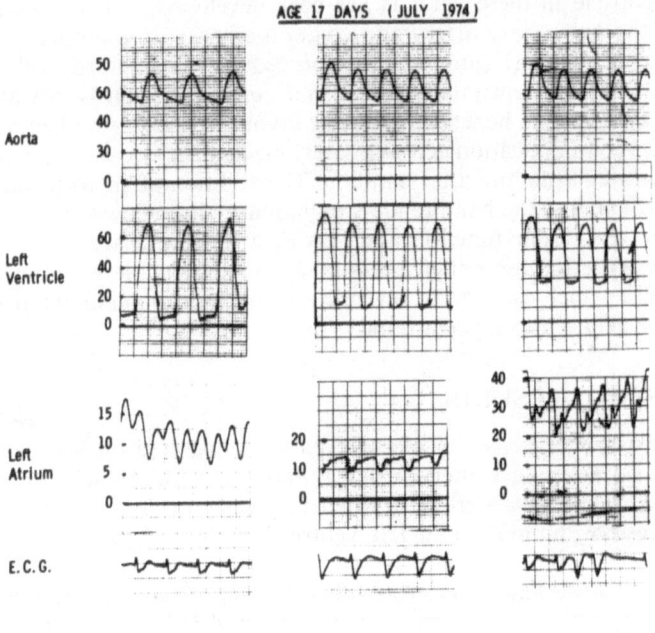

Figure 6 Anatomical correction of TGA and intact septum, age 17 days (July 1974)

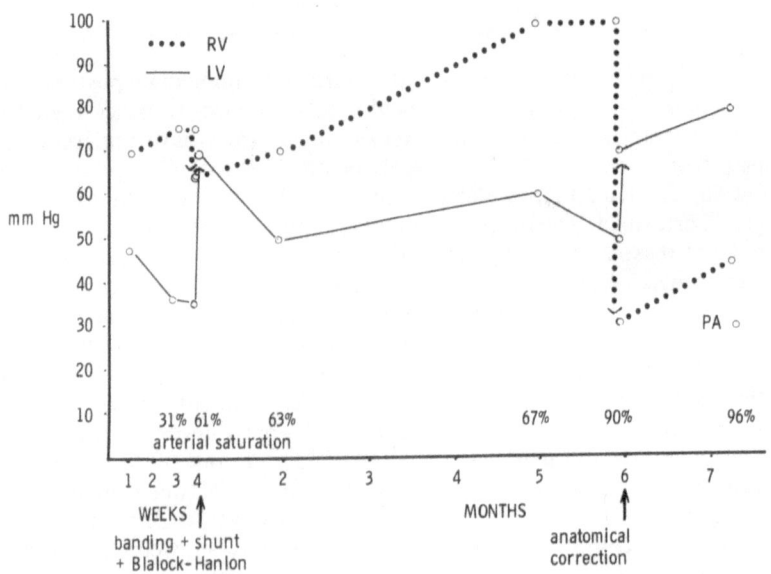

Figure 7 Anatomical correction of TGA with intact septum pressures

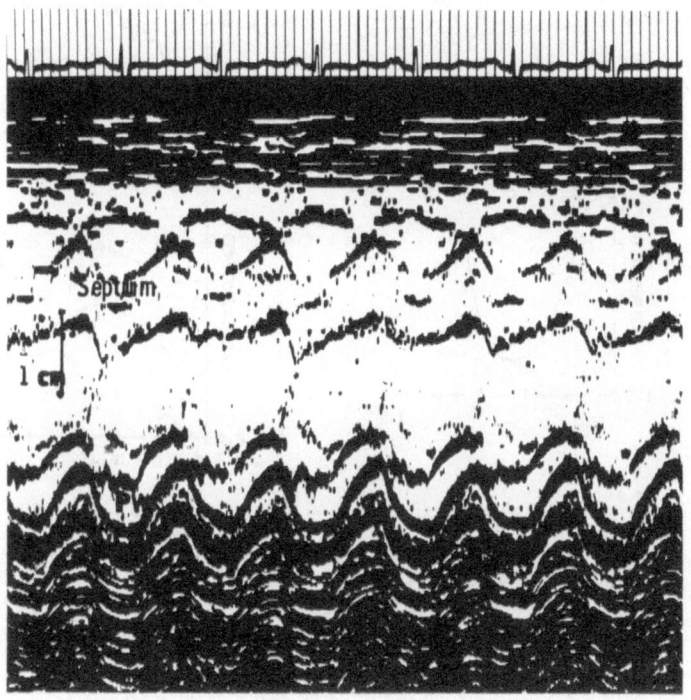

Figure 8 Postoperative echo in a patient who has had a 'switch' operation for TGA showing normal movement of left ventricular wall

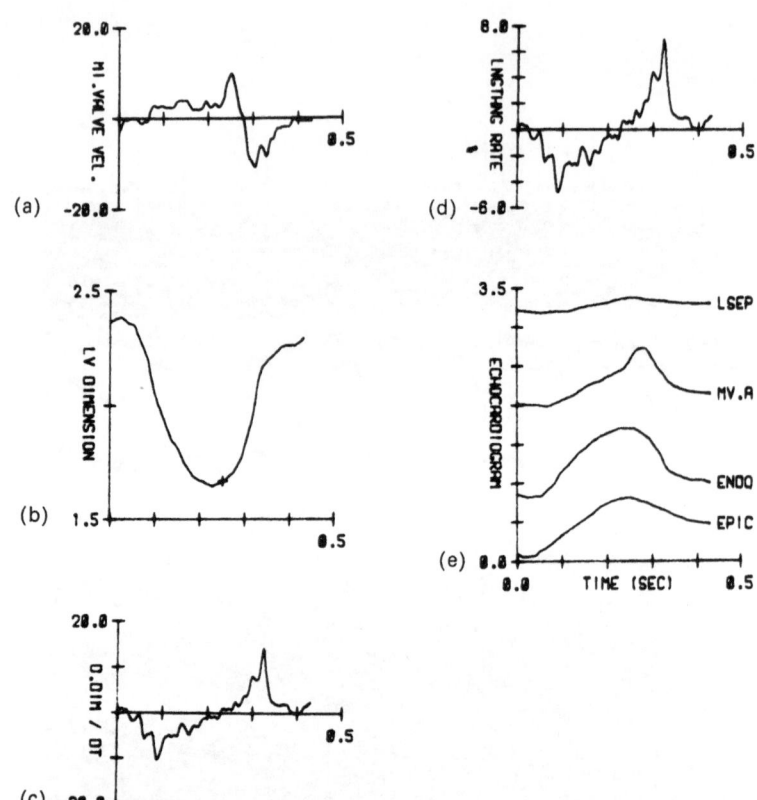

Figure 9 Computer output of left ventricular echocardiogram 2 weeks after anatomical correction. (a) Digitized echocardiogram from right and left sides of septum and endocardial and epicardial surfaces of posterior wall and anterior mitral valve (MV) cusp. (b) Changes in left ventricular dimension. X on LV dimension represents time MV opening coinciding with minimum dimension. (c) Rate of change in dimension (D.Dim./D.T.). (d) Lengthening rate or velocity of circumferential fibre shortening. (e) Rate of change of position of anterior MV cusp.

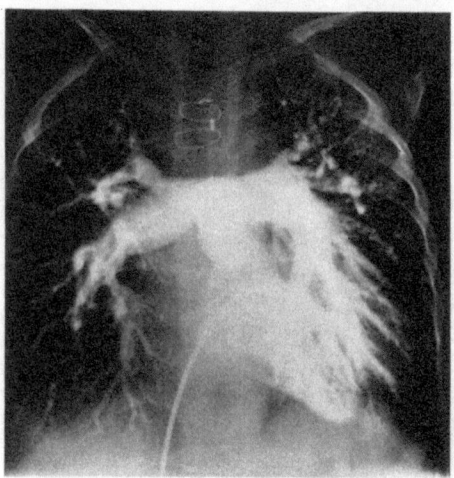

Figure 10a Postoperative angiography showing normal appearance of anterior outflow tract to the lungs

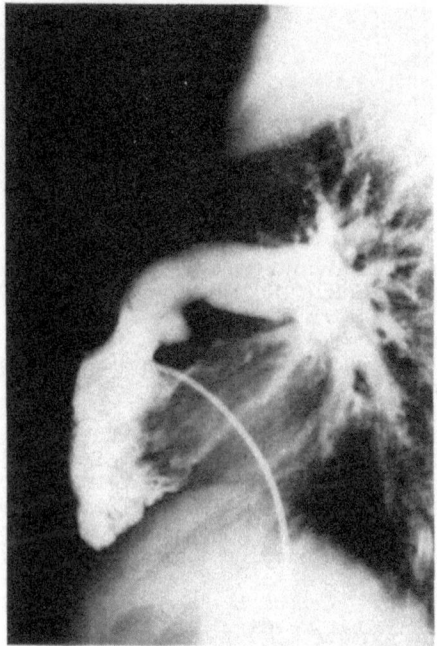

Figure 10b Postoperative angiography showing normal appearance of anterior outflow tract to the lungs (lateral view)

The results in this series show that anatomical correction of transposition of the great arteries can give encouraging early results and can be applied in patients with intact septum. The role of the operation, however, is still not established and further experience is required to determine its late result.

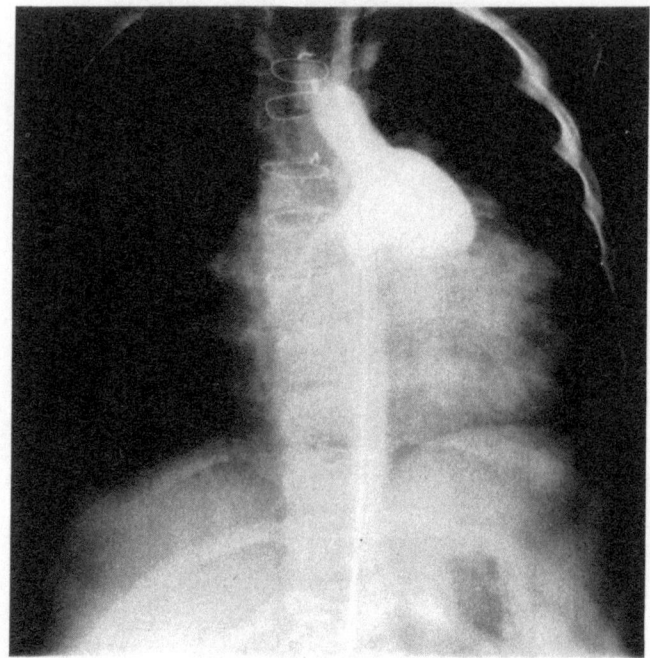

Figure 11   Angiography in a patient who had a previous banding operation

References

1. Rashkind, W. J. and Miller, W. W., (1966). *J. Am. Med. Assoc.*, **196**, 991
2. Blalock, A. and Hanlon, C. R. (1950). *Surg. Gynecol. Obstet.*, **90**, 1
3. Mustard, W. T. (1964). *Surgery*, **55**, 469
4. Senning, A. (1959). *ibid.* **45**, 966
5. Tynan, M., Aberdeen, E. and Stark, J. (1972). *Circulation*, **45**, suppl. 1, p.3
6. Stark, J., *et al.* (1972). *ibid.* 45/46, suppl. 1, p. 116
7. El Said, G. *et al.* (1972). *Am. J. Cardiol.*, **30**, 526
8. Jatene, A. D., Fontes, V. F., Paulista, P. P., Souza, L. C. B., Negar, F., Gelantier, H. and Saura, J. E. M. R. (1976). *J. Thorac, Cardiovasc. Surg.*, **72**, 364
9. Yacoub, M. H., Radley-Smith, R. and Hilton, C. J. (1976). *Br. Med. J.*, **1**, 112
10. Ross, D. N., Rickards, A. and Somerville, J. (1976). *ibid.* **1**, 1109
11. Yacoub, M., Radley-Smith, R. (197). Anatomy of the coronary arteries in transposition of the great arteries and methods for their transfer in anatomical correction. *Thorax*
12. Lev, M. *et al.* (1969). *Am. J. Cardiol.*, **23**, 409
13. Tynan, M. (1972). *Circulation*, **46**, 809
14. Editorial. 1976, *Br. Med. J.* **1**, 1104
15. Yacoub, M., Radley-Smith, R. and Maclaurin, R. *Lancet*, (1977), **i**, 1275
16. Gibson, D. G. and Brown, D. J. (1973) *Br. Heart J.*, **35**, 1145

Section VII
Left ventricular function and protection

36

Non-invasive study of left ventricular function

D. G. GIBSON

The first use of echocardiography in studying left ventricular function was to measure the cavity size[1,2], and there is a considerable body of evidence to suggest that reliable estimates of a minor diameter can be made using this method. More recently, a second index of left ventricular function, the rate of change of dimension, has been studied and taken to indicate the myocardial fibre-shortening rate[3,4]. Measurements can be made in absolute terms, expressed in cm/s, or normalized to refer to unit length of dimension, when they are referred to as Vcf or velocity of circumferential fibre-shortening. Mean values of shortening rate have been estimated and shown to correlate with corresponding values derived from angiograms in the same patients.

The measurements described above are based on only two determinations of cavity size in each cardiac cycle, made at end-diastole and end-systole. Currently available echocardiographs, however, have a repetition frequency of 1000/s, and so have the potential of studying left ventricular wall motion continuously, with considerably better resolution in time than that obtainable with angiographic methods. Although left ventricular dimension can be measured manually throughout the cardiac cycle, this is very laborious, and the process can be greatly speeded up using a simple computer technique. In order to do this, the echocardiogram to be studied is placed on a digitizing table, and a cursor is run along each of the echoes to be measured. The position of the cursor is detected electronically, and converted into a series of digital coordinates, up to 100 per cardiac cycle being generated for each echo and stored in the computer. This process can be applied to echoes from the right and left sides of the septum, the anterior cusp of the mitral valve and endocardial and epicardial surfaces of the posterior wall. It is also possible to digitize any other continuous signal such as the apex-cardiogram or left ventricular pressure trace. Once these have been digitized, the computer can plot them unchanged, or can perform further manoeuvres on them. For

245

example, the coordinates of the left side of the septum can be subtracted from those of the endocardial surface of the posterior wall to give a continuous measure of transverse dimension, or those of endocardium be subtracted from epicardium to give a curve of left ventricular wall thickness. It is also possible to differentiate a trace with respect to time, so that its rate of change can be calculated. An example of such a plot, taken from the echocardiogram of a normal subject, is shown in Figure 1. The original information has been plotted unchanged in the lowest panel. In the middle panel is shown left ventricular dimension, which falls during systole, and increases rapidly at first during the early phase of ventricular filling, and then more slowly during

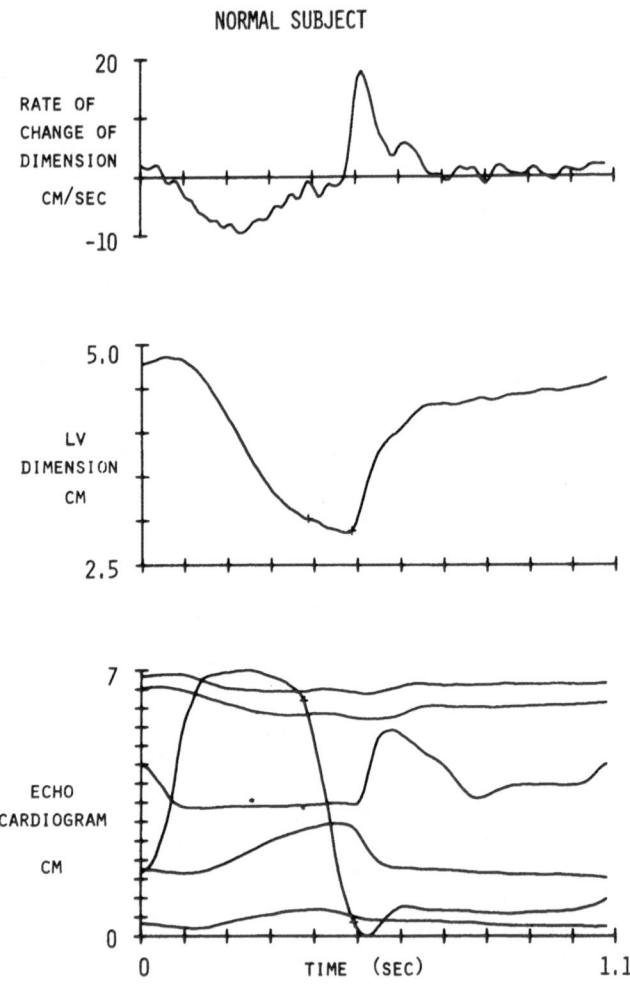

Figure 1   Computer output of the echocardiogram of a normal subject

the period of diastasis. The timing of aortic valve closure and mitral valve opening are superimposed, as two crosses, on this trace since they define the period of isovolumic relaxation, and it will be seen that there has been little change in dimension at this time. It is also apparent that mitral valve opening coincides closely with minimum dimension, suggesting that the increase occurring during diastole is due to ventricular filling. Finally, the top trace gives the rate of change of dimension, which reaches approximately 10 cm/s during systole and 20 cm/s during diastole. These estimates of peak rates of wall movement have been compared with the corresponding values from angiograms in the same patients, and satisfactory agreement between the two has been confirmed[5].

It is a limitation of standard M-mode echocardiography, however, that only a small part of the left ventricular cavity can be studied directly, so that if attempts are made to extrapolate values obtained in this way to the cavity as a whole, serious errors may result if incoordinate left ventricular function is present. It has been widely assumed, therefore, that M-mode methods are of little value in assessing left ventricular contraction or relaxation patterns unless overall function is known to be uniform, an assurance that may be difficult to supply under many clinical conditions. It is the purpose of the present paper to describe methods whereby the scope of M-mode echo-cardiography can be extended to detect incoordinate left ventricular function. It also seems possible that these methods may give information about some of the disturbances that can interfere with the highly organized processes constituting normal contraction and relaxation. In order to do this, it must be accepted that the echo dimension cannot reflect overall left ventricular function, but merely local behaviour in the region studied. If contraction is coordinate, local and general function will be in phase with one another, but if contraction patterns are disturbed, then this is no longer the case. Such abnormalities might be detected, therefore, by comparison of changes in echo dimension with some measure of overall function. A number can be used, of which the most general is the left ventricular pressure trace[6]. The results can be plotted as a pressure–dimension loop, an example from a normal subject being shown in Figure 2. Four phases can be recognized: isovolumic contraction, when pressure increases at constant dimension; ejection, when dimension falls, again at constant dimension; and finally filling. The area of the loop represents stroke work done by the myocardium in the region studied by the echo beam on the blood within the ventricle, and the fact that it is rectangular shows that this process of energy transfer from myocardium to circulation is mechanically efficient. The loop from a patient with ischaemic heart disease is shown in Figure 3. It is distorted, so that its area is reduced, and contraction correspondingly less efficient. This loss of efficiency caused by incoordinate contraction can be seen to be due to abnormal dimension changes as the ventricular pressure rises and falls, i.e. during isovolumic contraction and relaxation. This is fortunate if one wishes to study left ventricular function with M-mode echocardiography, since during these periods when the volume of the ventricle is constant, it is not possible for a single localized wall movement to occur. If outward movement occurs at this time in one region, then equal and opposite inward movement must occur

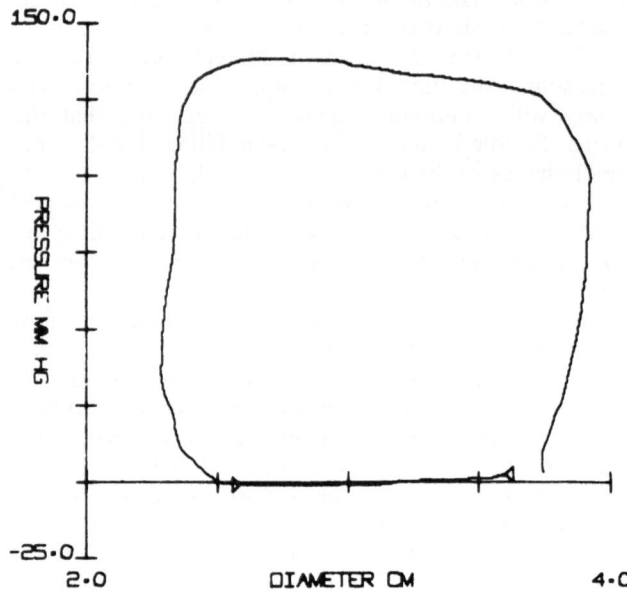

Figure 2 Left ventricular pressure–dimension loop from a normal subject. The loop is approximately rectangular

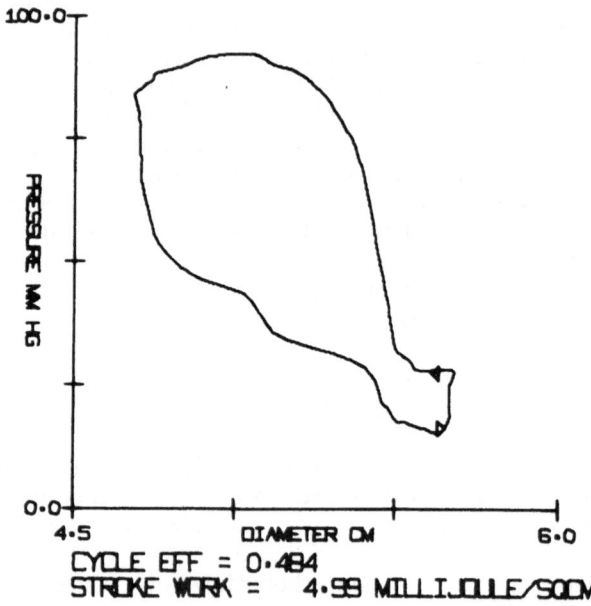

CYCLE EFF = 0·484
STROKE WORK = 4·99 MILLIJOULE/SQCM

Figure 3 Left ventricular pressure–dimension loop from a patient with ischaemic heart disease. The loop is distorted by abnormal wall movement during isovolumic contraction and relaxation

elsewhere in order to maintain the cavity volume constant. M-mode echo-cardiography, although showing only regional function, is very sensitive in detecting abnormal wall movement during the two isovolumic periods, that is, those times in the cardiac cycle when such movement has its greatest effect on the overall efficiency of the heart as a pump.

These ideas can be extended to employ purely non-invasive techniques. Figure 4 shows the echocardiogram of a patient who developed a low cardiac output state after open-heart surgery. It will be seen that outward movement of the posterior wall is virtually complete before the onset of opening of the mitral valve, that is, it has occurred in the period of isovolumic relaxation. This is very abnormal, and indicates severe localized left ventricular dysfunction, due in this case to an anterior descending coronary artery embolus. The use of the mitral valve echo in this way to detect incoordinate wall movement has been described in detail elsewhere[7].

A second approach has been to use the apex-cardiogram, a non-invasive record of movement of the apex of the heart[8]. During the upstroke and downstroke, this record is synchronous with the corresponding periods of the left ventricular pressure trace[9]. The results of this investigation can thus be plotted as an apex-cardiogram–echo dimension loop, in exactly the same way as a pressure–dimension loop. Normally, there is little change in dimension during the upstroke or downstroke of the apex-cardiogram, as

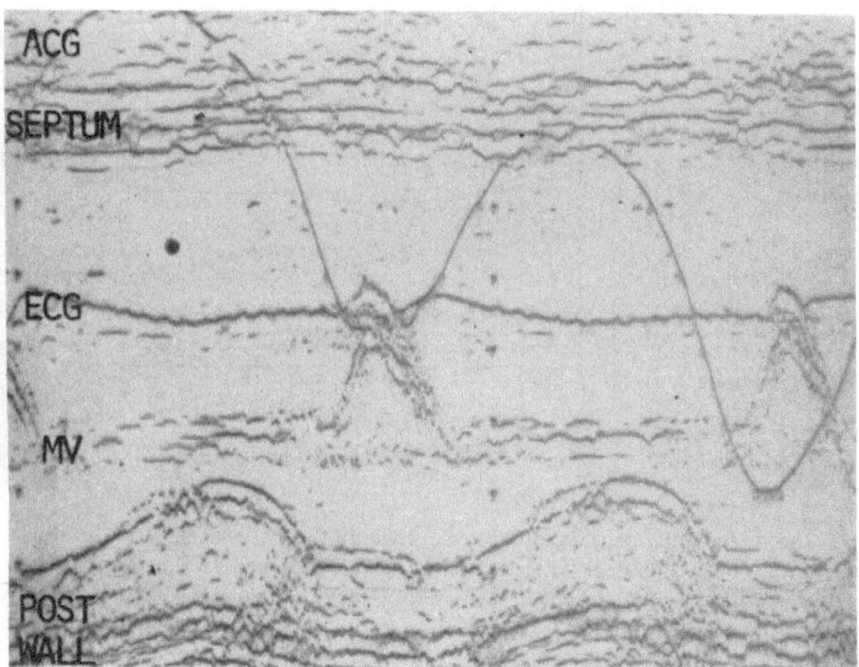

Figure 4 Left ventricular echocardiogram of a patient with a postoperative low cardiac output state. Outward wall movement is almost complete before the onset of mitral valve opening

shown in Figure 5. By contrast, in Figure 6 from a patient with ischaemic heart disease, there is an abnormal reduction in dimension during the up-stroke, and an abnormal increase in dimension during the downstroke. An abnormal reduction in dimension in one region of the heart during isovolumic contraction implies an aneurysmal increase elsewhere in the ventricle. It thus follows that the region observed by the echo beam is functioning normally,

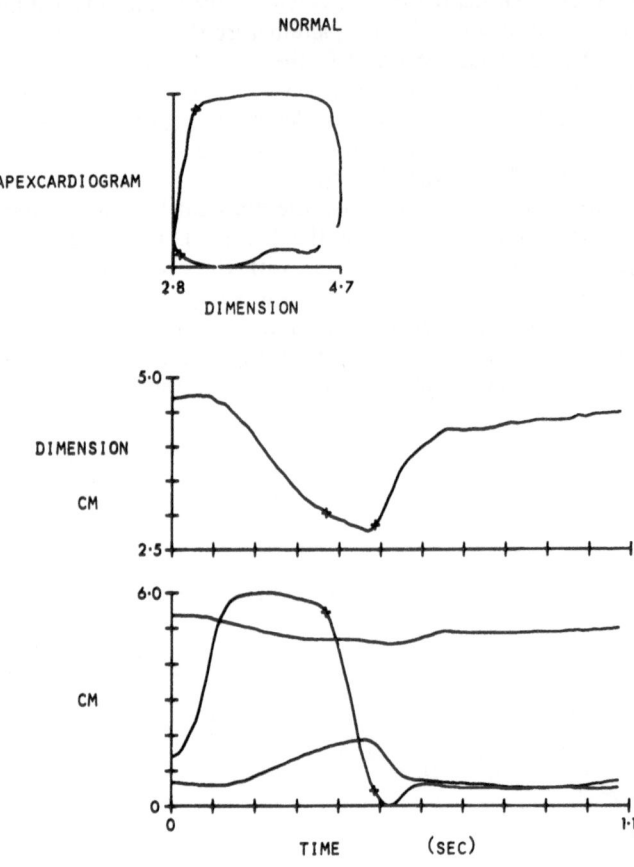

Figure 5 Relation between left ventricular dimension and apex-cardiogram in a normal subject

but that there must be a region elsewhere where the onset of tension develop-ment has been delayed. This deduction was confirmed by left ventriculo-graphy, which demonstrated apical dyskinesia. A dimension increase during isovolumic relaxation also appears to be the behaviour of normal myo-cardium in an abnormal ventricle: localized ischaemia causes delayed re-laxation in the affected area, and thus a further reduction in dimension while the rest of the ventricle is relaxing. Angiographic methods of displaying these abnormalities have been described in detail elsewhere.

STUDY OF LEFT VENTRICULAR FUNCTION

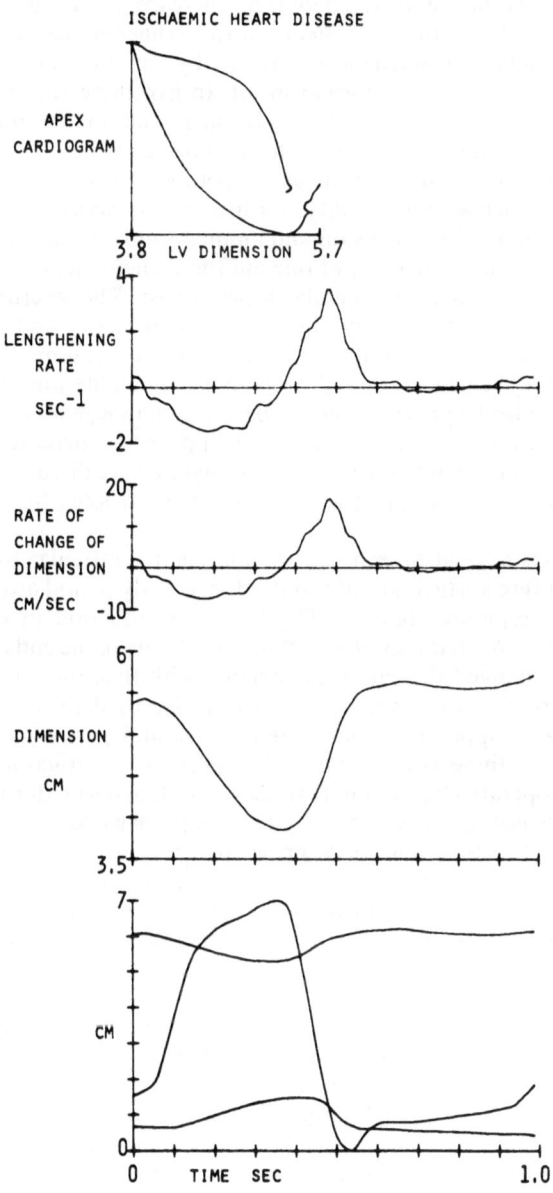

ISCHAEMIC HEART DISEASE

APEX CARDIOGRAM

3.8 LV DIMENSION 5.7

LENGTHENING RATE SEC^{-1}

RATE OF CHANGE OF DIMENSION CM/SEC

DIMENSION CM

CM

0 TIME SEC 1.0

Figure 6 Relation between echocardiogram and apex-cardiogram in a patient with apical dyskinesia due to ischaemic heart disease

The picture obtained when the region studied by the echo beam is itself abnormal is shown in Figure 7. There is an increase in dimension during the isovolumic relaxation. In 20 patients with ischaemic heart disease and regional contraction disturbances shown by angiography, echo–apex-cardiogram relations were abnormal in all. In five these suggested that the primarily abnormal region was being studied, and in the remainder the changes appeared compensatory to abnormalities elsewhere.

It is thus possible to use non-invasive methods to detect three different types of left ventricular abnormality: an increase in cavity size, a reduction in peak rate of change of dimension and an incoordinate contraction pattern. These can all vary independently of one another. These methods can be used preoperatively in patients with valvular heart disease. The severity of valvular regurgitation is reflected in cavity dimension at end-systole and end-diastole. Mitral valve disease, as described elsewhere in this volume, modifies the pattern of wall movement during diastole in a predictable way. Incoordinate contraction can also be present, and can be detected independently of changes due to valve disease; and when present, it appears to increase the risks of surgery. Although it is sometimes due to coronary artery disease, it frequently is not, and may reflect the presence of severe hypertrophy, fibrosis or small vessel disease.

These methods have also been used to study left ventricular function after correction of severe aortic regurgitation[10]. In the early period after operation, there are three separate changes. The first is a reduction in end-diastolic cavity dimension, which is apparent within a few hours of the end of operation, and persists unchanged thereafter. Associated with this, there is a reduction in peak Vcf from normal values preoperatively, to depressed ones post-operatively, again apparent within a few hours and persisting unchanged. Superimposed on these is a period of incoordinate contraction, maximum 2–3 days postoperatively, which regresses spontaneously during the next 1–2 weeks. This last appears to represent a temporary effect of operation on left ventricular function and may prove to be a satisfactory method of monitoring the quality of myocardial preservation. It may summate with incoordinate contraction present preoperatively, leading to the development of severe impairment of overall left ventricular function in the early post-operative period.

These results indicate that it is not appropriate to consider left ventricular function as a single entity. After aortic valve replacement, left ventricular dimension falls, which is an improvement, Vcf falls, which is a deterioration, and superimposed on these are changes in contraction pattern which vary with time. Rather, impaired left ventricular function should be investigated in detail to determine its precise mechanism in individual patients, instead of ascribing it to reduction in a single 'parameter' whenever it occurs.

In surgical practice, incoordinate contraction may have particular signifi-cance, since it appears to be caused to a greater or lesser extent by all bypass operations, and since it cannot be treated pharmacologically. The only possible approaches are to reduce its incidence to a minimum by careful myocardial preservation, and to avoid aggravating it by inappropriate pharmacological manoeuvres postoperatively.

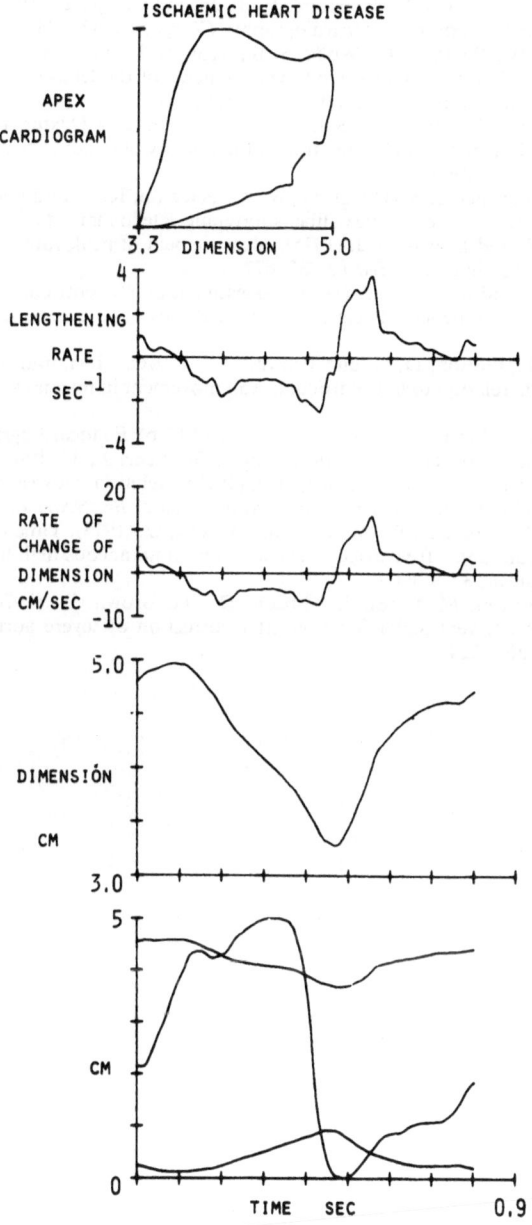

Figure 7 Relation between echocardiogram and apex-cardiogram in a patient with a posterior aneurysm due to ischaemic heart disease

References

1. Fortuin, M. J., Sherman, M. E., Hood, W. P. Jr. and Craige, E. (1970). Evaluation of left ventricular function by echocardiography. *Circulation*, **42**, 111
2. Feigenbaum, H., Popp, R. L., Wolfe, S. B., Troy, B. L., Pombo, J. F., Haine, C. L., and Dodge, H. T. (1972). Ultrasound measurements of the left ventricle: a correlative study with angiography. *Arch. Intern. Med.*, **129**, 641
3. Paraskos, J. A., Grossman, W, Soltz, S., Dalen, J. E. and Dexter, I. (1971). A noninvasive technique for the determination of the velocity of circumferential fiber shortening. *Circulat. Res.*, **29**, 610
4. Cooper, R., Karliner, J. S., O'Rourke, R. A., Peterson, K. L. and Leopold, C. (1972). Ultrasound determination of mean fiber shortening rate in man. *Am. J. Cardiol.*, **29**, 257
5. Gibson, D. G. and Brown, D. J. (1975). Measurement of peak rates of left ventricular wall movement in man. *Br. Heart J.*, **37**, 677
6. Gibson, D. G. and Brown, D. J. (1976): Assessment of left ventricular systolic function in man from simultaneous echocardiographic and pressure measurements. *Br. Heart J.*, **38**, 8
7a. Upton, M. T., Gibson, D. G. and Brown, D. J. (1976a). Instantaneous mitral leaflet velocity and its relation to left ventricular wall movement in normal subjects. *Br. Heart J.*, **38**, 51
7b. Upton, M. T., Gibson, D. G. and Brown, D. J. (1976b). Echocardiographic assessment of abnormal left ventricular relaxation in man. *Br. Heart J.*, **38**, 1001
8. Venco, A, Gibson, D. G. and Brown, D. J. (1977). Relation between apex-cardiogram and changes in left ventricular pressure and dimension. *Br. Heart J.*, **39**, 117
9. Manolas, J., Rutishauser, W., Wirz, P. and Arbenz, U. (1975). Time relations between apex-cardiogram and left ventricular events using simultaneous high fidelity tracings in man. *Br. Heart J.*, **37**, 1263
10. Venco, A., Sutton, M. G. St. J., Gibson, D. and Brown, D. (1976). Non-invasive assessment of left ventricular function after correction of severe aortic regurgitation. *Br. Heart J.*, **38**, 1324

37

Factors affecting left ventricular performance

W. G. NAYLER AND A. M. SLADE

Mammalian heart muscle is exquisitely sensitive to oxygen, and if for any reason the supply of oxygen is limited, the mechanical performance of the muscle and the integrity of its ultrastructure are severely compromised. The availability of an adequate supply of oxygen is, of course, only one of many factors that affect ventricular function. Other factors affecting ventricular function include substrate supply, heart rate, end-diastolic volume—and hence fibre length, pH, activation of the sympathetic nervous system, thyrotoxicosis, etc. An explanation of how these factors modify ventricular performance is, perhaps, most easily understood if the explanation is presented in terms of the subcellular organelles that are involved, and the sequence of events involved in the transition between diastole → systole → diastole.

ULTRASTRUCTURE OF VENTRICULAR MUSCLE

Mitochondria and energy supply

Approximately 40% of cardiac muscle is made up by mitochondria, which, as Figure 1 shows, lie sandwiched between the myofibrils. The mitochondria have a characteristic appearance, with a relatively simple outer membrane and a more complex (Figure 2) inner membrane which folds repeatedly, thereby providing a relatively large surface area on which many of the mitochondrial enzymes are located. The occurrence of small electron-dense deposits within the mitochondria is a normal finding and (Figure 2) should not be confused with the relatively larger and more diffuse deposits of electron-dense materials found in the mitochondria[1] of damaged cells. Whereas the mitochondria of well-oxygenated heart muscle are fairly uniform in their appearance, an inadequate supply of oxygen, particularly if it is accompanied by substrate withdrawal, causes the mitochondria to assume different and

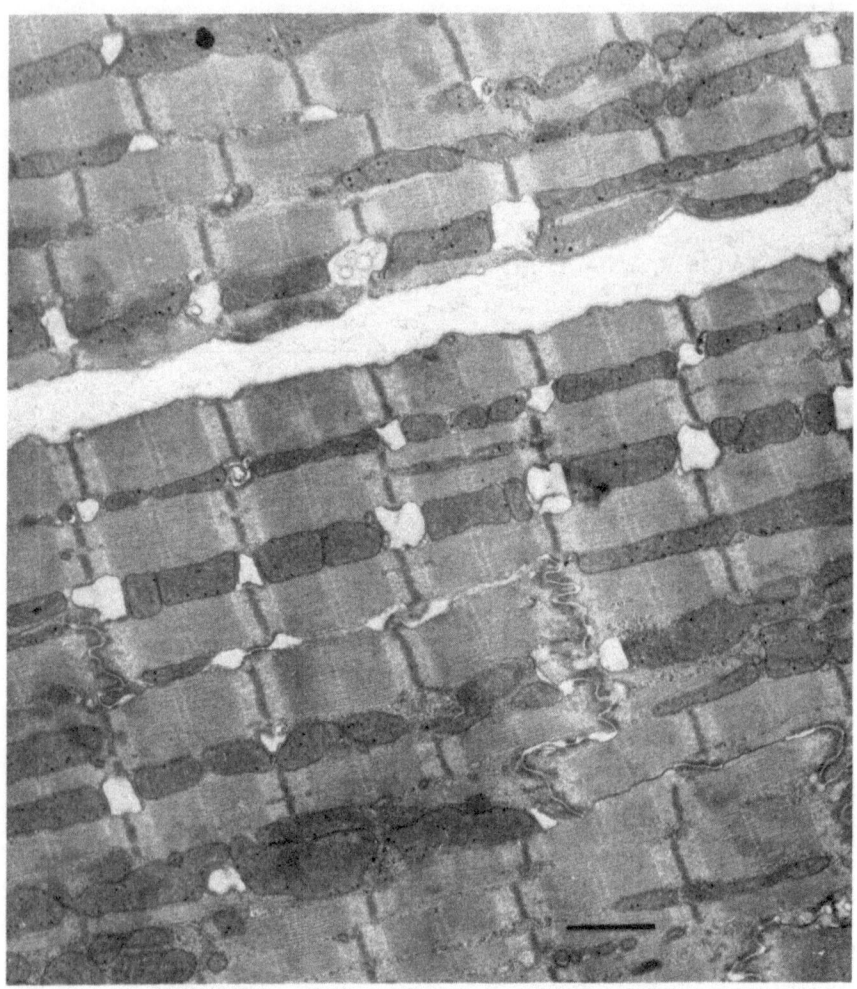

Figure 1 Longitudinal section of rabbit heart muscle (× 11 850). Note the numerous mitochondria sandwiched, in rows, between the myofilaments. The space in between the two cells is filled with extracellular fluid. Marker bar, 1 μm

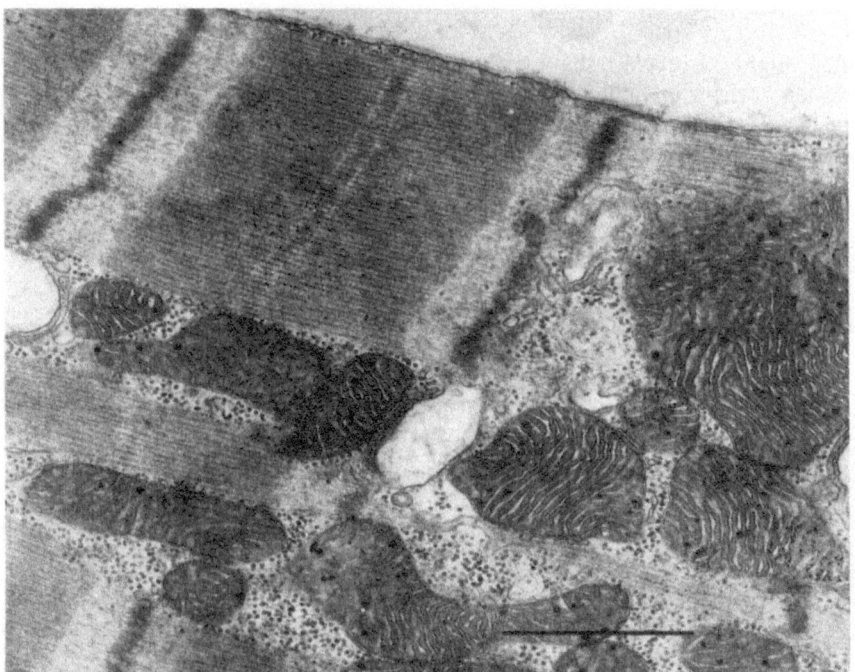

Figure 2 Longitudinal section of rabbit heart muscle ($\times$ 25 600). Marker bar, 1 μm. Note the detailed structure of the mitochondria. The granules in the cytosol are glycogen

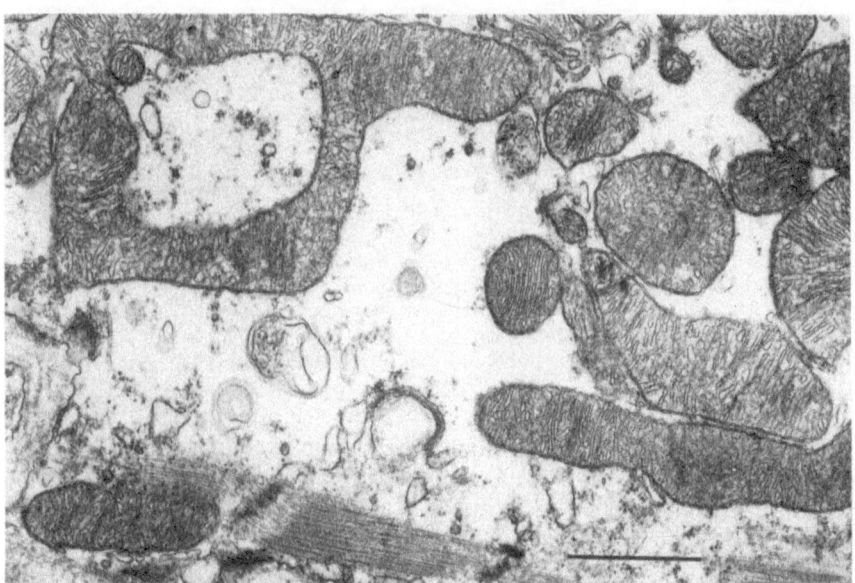

Figure 3 Longitudinal section of rabbit heart muscle perfusion fixed after hypoxic ($pO_2 < 6$ mmHg) perfusion ($\times$ 18 000). Note the presence of oedema and of swollen, invaginated mitochondria. Marker bar, 1 μm

often highly irregular shapes[1,2]. Some mitochondria (Figure 3) become swollen; others invaginate. Electron-dense bars form (Figure 4) and often crysteolysis takes place (Figures 3 and 4) resulting in the partial lysis or destruction of the inner membrane (cristae).

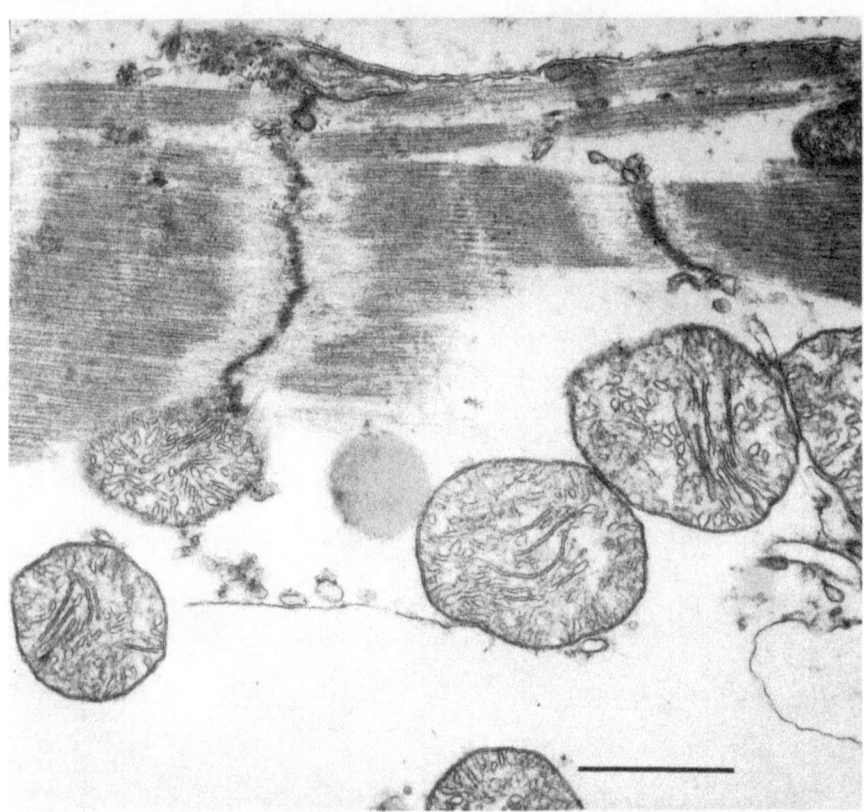

Figure 4 Longitudinal section of rabbit heart muscle perfusion fixed after hypoxic ($pO_2 < 6$ mmHg) instead of aerobic ($pO_2 > 600$ mmHg) perfusion ($\times$ 21 000). Marker bar, 1 μm. Note swollen mitochondria, and the presence of electron-dense bars in the mitochondria. The myofilaments are disrupted and the cell membrane is disrupted so that a mitochondrion is passing from the intracellular to the extracellular phase

During normal aerobic metabolism the mitochondria utilize O_2, to rephosphorylate ADP $\rightarrow$ ATP. Conventionally the capacity of mitochondria to utilize O_2 is expressed in terms of n atoms O_2 used/mg mitochondrial protein/min—the QO_2 value. Whereas mitochondria isolated from aerobically perfused hearts ($pO_2 > 600$ mmHg) utilize O_2 at a rate in excess of 100 n atoms O_2/mg protein/min, mitochondria (Figure 5b) isolated from heart muscle after it has been perfused in the presence of a relatively low pO_2 utilize O_2 relatively ($p < 0.001$) slowly[3,4]. At the same time these hypoxic damaged mitochondria (Figure 5a) accumulate ionized calcium at a relatively rapid rate. This rapid accumulation of Ca^{2+} by hypoxic damaged mitochondria leads to a further deterioration[5] in function, because Ca^{2+} accumulation takes place in preference to rephosphorylating[1] ADP → ATP.

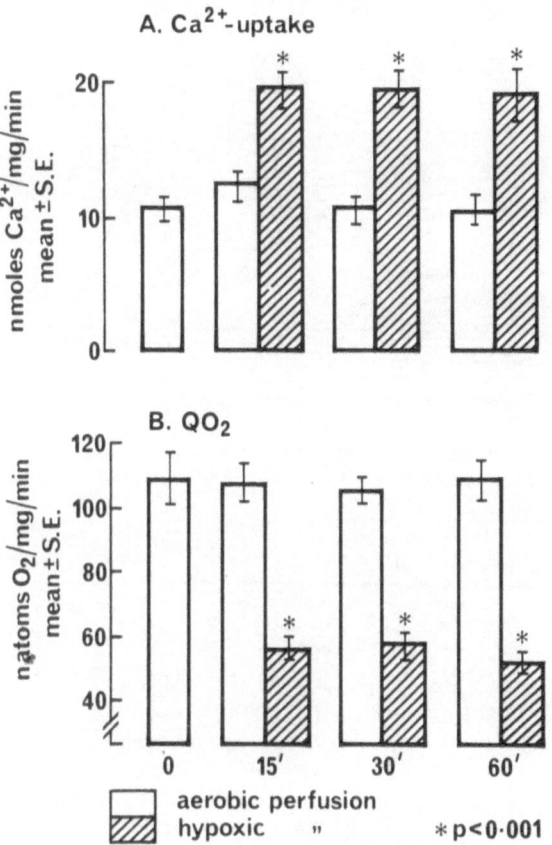

Figure 5 Effect of hypoxic perfusion on the ability of cardiac mitochondria to accumulate Ca^{2+} (A) and utilize O_2 (B). The isolated Langendorff perfused hearts were perfused either aerobically or under hypoxic conditions for the indicated times before the mitochondria were harvested. Aerobic conditions (pO_2 > 600 mmHg) obtained by gassing the perfusate buffer with 95% O_2 + 5% CO_2. Hypoxic conditions (pO_2 < 6 mmHg) were obtained by gassing the perfusate with 95% N_2 + 5% CO_2. Each result is mean ± SE of six separate experiments

The contractile proteins

Basically the contractile proteins can be divided into two major types[6]—the thick, enzymatically active myosin filaments and the relatively thin actin filaments. These two sets of filaments interdigitate, as shown in Figure 2, and schematically in Figure 6. When contraction occurs the myosin filaments remain at a fixed length, and the relatively thin actin filaments are displaced relative to the fixed-length myosin filaments. The Z bands, which define the

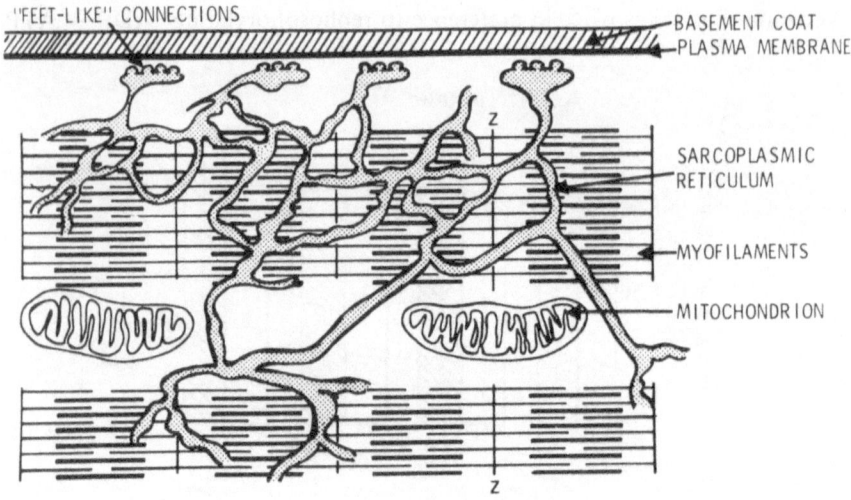

Figure 6 Schematic representation of the ultrastructure of a cardiac muscle cell, showing the interdigitating arrangement of the thin actin and thick myosin filaments

ACTIVATION OF CONTRACTION INVOLVES

1. INTRACELLULAR $Ca^{2+} > 10^{-7}$ M

2. REMOVAL OF INHIBITORY INFLUENCE OF THE TROPONIN - TROPOMYOSIN COMPLEX ON ACTIN - MYOSIN INTERACTION

3. ACTIN - INDUCED ACTIVATION OF MYOSIN ATPase

$$ATP \rightleftharpoons ADP + P_i + ENERGY$$

4. ACTIVATION OF CROSS BRIDGES BETWEEN ACTIN AND MYOSIN

5. DISPLACEMENT OF THE ACTIN RELATIVE TO THE MYOSIN FILAMENTS

6. CONTRACTION

Figure 7 Schematic representation of the events involved in excitation–contraction coupling in heart muscle

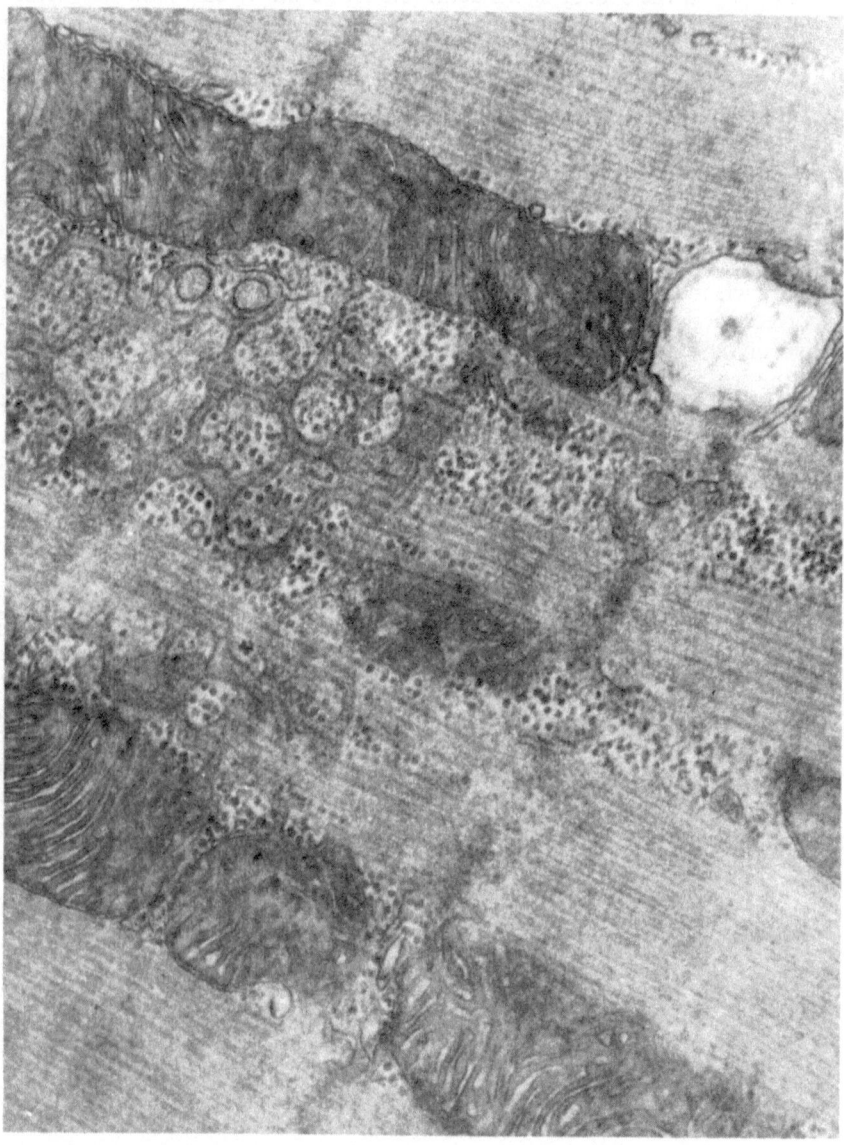

Figure 8 Longitudinal section of guinea pig cardiac muscle showing the lace-like appearance of the sarcoplasmic reticulum, mapping around the myofilaments ($\times$ 54 600)

fundamental unit of muscle—the sarcomere, being the distance between two adjacent Z bands, probably hold the whole system in register. It is generally believed that the sliding of the actin relative to the myosin filaments involves the cyclic making and breaking of cross-bridges between the thin actin and thick myosin filaments[6]. The energy required for this process is supplied, in the form of ATP, by the mitochondria. In addition to ATP, there is a requirement for Mg^{2+}, a co-factor for the ATPase enzyme, and Ca^{2+}, in excess of 10^{-7} M. This requirement[7] for Ca^{2+} can most easily be explained by remembering that another protein complex – the troponin–tropomyosin complex[8] – occurs at regular intervals, about every 380 Å, along the actin filament. When *not* occupied by Ca^{2+} the troponin–tropomyosin complex prevents the actin filaments from approaching the myosin. If actin does approach the myosin complex it can, provided that the ionic conditions are correct, activate a latent myosin ATPase enzyme, thereby facilitating the hydrolysis of sufficient ATP to provide the energy needed for the activation of the cross bridges, and hence for contraction. Hence when Ca^{2+} is available in the immediate vicinity of the myofilaments it associates with the troponin complex, and in so doing suppresses the inhibitory effect Ca^{2+}-free troponin exerts on the actin-induced activation of the myosin ATPase enzyme. For convenience this activation process has been summarized in Figure 7.

The sarcoplasmic reticulum

If the activation of contraction requires a raised cytosolic Ca^{2+} it is not surprising that the reverse process – the transition from systole to diastole – requires the removal of Ca^{2+} from the vicinity of the troponin complex. This retrieval of Ca^{2+} is achieved largely via the sarcoplasmic reticulum which, as Figures 6 and 8 show, is a fine membrane-like system of tubules[9,10] that wraps around the myofilaments and which has the capacity to accumulate Ca^{2+} against relatively large concentration gradients. This retrieval

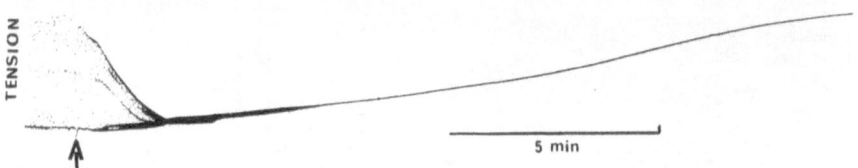

5 min

Figure 9 Mechanogram showing tension recorded from an isolated heart perfused initially under aerobic conditions. At the arrow hypoxic ($pO_2 < 6$ mmHg) conditions were introduced. Tension is recorded as an upwards deflection. Note that hypoxia causes a decline in peak developed tension and a raised resting tension

process is, however, energy-dependent and requires ATP. Hence we have ATP being required as the energy source for contraction, and ATP being required as the energy source for relaxation. The failure of the mitochondria to provide sufficient ATP to meet the requirements of cardiac muscle will, therefore, theoretically result in a decline in peak developed tension, and a raised resting tension. The mechanogram shown in Figure 9 shows that this is exactly what happens when heart muscle becomes hypoxic: developed tension declines, and resting tension increases.

The cell membrane

Each cardiac muscle cell is limited by a 75–90 Å thick plasma membrane[11], which provides the cell with its relatively permeable barrier[12]. The distribution of this membrane is complex mainly, as we have described elsewhere[10,11], because it invaginates to form a series of slender branching tubules (Figure 10) – T-tubules, which penetrate deep into the myofilaments, particularly in the vicinity of the Z bands.

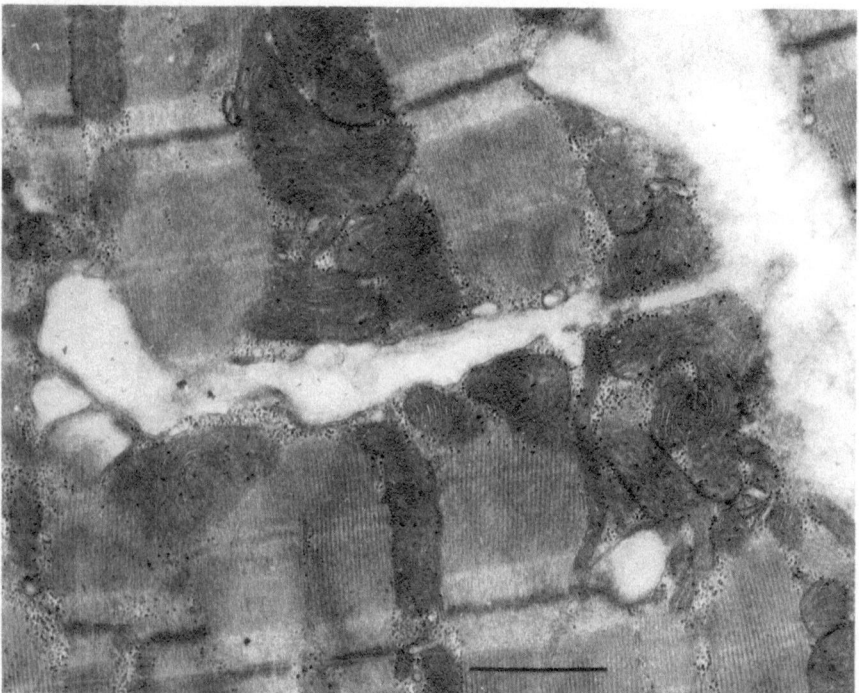

Figure 10 . Longitudinal section of heart muscle showing the T-tubule invagination of the cell membrane ($\times$ 18 300)

Maintenance of both the cell membrane and these T-tubular extensions requires energy, and if the supply of oxygen to the heart becomes limited then we consistently find damage to the membrane such that intracellular enzymes,[13,14] and sometimes intracellular organelles are free to diffuse into the extracellular space (Figure 11). The more prolonged the period of hypoxia, the greater is the extent of the membrane damage, until finally we find cells in which the membrane damage is so extensive (Figure 4) that even intact mitochondria enter the extracellular space.

Maintenance of the integrity of the cell membrane is, of course, vitally important. The cell membrane provides the semipermeable barrier that enables the intracellular ionic environment to be maintained correctly for the functioning of the various intracellular organelles, including the myofilaments; in addition the cell membrane allows for the rapid distribution of the excitatory stimulus[12].

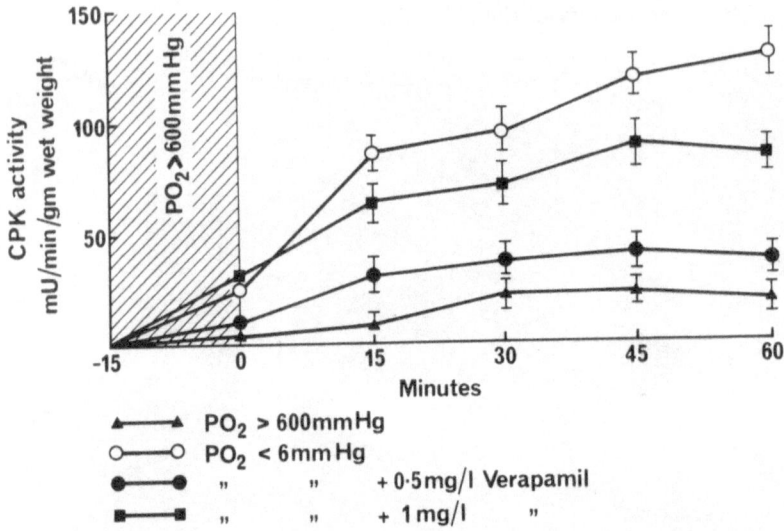

Figure 11 CPK activity detected in the coronary effluent of isolated rabbit hearts perfused either aerobically ($pO_2 > 600$ mmHg) or under hypoxic conditions ($pO_2 < 6$ mmHg) with and without verapamil. Note that verapamil protected the heart against the hypoxic-induced increase in CPK release

Excitation of the cell membrane involves a complex sequence of events resulting, we believe[10], in a raised myoplasmic concentration of Ca^{2+}, provided that the extracellular phase contains Ca^{2+}. During the action potential there is a small inwards displacement of Ca^{2+}, the magnitude of which is inadequate to account for the initiation of contraction unless an additional amount of Ca^{2+} can be released from the internal stores. Intracellularly stored Ca^{2+} is available for release from within the sarcoplasmic reticulum and recent studies[15] have shown that in cardiac muscle the signal for this secondary release of Ca^{2+} may be the Ca^{2+} that is displaced inwards during the plateau phase of the action potential. Because peak tension developed during contraction is a direct function of the rate at which the myosin ATPase enzyme hydrolyses ATP, and this in turn depends upon the amount of Ca^{2+} that is available to occupy the troponin sites (thereby repressing their inhibition of the actin-induced activation of the myosin

264

ATPase), it follows that there is a correlation between the amount of Ca^{2+} that enters the cell during the plateau phase of the action potential and peak tension developed during contraction.

If excitation–contraction coupling involves an inwards displacement of Ca^{2+} from the extracellular to the intracellular phase, this same amount of Ca^{2+} must be returned to the extracellular phase either during the transition from systole to diastole, or during diastole. Comparably little is known about the transport system that is responsible for 'pumping' Ca^{2+} out of the cell. A $Ca^{2+}:Na^+$ exchange system may be involved, or it may be an energy-dependent system involving the Ca^{2+}-activated ATPase enzyme in the cell membrane[16].

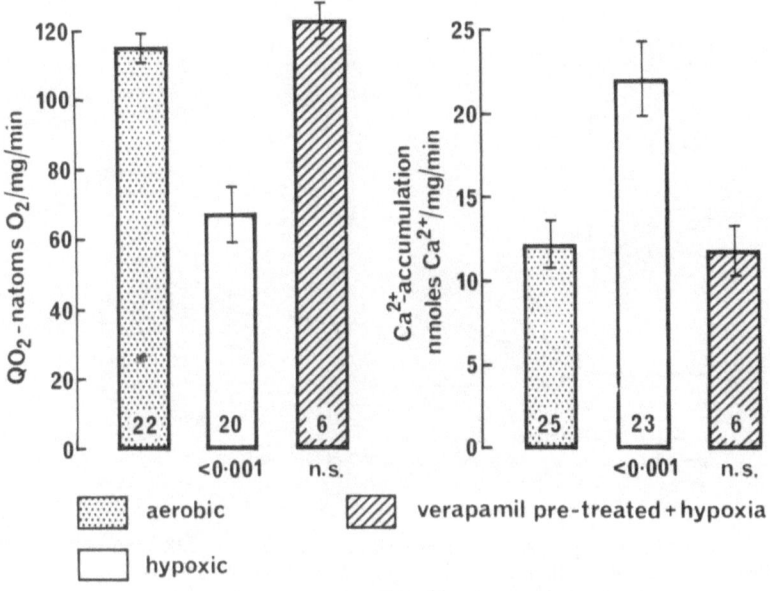

Figure 12 The rabbits were protected with placebo or verapamil for 5 days before the hearts were isolated and perfused under either aerobic or hypoxic conditions. The mitochondria were then harvested and assayed for QO_2 and Ca^{2+}-accumulating activity. Note that pretreatment of the rabbits with verapamil protected the hearts against the damage caused by hypoxic conditions. Results are mean ± SE of the indicated numbers of experiments

Because the return of Ca^{2+} to the extracellular phase is slow, relative to the speed at which Ca^{2+} is transported into the cell, a sudden increase in heart rate will result in a raised cytosolic Ca^{2+}, and hence an increase in force of contraction. If the amount of contraction that occurs is proportional to the number of calcium ions that enter the cells during excitation, then it is fairly obvious that we can modify the extracellular phase by loading it up with calcium or by taking it out and thereby altering the amount of contraction that occurs. Every surgeon who has used potassium citrate to induce cardiac arrest has unwittingly lowered the calcium concentration in the perfusate, because citrate is in fact a superb chelator for calcium. He thought he was using the potassium to arrest; he was in part, but also he was removing the calcium from the extracellular phase. This of course is one of the reasons why potassium citrate arrest caused damage to the myocardium, because we know calcium is required for the maintenance of membrane structure[17].

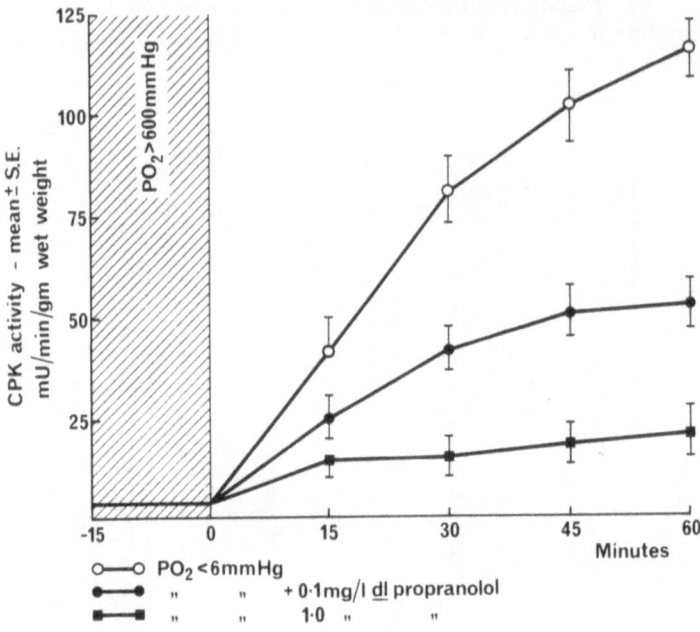

Figure 13 Effect of propranolol on the hypoxic-induced release of CPK from isolated rabbit hearts. Each point is the mean ± SE of six experiments. The drug was added directly to the perfusate, coincident with the introduction of the hypoxic conditions

Drugs can be used to modify contractile force. For example verapamil – a drug which acts at the cell membrane to impede the entry of calcium during the action potential – depresses left ventricular function[18]. This compound, probably because it does decrease cardiac work, has an O_2-sparing effect on the myocardium and therefore can protect the heart against the deleterious effects of hypoxia[9]. Evidence of this protection comes from ultrastructural studies[2], and from biochemical studies showing preservation of mitochondrial function[3] (Figure 12) and delayed CPK[2] release (Figure 13). Conversely drugs that increase cardiac work, – for example digoxin, cause an exacerbation of enzyme release. Evidence of this exacerbation of hypoxic-induced damage being caused by agents that increase cardiac work is provided by the data shown in Figure 14, where endiastolic resting tension was used as a monitor of the hypoxic-induced damage.

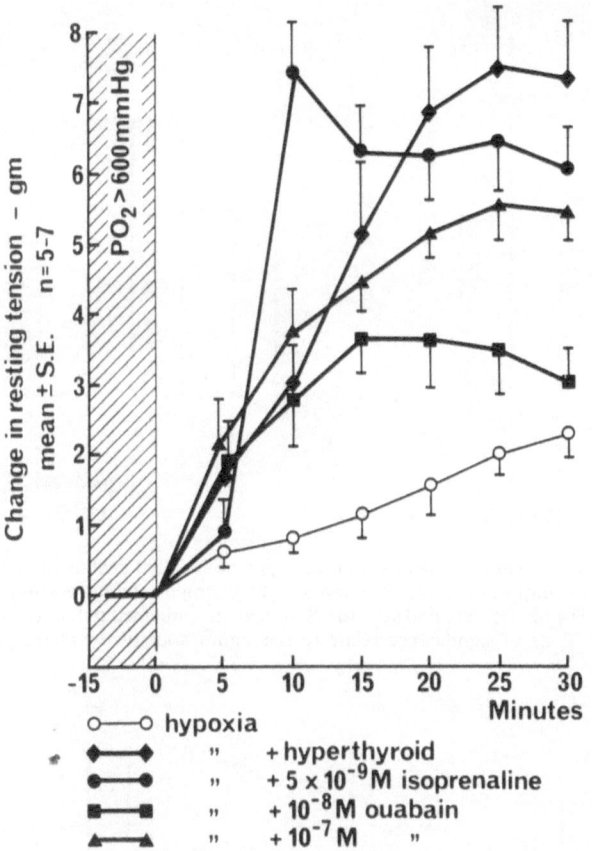

Figure 14 Effect of various positive inotropic agents on the hypoxic-induced increase in resting tension developed by isolated perfused hearts paced to beat at a regular rate

PROTECTIVE PROCEDURES

In conclusion, we can speculate now on the possible ways in which the myocardium can be protected if the availability of oxygen is limited. Certainly drugs such as verapamil, that decrease cardiac work, provide protection. Vasodilator agents that decrease resistance in the arterial system will also reduce the oxygen requirements of the heart and therefore, indirectly, protect the myocardium. Cardiac work can also be decreased by decreasing pH. Recent experiments in our own laboratories have shown that the introduction of a mild respiratory acidosis protects hypoxic heart muscle, evidence of this protection being obtained in terms of the maintenance of the cellular stores of ATP and CP (Figure 15), the maintenance of mitochondrial function assessed in terms of QO_2 and Ca^{2+}-accumulation (Figure 16) and a delayed release of intracellular enzymes (Figure 17). In these studies the perfusate pH was decreased from 7.4 to 6.9. A further decrease in pH, to 6.6, was

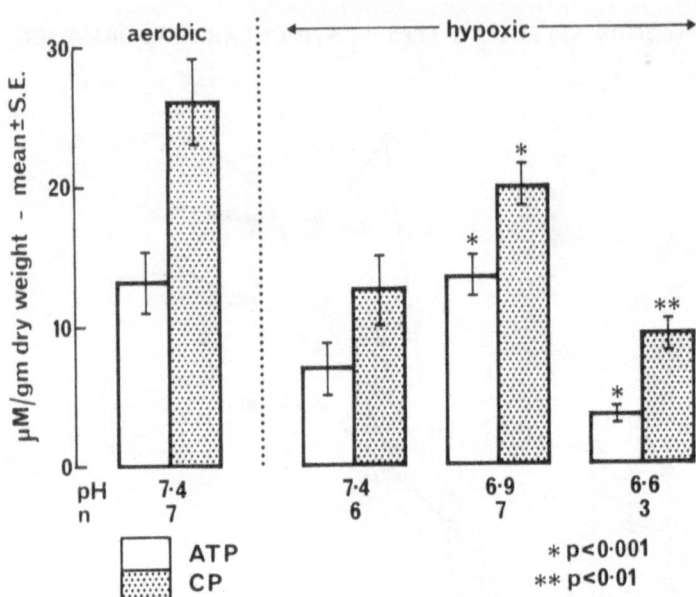

Figure 15 Effect of a respiratory acidosis on the hypoxic-induced decline in cardiac stores of ATP and CP. Respiratory acidosis was induced by changing the proportion of CO_2 in the gas mixtures. The hearts were perfused for 30 min at the indicated pH, and then assayed for ATP and CP. Tests of significance relate to the significance of the change caused by altering the pH

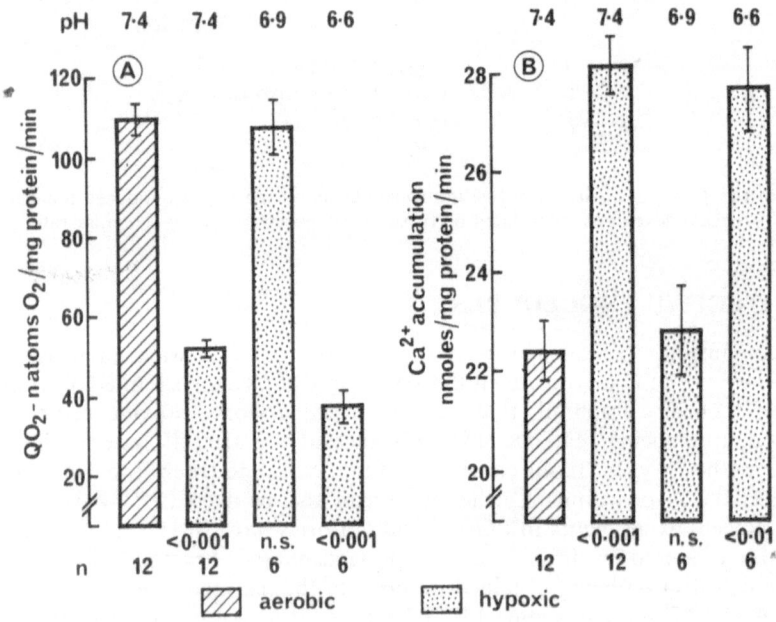

Figure 16 QO_2 and Ca^{2+}-accumulating activity of mitochondria isolated from hearts perfused under either aerobic conditions at pH 7.4, or under hypoxic conditions at pH 7.4, 6.9 and 6.6. Note that a pH of 6.9 protected the mitochondria of the hypoxic perfused hearts

detrimental. If a mild acidosis is to be considered for this purpose then one other factor must be considered – that is the pH sensitivity of the pacemaker tissue.

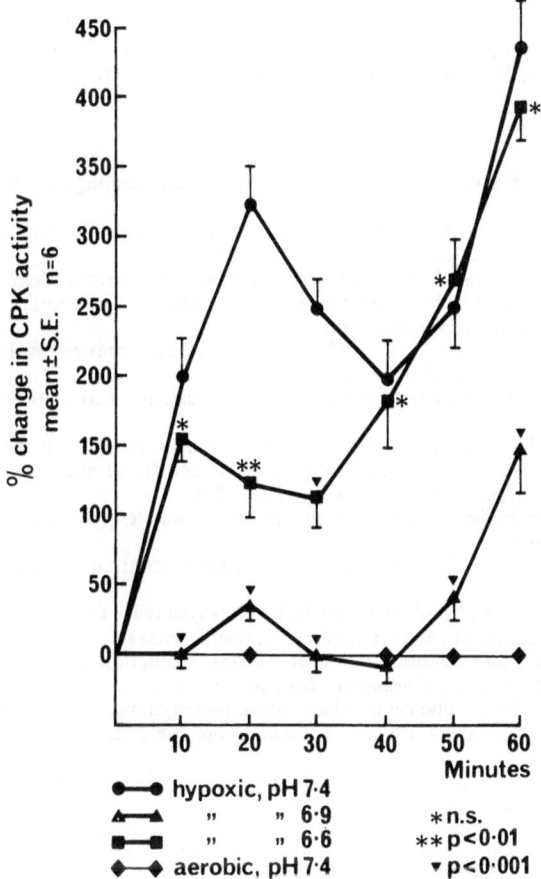

Figure 17   CPK released into the coronary effluent from rabbit hearts perfused aerobically, or under hypoxic conditions at pH 7.4, 6.9 and 6.6. The respiratory acidosis was induced by gassing the perfusate with the required CO_2/N_2 mixtures

B-adrenoceptor antagonists can, of course, provide protection[19] perhaps because of their membrane-stabilizing activity but more likely because of their ability to block the increase in cardiac work caused by the release[20] of endogenously stored catecholamines in response to an hypoxic insult.

CONCLUSION

An understanding of the ultrastructure of heart muscle, and of the requirement of heart muscle for energy in the form of ATP provides a possible basis for experiments aimed at elucidating which procedures can be used to protect the heart when it is deprived of O_2.

Acknowledgment

This work was supported by the Clinical Research Fund of the National Heart and Chest Hospitals and by the Medical Research Council.

References

1. Ganote, C. E., Seabra-Gomes, R., Nayler, W. G. and Jennings, R. B. (1975). *Am. J. Pathol.*, **80**, 419
2. Nayler, W. G., Grau, A. and Slade, A. M. (1976). A protective effect of verapamil on hypoxic heart muscle. *Cardiovasc. Res.*, **10**, 650
3. Nayler, W. G., Fassold, E. and Yepez, C. (In press). The pharmacological protection of mitochondrial function in hypoxic heart muscle: effect of verapamil, propranolol and methylprednisolone. *Cardiovasc. Res.*
4. Nayler, W. G. and Fassold, E. (1977). Hypoxic-induced changes in the ultrastructure of cardiac muscle. *J. Mol. Med.*, **2**, 299
5. Chance, B. (1965). The energy-linked reaction of calcium with mitochondria. *J. Biol. Chem.*, **240**, 2729
6. Katz, A. M. (1970). Contractile proteins of the heart. *Physiol. Rev.*, **50**, 63
7. Weber, A. (1959). On the role of calcium in the activity of adenosine 5-triphosphate hydrolysis by actomyosin. *J. Biol. Chem.*, **234**, 2764
8. Ebashi, S. and Endo, M. (1968). Calcium ion in muscle contraction. *Prog. Biophys Mol. Biol.*, **18**, 125
9. Peachey, L. D. (1965). Tranverse tubules in excitation–contraction coupling. *Fed. Proc.*, **24**, 1124
10. Nayler, W. G. (1975). The cardiac cell. In W. G. Nayler (ed.). *Contraction and Relaxation in the Myocardium.*, pp. 1–28. (London: Academic Press)
11. Nayler, W. G. and Seabra-Gomes, R. (1975). Excitation–contraction coupling in cardiac muscle. *Prog. in Cardiovasc. Dis.*, **14**, 75
12. Nayler, W. G. (1975). The cellular basis for anti-arrhythmic therapy. In D. M. Krikler and J. F. Goodwin (eds.). *Cardiac Arrythmias*, pp. 208–222. (London: W. B. Saunders Company)
13. Sobel, B. E. (1972). Serum enzyme determinations in the diagnosis and assessment of myocardial infarction. *Circulation*, **45**, 471
14. Hearse, D. J. and Humphrey, S. M. (1975). Enzyme release during myocardial anoxia: a study of metabolic protection. *J. Mol. Cell. Cardiol.*, **7**, 463
15. Dunnett, J. and Nayler, W. G. (1976). Dependence of calcium efflux rate from cardiac sarcoplasmic reticulum vesicles on external calcium concentrations. *J. Physiol.*, **266**, 79P
16. Nayler, W. G., Dunnett, J. and Sullivan, A. (1976). Drug-induced changes in the superficially-located stores of calcium in heart sarcolemma. *Recent Adv. Stud. Card. Struct. Metab.*, **9**, 53
17. Zimmerman, A. N. E. and Hülsmann, W. C. (1966). Paradoxical influence of calcium ions on the permeability of the cell membrane of the isolated rat heart. *Nature (Lond.)*, **211**, 646
18. Nayler, W. G. and Szeto, J. (1972). Effect of verapamil on contractility, oxygen utilization and calcium exchangeability in mammalian heart muscle. *Cardiovasc. Res.*, **6**, 120
19. Sakai, K. and Spieckermann, P. G. (1973). Effects of reserpine and propranolol on anoxia-induced enzyme release from the isolated perfused guinea-pig heart. *Naunyn Schmiedeberg's Arch. Pharmacol.*, **291**, 123
20. Shahab, L. and Wollenberger, A., (1967). Friesetzung von Noradrenaline aus dem isolierten durchströmten Herzen bei akuter Anoxia und nach Gabe von Stoffwechsel-giften. *Acta Biol. Med. Germ.*, **19**, 939

38

Elective cardiac arrest: historical perspective

D. G. MELROSE

I want first to set the scene. Consider a group of people practising in animals the management of an open heart operation. Remember the clumsy perfusion equipment, primitive anaesthesia, little or no measuring equipment, a host of mysteries gradually overcome, and then the first attempt at clinical application. Suddenly the rules established are completely without validity, drowned in a torrent of blood streaming into the opened heart from a patent ductus, a large bronchial anastomosis or an incompetent aortic valve above the septal defect. Clarence Dennis who perhaps did the first clinical case was overwhelmed in this way in 1951[1]. No animal practice had provided the abnormal conditions which justified the operation.

Thus the direction of work changed perceptibly. The establishment of a satisfactory whole-body perfusion obviously did not ensure a 'dry heart' or even adequate surgical vision. A quote from that time reads 'The ideal situation will be reached only when the surgeon is able to work on hearts from which all blood flow is excluded and which are quite flaccid'.

Added to this was the new danger of air trapped within the cardiac cavities after cardiotomy. So real was this that in 1953 Senning[2] suggested that it was safer to induce ventricular fibrillation with the risk entailed of failure to restore normal beating rather than allow the ventricle to beat, and Swan et al.[3] was filling the whole chest with Ringer solution before closing the incision into the heart.

Remember too the intense competition between the hypothermia school and those who preferred to imitate the natural circulation mechanically. Lewis and Taufic in 1953[4] and Swan and Zeavin in 1954[5] had reported several successful intracardiac operations under direct vision using only surface cooling at a time when Gibbon had reported only the first successful use of a heart/lung machine[6].

It may seem absurd in retrospect but to sit on the fence by suggesting a combination of the two might be helpful was regarded at that time as a sign of intellectual and moral weakness. Most surgeons agreed at the time with

Bigelow's statement that from the standpoint of clinical application, it was apparent at present to be combining the risks of two dangerous procedures[7].

However, we in London were more fortunate in that a concurrent programme of the two schools existed and thus we had little difficulty in bridging the gap. We had been alerted to a possible role of potassium and calcium changes in hypothermia, and I quote, 'But since the calcium/potassium ratio rises in hypothermia and it has been shown that the heart is excessively sensitive to other cations at low body temperatures it may be that changes considered inconsequential at normal body temperature become lethal at a low temperature'[8], it was natural to pursue the possibility of manipulating deliberately the ionic environment of the myocardium. Using hypothermia or whole body perfusion in dogs we set out to prove that ideal conditions could be achieved. We chose potassium citrate to exaggerate the effect described by Ringer in 1883 where potassium inhibited and calcium stimulated the heart. By the middle of 1955 we were fairly confident we had a safe and reliable method tested in many species. Publication of a short preliminary communication[9] set off a burst of activity in the USA and by 1957 most of the really active centres in the USA were using potassium citrate arrest. Effler and Kolff operated on their first patient on 17 February 1956[10], a 17-month-old child. I quote, 'The simplicity of the technique and the ideal exposure it afforded convinced us that if unforeseen complications or toxicity did not materialise, this adjunct to cardiac surgery would be a very important advance'. And in 1957, 'The Melrose technique has now been employed in 96 patients and the results have given us no cause to employ or to search for any other cardioplegic drugs'[11]. Kirklin too, 'In any surgical endeavour there is wisdom in an attempt to define the need for further investigation. I would like to talk about the need for this in induced cardiac asystole or whatever one wants to call this state. We agree with everything said about asytole as described and we do not feel in need of improvements for operations within the ventricle. We feel that one has safe operating conditions for about thirty minutes, and probably reasonably safe conditions for forty minutes'[12].

It was no wonder that with such heady enthusiasm from these considerable authorities that almost everyone followed suit. At that time in answer to the question 'why potassium citrate?', our colleague J. S. Baker, who was a pharmacologist at Charing Cross Hospital said, 'It is probable that, from the point of view of protection of the myocardium, there is no particular virtue in potassium citrate as an arresting agent compared with others such as potassium chloride. Nor may there be much advantage if the only criteria is a flaccid diastolic arrest with no escape beats: but when to these is added the question of ventricular fibrillation it is clear that potassium citrate has much to offer'. He goes on to show that much lower concentrations of potassium citrate as compared to potassium chloride are needed and that ventricular fibrillation is exceptional during the recovery phase rather than the rule as with potassium chloride. He also emphasized the roles of both the potassium ion and citrate moieties in potassium citrate. An interesting section refers to hearts arrested with potassium citrate at 25 °C and maintained without flow for 30 min. These recovered after reperfusion to 100% by his criteria rather than to the 80% of the 37 °C controls[13].

And what of our contemporaries at the time? Unknown to us, in 1954 Lam was also experimenting with methods of stilling the heart to improve access. He began by filling the left ventricle with potassium chloride but found the method unreliable and by the end of 1955 had concluded that acetylcholine injected into the root of the aorta in a dose of 10 mg/kg (b.w.) was preferable. He said then, 'Although apparently in arrest the heart beats when the ventricular wall is stimulated mechanically by forceps. However, there is usually no activity during suturing of the interventricular septal defects or procedures on the heart valves. We ignore sporadic beats'[14]. He went on to say that he removed the aortic clamp before beginning to close the cardiac incision because the sutures could be easily put in with the heart beating and that he thought that such beating helped get rid of air.

It is interesting that in 1957 when he reported to the National Institute of Health meeting in Chicago he told us his mortality for VSDs repairs was 32% in 23 cases. As he was an expert and quick surgeon it gives a measure of the conditions of that time. Many were very small infants and it must be allowed that his mortality was among the best in the country for children over the age of 3. Lillehei supported him at that meeting and decried potassium citrate[15]. He had tried it twice in cases of severe aortic incompetence. In both cases asystole followed a large injection of 2.5% potassium citrate but no restoration of beat could be achieved. He stressed the distention of the heart which followed removal of the aortic clamp and his belief that the heart should beat in these circumstances to prevent the slightly regurgitant valves allowing the ventricle to distend. He confirmed Lam's results and indicated that he was prepared to use his technique. However he commented that 'The slowly beating ischaemic heart may be utilizing more energy than the completely still heart'[15], and warned that only very short periods should be allowed and that it should only be used when the cardiac reserve was reasonably good.

In spite of his support acetylcholine soon vanished from the list of agents used but work began in animal laboratories on a large variety of alternatives. Muscle relaxants were enjoying an anaesthetic vogue and were tried, antihistaminics, local anaesthetics, miscellaneous compounds of all sorts, and of course a wide variety of ions alone or in combination. None so obviously outshone potassium citrate that this was replaced in clinical practice.

You may wonder why the obvious combination of potassium and cold were not used. Again you must remember the spirit of the times. Bypass time was kept to the absolute bare minimum; ventricular fibrillation was still feared. The two schools were still separate. Fred Cross actually did the vital experiment at this time but it was ignored[16]. He showed that a very cold heart withstood ischaemia much better than a warm one and then showed that initial arrest with potassium citrate followed by washout with oxygenated blood at 0 °C further reduced oxygen consumption. But he concluded that 'We did not feel it was necessarily much better in the potassium plus cold heart', even though he adds that on reperfusion the heart takes over more quickly. His work was ignored.

To a question at that time on how we fixed the clinical dose I replied, 'Starting from the knowledge that to stop a heart effectively a concentration of 1 mg/ml of perfusate was required an informed guess as to the dilution involved indicated that we should increase this concentration—about 15-fold to allow for dilution and to ensure an adequate level throughout the myocardium'. And it was this guess which laid the foundation of the rejection of potassium citrate as a safe substance in elective arrest. The concentration of the stock salt solution was set at 25%. This is a high concentration and one difficult to maintain in perfect solution, especially in a refrigerator at 4 °C. We failed to take account of this and as the technique spread it was inevitable that changes occurred in the preparation of the solution and in how the technique was used. Suddenly the bubble burst. Two papers were published which drew attention to serious problems.

In 1959 Helmsworth, Kaplan, Leland Clark and others published a paper in the Annals of Surgery[17]. In it they concluded that in the circumstances of their technique in dogs with total perfusion some mild myocardial damage could be found, but that subsequent to induced asystole a serious degree of myocardial necrosis could always be found regardless of how well the animal appeared postoperatively.

Their paper was followed by others, and particularly one from Glen Morrow and his associates at the National Institute of Health[18]. In June 1960 they reported on the detailed pathological examination of 30 hearts from patients failing to survive open heart surgery; 19 of these had had potassium citrate arrest. In 15 (75%) of this group a destructive type of necrosis was found which had not occurred in the 11 in whom potassium citrate had not been used. The lesions varied from the trivial to massive. They examined the aetiology and remarked on the difference between using potassium citrate from a bulk solution and from freshly prepared ampoules, concluding that fresh preparations were the more damaging. Their conclusions were that the advantages were far outweighed by the hazards and that they had abandoned the method. So did everyone else, quite properly.

Thus ends this part of the story.

Poignant is a comment in a recent paper by Tyers and others[19] asking why we had not stuck to the best concentration of approximately 40 mEq potassium citrate. The answer is in the conditions prevailing at that time and the fact we were overwhelmed with the flood of new problems. Certainly 10–50 mEq gave excellent results in controlled conditions. In practice we diluted 2 ml of 25% potassium citrate in 30 ml of blood, giving a concentration of over 200 mEq. We were so concerned with the need to achieve rapidly complete arrest in spite of anatomical difficulties such as aortic incompetence, very large hearts etc., that we recommended a dose that eventually brought the technique into disrepute.

It brought to an end as well very many promising lines of work. At that time a much more thorough analysis of the mode of action of cardioplegic agents was going on in many laboratories. Had the impetus continued for but another year I am sure the fruits of such research would have naturally been fitted into clinical practice. Now that a decent interval has supervened these fruits are happily being gathered.

References

1. Dennis, C., Spreng, D. S. Jr., Nelson, G. F., Karlson, K. E. *et al.* (1951). *Ann. Surg.*, **134**, 709
2. Senning, A. (1953). *Acta Chir. Scand.*, **105**, 376
3. Swan, H., Zeavin, I., Blount, S. G. Jr. and Virtue, R. N. (1953). *J. Am. Med. Assoc.*, **153**, 1081
4. Lewis, F. J. and Taufic, M. (1953). *Surgery*, **33**, 52
5. Swan, H. and Zeavin, I. (1954). *Ann. Surg.*, **139**, 385
6. Gibbon, J. H. Jr. (1954). *Minnesota Med.*, **37**, 171
7. Bigelow, W. G. and McDirnie, J. E. (1953). *Ann. Surg.*, **137**, 361
8. McMillan, I. K. R., Melrose, D. G., Churchill-Davidson, H. C. and Lynn, R. B. (1955). *Ann. Roy. Coll. Surg. Engl.*, **16**, 186
9. Melrose, D. G., Dreyer, B., Bentall, H. H. and Baker, J. B. E. (1955). *Lancet*, **ii**, 21
10. Effler, D. B., Groves, L. K., Sane, F. M. Jr. and Kolff, W. J. (1956). *Cleveland Clin. Q.*, **23**, 105
11. Effler, D. B. and Groves, L. K. (1957). *Extracorporeal Circulation*, p. 459. (Springfield, Ill.: Charles C. Thomas)
12. Kirklin, J. W. (1957). *Extracorporeal Circulation*, p. 492. (Springfield, Ill.: Charles C. Thomas
13. Baker, J. B. E., Bentall, H. H., Dreyer, B. and Melrose, D. G. (1957). *Lancet*, **ii**, 555
14. Lam, C. R., Geoghegan, R. and Lepore, A. (1955). *J. Thoracic. Surg.*, **30**, 620
15. Lillehei, C. W., Goff, V. L., Sellers, R. D., Hodges, P. C. and Varco, R. L. (1957). *Extracorporeal Circulation*, p. 466. (Springfield, Ill.: Charles C. Thomas)
16. Cross, F. S. (1957). *Extracorporeal Circulation*, p. 491. (Springfield, Ill.: Charles C. Thomas)
17. Helmsworth, J. A., Kaplan, S., Clark, L. C. Jr., McAdams, A. J., Matthews, E. C. and Edwards, F. K. (1959). Myocardial injury associated with asystole induced with potassium citrate. *Ann. Surg.*, **149**(2), 200
18. Waldhausen, J. A., Braunwald, N. S., Bloodwell, R. D., Cornell, W. P. and Morrow, A. G. (1960). *J. Thoracic Cardiovasc. Surg.*, **39**, 799
19. Tyler, G. F., Todd, G. J., Niebauer, I. M., Manley, N. J. and Waldhausen, J. A. (1975). *Surgery*, **78**(1), 45

39

The role of electrolyte and temperature changes in myocardial protection

D. J. HEARSE

INTRODUCTION

From a number of our recent biochemical and functional studies[1-3] my colleagues and I have concluded that the effective protection of the ischaemic myocardium during elective cardiac arrest can be resolved into two distinct components:

1. First, and of great importance is the rapid induction of complete diastolic arrest. Although immediately following the onset of myocardial ischaemia there is an abrupt reduction of contractile activity, this is not complete and considerable contraction occurs for several minutes and may recur periodically during ischaemia. The abolition of this contractile activity and hence the conservation of vital cellular energy supplies for cellular maintenance and subsequent recovery, can have a major protective effect.
2. The second component of effective protection is to attempt to combat one or more of the many deleterious cellular changes which occur as a result of ischaemia.

Taking practical surgical considerations into account I believe that these two important criteria for the protection of the ischaemic myocardium can best be achieved by combining a subtle manipulation of the composition of the extracellular fluid with the careful control of myocardial temperature. In order to illustrate, both individually and in combination, the striking protection that may be afforded by chemical cardioplegia and hypothermia I would like to review some of the recent findings from my laboratories.

METHODS

Experimental model

The isolated perfused working heart rat model, which has already been described in detail[4], is a left heart preparation in which oxygenated perfusion medium (at 37 °C) enters the cannulated left atrium at a pressure of 20 cmH$_2$O and is passed to the ventricle from which it is spontaneously ejected (electrical pacing was not used in this study) at a rate of 40–55 ml/min, via an aortic cannula, against a hydrostatic pressure of 100 cmH$_2$O. Coronary effluent can be sampled for biochemical analysis or pooled and recirculated with the aortic outflow.

Total cardiopulmonary bypass with maintained coronary perfusion may be simulated by clamping the left atrial cannula and introducing perfusion fluid at 37 °C into the aorta from a reservoir located 100 cm above the heart. This preparation, which is essentially that described by Langendorff[5], will continue to beat but does not perform any external work. Ischaemic cardiac arrest may be induced in this preparation by clamping the aortic cannula. Short periods of preischaemic *coronary infusion* (at 37 °C or any desired degree of hypothermia) of protective or cardioplegic solutions may be achieved using a reservoir (located 60 cm above the heart) attached to a side arm of the aortic cannula.

Experimental time course

Immediately after excision of the heart the aorta was connected to the aortic cannula and Langendorff perfusion initiated for a 5 min washout and equilibration period (Figure 1). During this 5 min period left atrial cannulation was completed and also control values for coronary flow in this

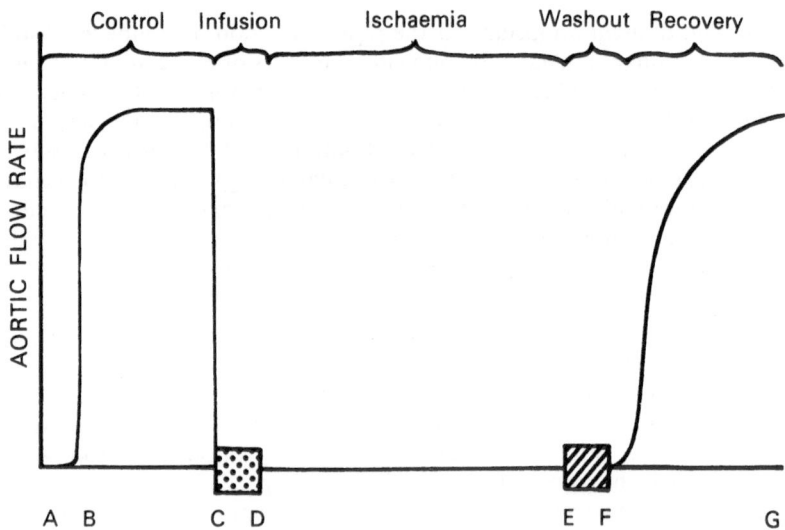

Figure 1 Experimental time-course. Hearts were perfused in the Langendorff mode between A and B (5 min), were converted to working preparations between B and C (15 min), were subjected to coronary infusion of various solutions between C and D (2 min) and were subjected to ischaemia between D and E (various times and temperatures). Hearts were reperfused at point E, initially as a Langendorff preparation (2 min) and were converted at point F to a working preparation

Langendorff preparation recorded. During this and subsequent perfusion periods the circulating fluid was Krebs–Hanseleit bicarbonate buffer[3,4,6], pH 7.4, containing 11.1 mmol/1 glucose and gassed with 95% oxygen and 5% carbon dioxide. The heart was then converted to a working preparation by terminating the retrograde aortic perfusion and initiating left atrial perfusion, and over a 15 min period control values for aortic and coronary flow rates, peak aortic pressure and heart rate were recorded. At the end of this control period the atrial and aortic cannulae were clamped and the heart was subjected to a 2 min period of coronary infusion with the protective solution under study. Infusion was then terminated and the entire heart was maintained in an ischaemic state for a fixed period of time. Although the hearts were perfused at 37 °C during the control and subsequent recovery period, the use of dual temperature circuits permitted the infusion of cardioplegic or protective solutions at 37 °C or at any desired degree of hypothermia. Similarly the hearts could be maintained at any desired temperature throughout the period of ischaemia.

After a suitable period of ischaemia the hearts were subjected to reperfusion at 37 °C. Initially reperfusion was in the Langendorff mode for 2 min during which time non-recirculating perfusion allowed washout and elimination of the residual cardioplegic infusate. Left atrial perfusion was then reinstated for a 20 min period and the recovery of various parameters of cardiac function recorded.

Solutions for coronary infusion

These solutions were all based upon the Krebs–Hanseleit bicarbonate buffer which was used as the basic perfusion fluid. Following various additions particular attention was paid to the correction of osmolarity (300 mosmol/kgH$_2$O); e.g., any increase in potassium ion concentration was matched by the appropriate reduction of sodium ion concentration, correction of pH (7.4), and in addition, precautions[7] were taken to prevent the precipitation of calcium in all media containing calcium and phosphate. All infusates were filtered through a cellulose acetate membrane (pore size 5μm) just before use and were gassed with 95% oxygen and 5% carbon dioxide prior to their introduction into the coronary circulation.

Expression of results

The absolute recovery values for various parameters of cardiac function in individual hearts were compared and expressed in terms of a percentage of those values obtained during the preischaemic control period. In addition to eliminating any inherent variability between individual hearts, this allowed the recovery of each parameter of function to be expressed as a percentage and to be related to the nature of the coronary infusate and to the duration and temperature of the period of ischaemic arrest. At least six hearts were used for each condition studied and all data were expressed as the mean ± standard error. Comparison between groups was by standard Student t-test.

RESULTS

Normothermic ischaemic arrest without coronary infusion

To provide a comparative baseline for the subsequent studies hearts ($n = 6$) were subjected to 30 min of ischaemic arrest at 37 °C without any prior coronary infusion. The results (Table 1) revealed extensive damage such that after 20 min of the recovery period aortic flow had recovered to only 3% $\pm$ 1.0% of its preischaemic value. A comparable impairment of other parameters of myocardial function was also observed.

Table 1 The effect of the composition of the preischaemic coronary infusate upon the final postischaemic recovery of aortic flow rate*

Infusate	Percentage recovery of aortic flow rate
None	3.0 ± 1.0
Buffer + 16 mmol/l KCl	29.9 ± 8.0
Buffer + 16 mmol/l K aspartate	28.1 ± 7.6
Buffer + 16 mmol/l K citrate	11.1 ± 5.4
Buffer + 16 mmol/l KCl + 16 mmol/l MgCl$_2$	68.1 ± 5.7
Buffer + 16 mmol/l KCl + 16 mmol/l Mg aspartate	73.6 ± 5.1
Buffer + 71 mmol/l acetylcholine	22.2 ± 10.2
Buffer + 7.4 mmol/l procaine	26.6 ± 10.4
Buffer + 16 mmol/l KCl + 16 mmol/l MgCl$_2$ + 11.1 mmol/l glucose	66.5 ± 8.1
Buffer + 16 mmol/l KCl + 16 mmol/l MgCl$_2$ + 11.1 mmol/l glucose + 0.01 iu/ml insulin	65.8 ± 3.1
Buffer + 16 mmol/l KCl + 16 mmol/l MgCl$_2$ + 10 mmol/l ATP	86.8 ± 0.9
Buffer + 16 mmol/l KCl + 16 mmol/l MgCl$_2$ + 10 mmol/l ATP + 10 mmol/l CP + 7.4 mmol/l procaine	93.6 ± 1.1

* All hearts were subjected to 30 min ischaemia at 37 °C

The efficacy of coronary infusion

Anionic and cationic effects

In an attempt to improve the functional recovery from normothermic ischaemia an attempt was made to modify the ionic composition of the extracellular fluid at the onset of ischaemia. Hearts were therefore subjected to a 2 min preischaemic period of coronary infusion with a variety of solutions containing elevated concentrations of one or more of the following: potassium chloride, potassium citrate, potassium aspartate and magnesium chloride.

The results, shown in Table 1, revealed that trapping infusate containing 16 mmol/l potassium chloride in the coronary tree caused a very rapid induction of cardiac arrest and improved postischaemic recovery such that hearts ($n = 6$) subjected to 30 min ischaemia recovered to 29.9 $\pm$ 8.0% of their control aortic flow rate. In additional experiments ($n = 6$ for each group) the 16 mmol/l potassium chloride was replaced by 16 mmol/l potassium aspartate or 16 mmol/l potassium citrate. The recoveries were 28.1 $\pm$ 7.6% and 11.1 $\pm$ 5.4% respectively. In a further series of experiments ($n = 6$ hearts for each group) hearts were subjected to preischaemic perfusion with solutions containing 16 mmol/l potassium chloride plus 16 mmol/l magnesium chloride or 16 mmol/l potassium chloride plus 16 mmol/l magnesium aspartate. The hearts were subjected to 30 min ischaemia and after 20 min of the recovery period the hearts had recovered to 68.1 $\pm$ 5.7% and 73.6 $\pm$ 5.1% of the control aortic flow rate.

These combined results for the recovery of aortic flow (but which were also representative for heart rate and peak aortic pressure) illustrate the marked protective action of both potassium and magnesium and show that their effects are additive. However, contrary to the suggestions of Bretschneider[8] and Kirsch[9,10] the inclusion of aspartate does not significantly improve protection and recovery. The inclusion of citrate, which may have a potential damaging effect through its ability to chelate calcium or inhibit anaerobic glycolysis, significantly reduced the protection afforded by potassium.

Electrical effects
High concentrations of procaine and acetylcholine have each been suggested as effective cardioplegic agents[10,11] and possibly also act as protective agents through their rapid induction of arrest and prevention of ischaemic beating. The ability of residual procaine to combat any rhythmic disturbance during recovery may add to its potential value. Hearts ($n = 6$ for each group) were therefore infused, prior to ischaemia, with perfusion fluid containing either 71 mmol/l acetylcholine or 7.4 mmol/l procaine. The recoveries for aortic flow were 22.2 $\pm$ 10.2% and 26.6 $\pm$ 10.4% respectively. Since in the absence of these compounds there was a very poor (3%) recovery, both procaine and acetylcholine must exert a protective effect.

Metabolic effects
The controversy over the alleged protective properties of glucose and possibly insulin in the oxygen-deficient heart has been well documented[12,13]. In general it appears that glucose can offer considerable protection to the anoxic or hypoxic[14-16] heart (where coronary flow is near normal, lactate accumulation, acidosis, and the inhibition of glycolysis may not occur) but is less able to offer protection to the ischaemic heart where coronary flow and toxic metabolite removal are severely impaired and anaerobic energy production is rapidly inhibited[17]. Studies were therefore carried out to determine whether glucose and insulin could afford any protection to the ischaemic myocardium. Hearts ($n = 6$ for each group) were subjected to preischaemic infusion with a solution in which the concentrations of potassium and magnesium had both been raised to 16 mmol/l and to which glucose

(11.1 mmol/l) and insulin (0.01 iu/ml) had been added. The results (Table 1) reveal that the inclusion of glucose reduced the recovery from 68.1% to 66.5 $\pm$ 8.1% and the inclusion of glucose and insulin led to a recovery of 65.8 $\pm$ 3.1%. Since the inclusion of glucose or glucose and insulin did not improve postischaemic recoveries these compounds were omitted from all future infusates.

Equally controversial as the protective properties of glucose and insulin are the alleged protective properties of extracellular high energy phosphates [18-20]. The potential protective effects of extracellular creatine phosphate and adenosine triphosphate were therefore investigated. Thus if adenosine triphosphate (10 mmol/l) was included in the buffer containing 16 mmol/l each of potassium and magnesium, the recovery of aortic flow was increased from 68.1 to 86.8 $\pm$ 0.9%, and if creatine phosphate (10 mmol/l) and procaine (7.4 mmol/l) were also included in the infusate, the recovery was further improved to 93.6 $\pm$ 1.1%.

Thus the additive protective effects of potassium, magnesium, adenosine triphosphate, creatine phosphate and procaine, permitted hearts, which would normally recover only 3% of their function after a period of normo-thermic arrest, to recover greater than 90% of their preischaemic functional capacity. Further studies revealed that if the hearts had been maintained at 28 °C instead of 37 °C for the duration of ischaemia the recovery could have been increased to 99.2 $\pm$ 0.6%. Investigations were therefore carried out to assess the degree of protection that may be afforded by hypothermia.

The efficacy of hypothermia

The protective effect of hypothermia and the relationship between protection and degree of hypothermia was investigated in a series of studies in which hearts were infused with the Krebs–Hanseleit solution containing potassium, magnesium, adenosine triphosphate, creatine phosphate and procaine, and

Table 2   The effect of the degree of hypothermia upon the final recovery of aortic flow rate following 60 min of ischaemic arrest*

Myocardial temperature during ischaemia	Percentage of postischaemic recovery of aortic flow rate
37 °C	3
33 °C	10
30 °C	58
28 °C	75
25 °C	84
20 °C	87
12 °C	95
4 °C	98

* Hearts were subjected to a 2 min period of coronary infusion immediately prior to the induction of cardiac arrest. The infusate was a Krebs–Hanseleit bicarbonate buffer in which the potassium and magnesium concentrations were each raised to 16 mmol/l and to which had been added 10 mmol/l each of adenosine triphosphate and creatine phosphate and 7.4 mmol/l procaine.

the hearts were then maintained at various degrees of hypothermia for a 60 min period of ischaemia. The results (Table 2) illustrate that as the myocardial temperature falls there is a progressive (but non-linear—see reference[3]) improvement in protection and postischaemic recovery.

DISCUSSION

The preceding results illustrate the striking protective properties of hypothermia and various chemical cardioplegic agents. These agents, through their ability to induce immediate diastolic arrest, reduce metabolic rate and degradative processes and prevent or delay the onset of various deleterious cellular changes, thus allowing a major extension in the period of ischaemic arrest that can be tolerated by the myocardium. While both hypothermia and chemical cardioplegia may exert a powerful protective effect in their own right the above and other results[3,21] would suggest that their effects are additive. While it could be argued that an extreme hypothermia of say 4 °C can confer sufficient tissue protection for the usual duration of ischaemic arrest it must be appreciated that in practical terms it is extremely difficult to *obtain* and *maintain* a rapid and uniform cooling of the myocardium to such a low temperature. This problem together with the possibility that severe hypothermia may induce some form of tissue damage, can be simply overcome and a comparable degree of protection achieved by combining moderate hypothermia with chemical cardioplegia.

Finally, in addition to avoiding extremes of temperature I would suggest that the composition of any coronary infusate should avoid extremes of concentration, osmolarity or pH. The problems resulting from unnecessarily high concentrations of potassium are well known, the dangers of infusing hearts with calcium-free media are emerging[22], and until we understand more fully the implications of cardioplegia and myocardial protection we should perhaps design our cardioplegic solutions to deviate as little as possible from the composition of normal extracellular fluid.

Acknowledgments

This work was supported in part by grants from the Wellcome Trust and the British Heart Foundation.

References

1. Hearse, D. J., Stewart, D. A. and Chain, E. B. (1974). Recovery from cardiac bypass and elective cardiac arrest: Metabolic consequences of various cardioplegic procedures in the isolated rat heart. *Circ. Res.*, **35**, 448
2. Hearse, D. J., Stewart, D. A. and Braimbridge, M. V. (1975). Hypothermic arrest and potassium arrest: Metabolic and myocardial protection during elective cardiac arrest. *Circ. Res.*, **36**, 481
3. Hearse, D. J., Stewart, D. A. and Braimbridge, M. V. (1976). Cellular protection during myocardial ischemia: the development and characterization of a procedure for the induction of reversible cardiac arrest. *Circulation* **54**, 193
4. Hearse, D. J., Stewart, D. A. and Braimbridge, M. V. (1977). Myocardial protection during bypass and arrest: a possible hazard with lactate-containing infusates. *J. Thoracic Cardiovasc. Surg.*, **72**, 880

5. Langendorff, O. (1895). Untersuchungen am aberlebenden Saugethierherzen *Pflueg Arch.*, **61**, 291

6. Krebs, H. A. and Hanseleit, K (1932). Untersuchungen uber die Harnstoffbildung im Tierkorper. *Hoppe Seyler's Z. Physiol. Chem.*, **210**, 33

7. Umbreit, W. W., Burris, R. H. and Stauffer, J. F. (1964). Preparation of Krebs–Ringer phosphate and bicarbonate solution. In *Manometric Techniques*, p. 132. (Minneapolis: Burgess)

8. Bretschneider, H. J. (1964). Uberlebenszeit und Wiederbelebungszeit des Herzens bei Normo- und Hypothermie. *Verh. Dtsch. Ges. Kreislaufforsch.*, **30**, 11

9. Kirsch, U., Rodewald, G. and Kalmar, P. (1972). Induced ischemic arrest. *J. Thoracic Cardiovasc. Surg.*, **63**, 121

10. Kirsch, U. (1970). Untersuchungen zum Eintritt der Totenstarre an ischaemischen Meerschweinchenherzen in Normothermie. Der Winfluss von Procaine, Kalium und Magnesium. *Arzheim, Forsch.*, **20**, 1071

11. Greenberg, J. J., Edmunds, L. H. and Brown, R. B. (1960). Myocardial metabolism and post-arrest function in the cold and chemically arrested heart. *Surgery*, **48**, 31

12. Opie, L. H. (1970). The glucose hypothesis: relation to acute myocardial ischemia. *J. Molec. Cell Cardiol.*, **1**, 107

13. Brachfeld, N. (1974). Ischemic myocardial metabolism and cell necrosis. *Bull. N.Y. Acad. Med.*, **50**, 261

14. Hearse, D. J. and Chain, E. B. (1972). The role of glucose in the survival and recovery of the anoxic isolated perfused rat heart. *Biochem. J.*, **128**, 1125

15. Hearse, D. J. and Humphrey, S. M. (1975). Enzyme release during myocardial anoxia: a study of metabolic protection. *J. Molec. Cell Cardiol.*, **7**, 463

16. Weissler, A. M., Kruger, G. A., Baba, N., Scarpelli, D. G., Leighton, R. D. and Gallimore, J. K. (1968). The role of anaerobic metabolism in the preservation of functional capacity and structure of anoxic myocardium. *J. Clin. Invest.*, **47**, 403

17. Rovetto, M. J., Whitmer, J. T. and Neely, J. R. (1973). Comparison of the effects of anoxia and whole heart ischemia on carbohydrate utilization in isolated rat hearts. *Circ. Res.*, **132**, 699

18. Wilkinson, J. H. and Robinson, J. M. (1974). Effects of energy-rich compounds on release of intracellular enzymes from human leukocytes and rat lymphocytes. *Clin. Chem.*, **20**, 1331

19. Parratt, J. R. and Marshall, R. J. The response of isolated cardiac muscle to acute anoxia: protective effect of adenosine triphosphate and creatine phosphate. *J. Pharm. Pharmac.*, **26**, 427

20. Fedelesova, M., Ziegelhoffer, A., Krause, E. G. and Wollenberger, A. (1969). Effect of exogenous adenosine triphosphate upon the metabolic state of the excised hypothermic dog heart. *Circ. Res.*, **24**, 617

21. Nelson, R. L., Goldstein, S. M., McConnell, D. H., Maloney, J. V. and Buckberg, G. (1976). Improved myocardial performance after aortic cross clamping by combining pharmacologic arrest with topical hypothermia. *Suppl. 3 to Circulation*, **54**, 11

40

Cold cardioplegia versus continuous coronary perfusion: clinical and cytochemical assessment

M. V. BRAIMBRIDGE, D. J. HEARSE, J. CHAYEN, L. BITENSKY AND S. ĆANKOVIĆ-DARRACOTT

INTRODUCTION

The best method of preserving myocardial integrity following aortic occlusion is still debatable 20 years after the beginning of open heart surgery. Occlusion of the aorta at normal temperatures[1] and the original potassium arrest cardioplegic method of Melrose et al.[2] have been abandoned because of unacceptable myocardial damage. Coronary artery perfusion with a beating heart has been the standard technique of myocardial preservation[3] but pericardial cooling[4], with or without the addition of a pump to circulate cold fluid faster[5], has recently become more widely adopted. 'Root cooling' of the heart[6], and the infusion of specially formulated cardioplegic solutions, such as those developed by Bretschneider[7] and Kirsch[8], have attracted much recent interest.

This study describes the results of a 4-year series of biopsies of the left ventricle in patients undergoing aortic and double valve replacements at St Thomas' Hospital. In the first group (1974–75), myocardial preservation was carried out with continuous coronary perfusion with a beating heart. In the second group (October 1975–77), the myocardium was preserved with cold cardioplegia with the St Thomas' Hospital Solution No. 1 (Table 1); 24 pairs of biopsies were obtained from each group and these were compared along with the clinical results from the entire population from which they were taken.

Assessment of the results was by clinical and cytochemical criteria. Assessment at cellular level of the effectiveness of myocardial preservation was made from full thickness left ventricular biopsies, taken at the beginning and end of bypass with an air-driven hollow needle[9]. These biopsies were graded cytochemically[10]. Biopsy was attempted in every aortic valve replacement but in

Table 1   Aortic valve replacement; St Thomas' Hospital techniques
of myocardial preservation

---

(1) Continuous coronary perfusion at 32 °C with a beating heart
    (a) Left coronary perfusion 70% of aortic clamp time
    (b) Right coronary perfusion 59% of aortic clamp time
(2) Cold cardioplegia
    (a) Coronary infusion with 1 litre 4 °C Ringer's solution with
                 16 mmol KCl
                 16 mmol $MgCl_2$
                 1 mmol procaine
    (b) Pericardial cooling, Hartmann's solution

---

some cases, for technical reasons, the biopsy was unsatisfactory or not obtained.

MATERIALS AND METHODS—CLINICAL SERIES

The series were primarily designed to compare biopsies taken from the left ventricles of patients undergoing aortic valve replacement at St Thomas' Hospital between 1974 and 1977 using two separate techniques of myocardial preservation—continuous coronary perfusion with a beating heart and cold cardioplegia (Table 1). An identical sequential number of biopsies (24) were compared from each group but they were taken from differing numbers of patients, as satisfactory pairs of biopsies taken both before and after bypass were not obtained for technical reasons from every patient operated on. The total population of patients operated on during the time the biopsies were being taken were compared clinically while the 24 pairs of biopsies were compared histochemically and biophysically.

Continuous coronary perfusion at 32 °C

Plastic coronary cannulae were fixed by purse-string sutures into each coronary artery; a Portex coronary cannula into the left coronary artery and a DeBakey into the right. The heart was kept beating with continuous perfusion of blood at 32 °C, except when the surgical procedure demanded a still field, at which time coronary perfusion was discontinued for periods not exceeding 4 min. Left coronary perfusion averaged 70% and right coronary perfusion 59% of the aortic occlusion time.

Of 60 patients in this group operated on between 1974 and October 1975, 47 underwent aortic valve replacement and 13 double (aortic and mitral) valve replacement.

Cold cardioplegic arrest

When the patient's temperature had been reduced on cardiopulmonary bypass to 30 °C, the aorta was occluded, the perfusion reduced from 2.4 to 1.5 l/m^2, and 1 litre of cardioplegic solution was infused into the coronary arteries over a period of 2–3 min.

The cardioplegic solution was the first solution developed from the experimental work of Hearse et al.[11], and is known locally as the St Thomas' Solution No. 1. This is distinguished from St Thomas' Solution No. 2 (reported by Jynge et al.[12]) by the absence of bicarbonate and phosphate and their associated buffering capacity. The root of the aorta below the aortic clamp was perfused for 2 min with 1 litre of Ringer's solution (4 °C), to which was added magnesium choride, potassium chloride and procaine hydrochloride (for composition see Table 2). All chemicals were ANALAR, obtained from the British Drug Houses, Parkstone, Poole, Dorset.

Infusion of the cardioplegic solution reduced the myocardial temperature to 8–16 °C as measured by a temperature probe inserted in the heart. The cardioplegic solution was usually infused by means of a cannula inserted through a purse-string suture into the root of the aorta, but in patients where aortic regurgitation was anything but slight, hand-held cannulae were inserted into each coronary artery orifice. The pericardium was then cooled with Hartmann's solution (4 °C) at a rate of 100 ml/min, the myocardial temperature being monitored throughout the period of cardiopulmonary bypass in order to maintain it below a maximum of 25 °C.

This group of 40 patients operated on between November 1975 and 1977 included 30 undergoing aortic valve replacement and ten undergoing double (aortic and mitral) valve replacements. Of the ten patients undergoing both aortic and mitral valve replacement, seven had a single infusion of the cardioplegic solution. In view of the cellular biochemical analyses obtained from these seven cases, it was decided to give a second infusion of the cardioplegic solution after insertion of the first valve. This was carried out in the remaining three patients.

BIOPSY TECHNIQUE

Full thickness needle biopsies (approximately 1.5 mm diameter) were obtained from the apex of the left ventricle by means of an air powered drill[9]. The biopsy was expelled onto a sterile swab in such a way that it was possible to identify the endomyocardial and epimyocardial zones. If the biopsy was of sufficient length it was bisected, and the two halves chilled separately in hexane which had been cooled to −70 °C. The tissue was processed on the day of sampling, sections being cut at 8 μm in a cryostat (cabinet temperature −30 °C).

QUANTITATIVE BIREFRINGENCE MEASUREMENTS

Quantitative birefringence measurements were made on freshly mounted sections by means of a Zeiss Universal Pol microscope to assess the response of the myosin to adenosine triphosphate (ATP)[10]. The section was first re-examined in air with the polarizer and analyser in the crossed position. The stage was rotated and the point of maximum brightness found by placing the stage midway between the two consecutive positions of extinction. A $\lambda/30$ Brace-Kohler rotating compensator was introduced between the specimens and the analyser and aligned with the polarizing system so that the

Table 2 Composition of cardioplegic solution

Composition of Ringer's solution		Additives		Final concentration	
Calcium chloride 2H$_2$O	0.33 g/l (2.25 mmol/l)	Magnesium chloride 6H$_2$O	3.25 g (15.99 mmol/l)	Calcium chloride 2H$_2$O	0.33 g/l (2.20 mmol/l)*
Potassium chloride	0.30 g/l (4.02 mmol/l)	Potassium chloride	1.19 g (15.96 mmol/l)	Potassium chloride	1.49 g/l (1.59 mmol/l)*
Sodium chloride	8.60 g/l (147.13 mmol/l)	Procaine hydrochloride	0.273 g (1 mmol/l)	Sodium chloride	8.60 g/l (144.25 mmol/l)*
Distilled water	1 l	Distilled water	20 ml	Magnesium chloride	3.25 g/l (15.68 mmol/l)*
				Procaine hydrochloride	0.273 g (0.98 mmol/l)*

* Concentration corrected for final volume of 1020 ml.

288

background was dark. Its reading was noted. The compensator was then rotated until the fibres under examination became dark; this reading was noted. The difference between the two readings was a measurement of the birefringence of the fibre. With the specimen unaltered in position, one drop of barbitone–sodium buffer (pH 9.4) containing 2 mM ATP and calcium chloride (0.036 M) was placed over the section and enclosed by a coverslip. An increase in birefringence invariably occurred, and a second series of readings was made. The values obtained were converted to absolute units of optical path difference (opd) by the equation $R_0 = R_c \sin 2\psi$ (R_0 = opd in the specimen measured in $m\mu$; R_c is a constant for the particular compensator used; ψ is the value measured by the process described). Since opd = birefringence × thickness, and the same area of the section was used for measuring the opd before and after the application of ATP, the subtraction of the first mean reading from the second gives a measure of the range of change in birefringence of the myofibrils.

Grading of biopsies

It has been found that the change in birefringence of experimentally produced ischaemic myocardium is consistently smaller than that of 'normal' myocardium[13]. Therefore a decrease in the range of change in birefringence of the myofibrils during bypass is an indication of declining function of the myocardium.

HISTOCHEMICAL TESTS

Histology of the tissue was demonstrated by haematoxylin and eosin staining, and serial sections were tested for the activity of succinate dehydrogenase, adenosine triphosphatase, cytochrome oxidase and monoamine oxidase by the methods of Chayen et al.[14,15] and Niles et al.[16]. The acid haematein stain was used as a test for the presence of freely available phospholipids[17]. Semi-quantitative gradings were ascribed to the activities manifested in each test[10,18] and the results were in parallel with the birefringence measurements.

CLINICAL RESULTS

Aortic valve replacement

The 24 pairs of biopsies in each group (48 in total) to be compared histochemically and biophysically were drawn from a population of 77 aortic valve replacements, 47 of whom were operated on using continuous coronary perfusion and 30 using cold cardioplegia to preserve the myocardium. The mean age was the same, but there were fewer females in the cardioplegic group (Table 3). Four of the first group had undergone previous surgery and two of the second (Table 4).

Aortic occlusion time was rather shorter (86 min compared with 100 min) in the cardioplegia group but the bypass time was almost identical, because of the longer recovery period necessary after electrolytic paralysis of the myocardium (Table 5).

Table 3   Aortic valve replacement 1974–77: age and sex distribution

	Total	Coronary perfusion 32 °C	Cardioplegia
Male	57	33	24
Female	20	14	6
	—	—	—
	77	47	30
Age		15–75	17–71
		(mean 52)	(mean 53)

Table 4   Aortic valve replacement 1974–77: previous operations (n = 77)

	Coronary perfusion 32 °C	Cardioplegia
Aortic valve replacement	3	2
Sinus of Valsalva aneurysm repair	1	0
	—	—
	4	2

Table 5   Aortic valve replacement 1974–77: bypass and aortic clamp time

	Coronary perfusion 32 °C	Cardioplegia
Bypass time (min)	80–270	83–245
	(mean 130)	(mean 123)
Aortic clamp time (min)	71–150	56–126
	(mean 100)	(mean 86)

Table 6   Aortic valve replacement 1974–77: hospital mortality (n = 77)

	Coronary perfusion 32°C	Cardioplegia
	(n = 47)	(n = 30)
Unperfused LAD coronary	1 (2%)	0
	(1.4%)	

There was one hospital death in the overall group of 77 patients (Table 6). This occurred in the coronary perfusion group and was due to an anterior myocardial infarct. A previous debridement of the calcified aortic valve had resulted, as is commonly the case, in the recurrent calcium spreading up the aortic wall and surrounding the left coronary artery orifice. No purse-string could be inserted to retain the coronary cannula and a balloon catheter was used. An unsuspected immediate division of the left coronary artery resulted in the left anterior descending coronary artery being unperfused throughout the procedure and the patient died.

Complications of coronary perfusion occurred in five (11%) of the patients in that group: the one death in the series, one dissected artery requiring saphenous vein bypass grafting, two lacerated coronary orifices which required careful suturing of the intima, and one patient whose dominant

Table 7 Aortic valve replacement 1974–77: complications of coronary perfusion ($n = 47$)

Death (unperfused LAD)	1
Dissected coronary artery (SVBG)	1
Lacerated coronary orifice	2
Poor perfusion right coronary artery	1
	5 (11%)

Table 8 Aortic valve replacement 1974–77: postoperative morbidity

	Coronary perfusion 32 °C ($n = 47$)	Cardioplegia ($n - 30$)
Supraventricular tachycardia	6 (13%)	first 12:6 (50%) last 18:2 (10%)
Cerebral confusion/visual defects	4 (8%)	2 (7%)
Haemorrhage	7 (15%)	0
Malaria	1 (2%)	0
Heart block	2 (4%)	1 (3%)

right coronary artery could not be adequately perfused (Table 7). This incidence of complications, due entirely to the myocardial preservation technique, prompted the change to cardioplegia.

Postoperative morbidity is shown in Table 8. Supraventricular tachycardia was particularly common in the first 12 patients in whom cardioplegia was used. It was then noted that the right atrium and appendage became dried out under the lights and a second catheter dripping cold Hartmann's solution was inserted into the right atrium, following which the incidence dropped to one-fifth. Significant postoperative haemorrhage did not occur in the cardio-plegic group, due perhaps to the fact that no pericardial blood was returned to the oxygenator.

Low cardiac output is discussed in relation to the biopsy results.

Double (aortic and mitral) valve replacement

The pairs of eight biopsies to be compared histochemically and biophysically were taken from a population of 23 double (aortic and mitral) valve replace-ments, 13 using continuous coronary perfusion and ten using cold cardio-plegia (Table 9). The mean ages of the two groups were identical but there was an increased predominance of females in the cardioplegic group. Almost half (six) of the 13 coronary perfusion group had had previous operations

Table 9 Aortic and mitral valve replacement 1974–77: age and sex distribution

	Total	Coronary perfusion 32 °C	Cardioplegia
Male	9	6	3
Female	14	7	7
Age	28–69 (mean 52)	28–64 (mean 52)	39–69 (mean 52)

compared with only a fifth (two) of the cardioplegic group. Three of the ten cardioplegic patients required tricuspid repair in addition to their aortic and mitral valve replacements, while only one did in the coronary perfusion group (Table 10).

Table 10   Aortic and mitral valve replacement 1974–77: additional procedures

	Coronary perfusion 32 °C	Cardioplegia
Tricuspid valvoplasty	1	3
Carpentier	0	2
De Vega	1	1
Subaortic resection	1	0

The aortic occlusion time in both groups was identical (Table 11), a little over 2 h in each instance. Bypass time also was almost the same.

Table 11   Aortic and mitral valve replacement 1974–77: bypass and aortic clamp time

	Coronary perfusion 32 °C	Cardioplegia
Bypass time (min)	145–198	136–178
	(mean 169)	(mean 156)
Aortic clamp time (min)	112–153	110–142
	(mean 129)	(mean 127)

There was one hospital death in each group, neither related to the myocardium (Table 12). One of the coronary perfusion group developed a cerebral embolus the day before she was to leave hospital and died 6 weeks later in another hospital. One of the cardioplegic group developed an acute and rapidly fatal *Klebsiella* pneumonia when on the point of being transferred to the ward from the intensive therapy unit.

Table 12   Aortic and mitral valve replacement 1974–77: hospital mortality

	Coronary perfusion 32 °C	Cardioplegia
Cerebral embolus	1	0
Klebsiella pneumonia	0	1
	—	—
	1 (8%)	1 (10%)

BIOPHYSICAL RESULTS

Aortic valve replacement

Of the 24 patients undergoing aortic valve replacement using continuous coronary perfusion at 32 °C who were biopsied, seven (29%) showed a decrease in birefringence values during bypass (Figure 1). Of these seven patients, two required significant amounts of inotropic support during the

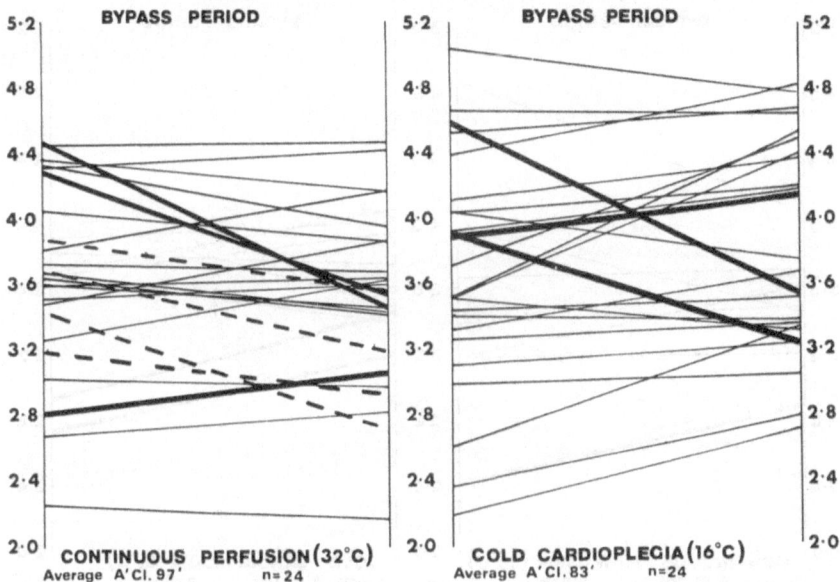

Figure 1 Changes in birefringence of the myocardium of patients undergoing aortic valve replacement (1). Values on the left vertical axis in each of the two groups refer to the birefringence range of myocardial fibres in left ventricular biopsies obtained from patients at the beginning of bypass. Birefringence values obtained from the same patient at the end of bypass are recorded on the right hand vertical axis. ———Light horizontal lines indicate patients who required no inotropic support postoperatively. ———Dark horizontal lines indicate patients who required inotropic support postoperatively. – – – Broken horizontal lines indicate patients who required inotropic support before bypass could be discontinued, but not in the postoperative period

postoperative period; four required support before bypass could be discontinued but did not require postoperative support; 17 (71%) patients showed no decrease in birefringence values during bypass and only one required significant inotropic support postoperatively (this patient had been in low cardiac output prior to bypass). No patient died in this group of patients biopsied (one of the unbiopsied patients died of complications of coronary perfusion).

Of the 24 patients undergoing aortic valve replacement using cold cardioplegic arrest who were biopsied, four (17%) showed a decrease in birefringence value during bypass (Figure 1) and two of these patients required significant amounts of inotropic support in the postoperative period. Of the 20 (83%) patients who showed no deterioration during bypass, only one required significant inotropic support postoperatively (this patient was also in low cardiac output prior to bypass). No patient died.

Aortic and mitral valve replacement

Of the eight patients undergoing aortic and mitral valve replacement with continuous coronary perfusion, two (25%) showed deterioration during

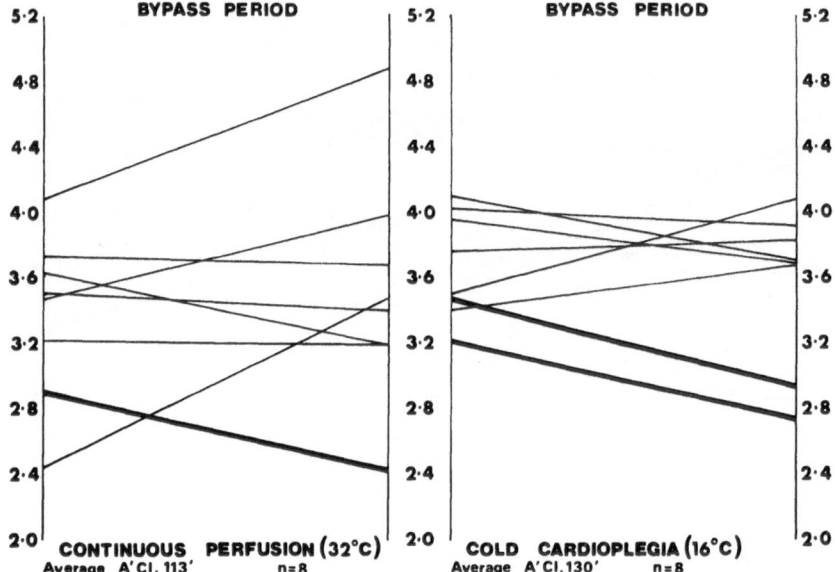

Figure 2 Changes in birefringence of the myocardium of patients undergoing aortic and mitral valve replacement (2). Values on the left vertical axis in each of the two groups refer to the birefringence range of myocardial fibres in left ventricular biopsies obtained from patients at the beginning of bypass. Birefringence values obtained from the same patient at the end of bypass are recorded on the right-hand vertical axis.————Light horizontal lines indicate patients who required no inotropic support postoperatively. ————Dark horizontal lines indicate patients who required inotropic support postoperatively

bypass (Figure 2), and one of these patients required significant inotropic support postoperatively. None died in the group of patients biopsied (one of the unbiopsied patients died of postoperative cerebral embolism).

Of the eight patients undergoing aortic and mitral valve replacement using cold cardioplegia who were biopsied, three (38%) showed deterioration during bypass, and two of these required significant inotropic support postoperatively. It was following these data that the second cardioplegic infusion was made after 1 h. No patient died in the group of patients biopsied (one of the unbiopsied patients died of *Klebsiella* pneumonia).

COMPARISON OF EPIMYOCARDIUM AND ENDOMYOCARDIUM

In 17 of the patients undergoing aortic valve replacement who were maintained by continuous coronary perfusion at 32 °C, the biopsy was sufficiently long to allow subdivision and comparison of endomyocardial and epimyocardial preservation (Figure 3). In 35% of the patients there was no deterioration in either half of the biopsy. In 53% the endomyocardial half of the full thickness biopsy deteriorated during bypass whilst the epimyocardium remained well preserved. In 12% the epimyocardial half deteriorated and the endomyocardial half was well preserved. Significant inotropic support was

294

required by one of the patients who had shown endomyocardial deterioration only.

Comparison of the endomyocardial and epimyocardial preservation was also made in 20 of the patients undergoing aortic valve replacement who were subjected to cold cardioplegic arrest (Figure 3). In 65% there was no de-

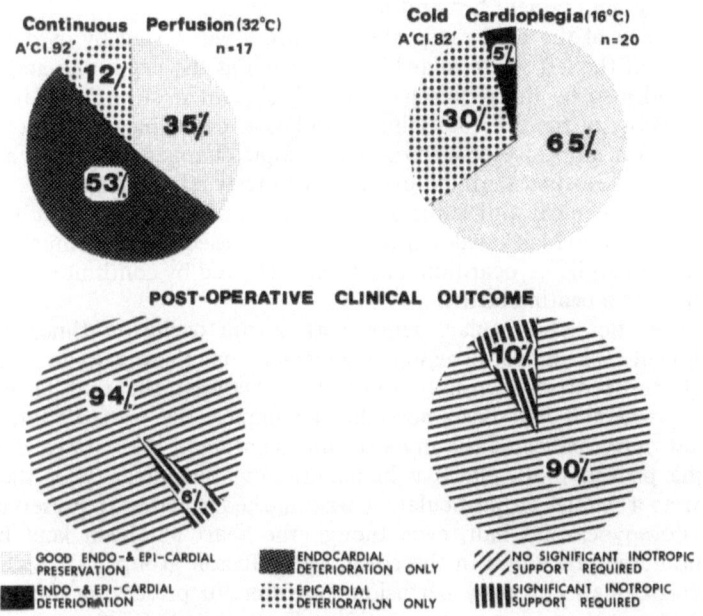

Figure 3 Cytochemical assessment of endocardial and epicardial preservation during aortic valve replacement (for explanation, see text)

terioration in either half of the biopsy. In 5% both halves of the biopsy showed deterioration. None showed solely endomyocardial deterioration, 30% showed epimyocardial deterioration with the endomyocardium well preserved. Two patients required substantial inotropic support postoperatively, one had shown epimyocardial deterioration only, and the other showed deterioration in both endomyocardial and epimyocardial halves of the biopsy.

DISCUSSION

The development of an effective protective cardioplegic solution which, if infused into the coronary circulation immediately prior to ischaemia would minimize the depletion of myocardial energy reserves, has been greatly stimulated by the work of Kirsch and Bretschneider in Germany[7,8,19–22].

The cold cardioplegic procedure adopted clinically at St Thomas' Hospital is based on experimental work by Hearse et al. in the isolated rat heart[11]. The first solution developed and described in this study (St Thomas' Solution

No. 1) consisted of 1 litre of a cold physiological medium with raised concentrations of potassium and magnesium to which had been added a small amount of procaine. It was not buffered. This solution differed from that of Kirsch in the larger volume and lower temperature used, and from that of both Kirsch and Bretschneider in that normal concentrations of sodium and calcium were maintained[23,24] and mannitol omitted.

The efficacy of the cold cardioplegic solution was tested by cytochemical assessment of the left ventricular biopsies taken at the beginning and end of bypass, and also by the requirement for significant postoperative inotropic support. Many of the previous clinical studies of cardioplegic solutions have been based on mortality or electronmicroscopic changes, both of which are markedly less sensitive than the cytochemical tests reported here.

Using cytochemical and clinical tests, groups of aortic and double valve replacements in which cold cardioplegia was used were compared with groups in which the myocardium had been preserved by continuous coronary perfusion with a beating heart.

In the aortic valve replacements, with aortic occlusion times of $1\frac{1}{2}$h, cytochemical and clinical assessment indicated that there was no difference in effectiveness of myocardial preservation between the two techniques. However, where it had been possible to compare the preservation of the inner and outer halves of the myocardium separately, the cold cardioplegic technique proved more effective in maintaining the integrity of the myocardium as a whole. In particular, it was markedly better at preserving the inner, endomyocardial half, even though the heart has been kept beating throughout the procedure in the coronary perfusion group[25]. It was rather less effective than coronary perfusion, however, in preserving the epimyocardial zone, perhaps due to the warming effect of the lights[26].

When the average aortic occlusion time was prolonged to more than 2 h in the double valve replacement groups, continuous coronary perfusion proved more effective than a single infusion of the cold cardioplegic solution. Adding a second infusion after 1 h, however, produced good preservation both cytochemically and clinically.

There was no mortality in the cardioplegic group of aortic valve replacement but one patient died in the double valve group. This compares favourably with the results from Kirsch's group (17%)[8] in which the aorta was occluded for 1 h, and those of Sondergaard's[27] group (6%) using the Bretschneider technique with the aorta occluded for $1\frac{1}{2}$h.

The advantage of cold cardioplegia to the surgeon is the markedly improved operative field when compared with coronary perfusion. The uninterrupted procedure in a still, relaxed, bloodless field should result in a reduced incidence of valve dehiscence and there is necessarily a total absence of complications of coronary perfusion itself.

Cytochemical assessment of myocardial preservation during aortic occlusion was of advantage to the surgeon over and above its research usefulness. The consistency with which deterioration of the myocardium during cardiopulmonary bypass was followed by the necessity for inotropic support enabled prediction of the type of postoperative course to be almost invariably made. The report on the myocardial biopsies was available to the surgeon on the evening of operation, which allowed modification of the ventilatory and other supportive management.

SUMMARY

Myocardial preservation by continuous coronary perfusion has been compared with cold cardioplegia. The 1 litre of St Thomas' cardioplegic protective solution' used for infusion into the coronary arteries was at 4 °C and had a normal electrolyte content except for raised concentrations of magnesium and potassium and the addition of procaine. Myocardial preservation was assessed by cytochemical grading of myocardial biopsies and also by the requirement for significant inotropic support postoperatively.

In aortic valve replacements with an aortic occlusion time of $1\frac{1}{2}$ h, both techniques afforded a similar degree of preservation, except that the inner half of the myocardium was markedly better preserved by cold cardioplegia. After 2 h in double valve replacements, a single cardioplegic infusion was not as effective as continuous coronary perfusion, but this could be corrected by a second infusion of the cardioplegic solution after 1 h.

Acknowledgments

This work was supported by a British Heart Foundation Grant and St Thomas' Hospital Endowment Fund. We would like to thank Miss Ann Hallinan of the Pharmacy Department for her technical assistance and advice, and also Mrs Christine Boles for her expert secretarial assistance.

References

1. Bloodwell, R. D., Kidd, J. N., Hallman, G. L., Burdette, W. J., McMurtrey, M. J. and Cooley, D. A. (1969). Cardiac valve replacement without coronary perfusion: Clinical and laboratory observations. In *Prosthetic Heart Valves*, p. 397. (Springfield, Ill.: Charles C. Thomas)
2. Melrose, D. G., Dreyer, B., Bentall, H. H. and Baker, J. B. (1955). Elective cardiac arrest. *Lancet*, **ii**, 21
3. Buckberg, G. D. and Hottenrott, C. E. (1975). Ventricular fibrillation. Its effect on myocardial flow distribution and performance. *Ann. Thoracic Surg.*, **20**, 76
4. Shumway, N. E., Lerver, R. R. and Stofer, R. C. (1959). Selective hypothermia of the heart in anoxic cardiac arrest. *Surg. Gynecol. Obstet.*, **109**, 750
5. Wheeldon, D. R., Bethune, D. W., Gill, R. D. and English, T. A. H. (1976). A simple cooling circuit for topical cardiac hypothermia. *Thorax*, **31**, 565
6. Sapsford, R. N., Blackstone, E. H., Kirklin, J., Karp, R. B., Kouchoukos, N. T., Pacifico, A. D., Roe, C. E. and Bradley, E. L. (1974). Coronary perfusion versus cold ischemic arrest during aortic valve replacement. *Circulation*, **49**, 1190
7. Bretschneider, H. J., Hubner, G., Knoll, D., Lohr, B., Nordbeck, H. and Spieckermann, P. G. (1975). Myocardial resistance and tolerance to ischaemia: Physiological and biochemical basis. *J. Cardiovasc. Surg.*, **16**, 241
8. Kirsch, U., Rodewald, G. and Kalmar, P. (1972). Induced ischemic arrest. Clinical experience with cardioplegia in open-heart surgery. *J. Thoracic Cardiovasc. Surg.*, **63**, 121
9. Braimbridge, M. V. and Niles, N. R. (1964). Left ventricular drill biopsy. *J. Thoracic Cardiovasc. Surg.*, **47**, 685
10. Čanković-Darracott, S., Braimbridge, M. V., Williams, B. T., Bitensky, L. and Chayen,

J. (1977). Myocardial preservation during aortic valve surgery. Assessment of five techniques by cellular chemical and biophysical methods. *J. Thoracic Cardiovasc. Surg.*, **73**, 699

11. Hearse, D. J., Stewart, D. A. and Braimbridge, M. V. (1976). Cellular protection during myocardial ischemia. The development and characterization of a procedure for the induction of reversible ischemic arrest. *Circulation*, **54**, 193

12. Jynge, P., Hearse, D. J. and Braimbridge, M. V. (1977). Myocardial protection during ischemic cardiac arrest: a possible hazard with calcium-free infusates. *J. Thoracic Cardiovasc. Surg.* **73**, 848

13. Chayen, J., Bitensky, L., Čanković-Darracott, S., and Braimbridge, M. V. (1978). Changes in birefringence induced by ATP acting on cardiac muscle. (In press)

14. Chayen, J., Altmann, P., Bitensky, L., Braimbridge, M. V., Kadas, T. and Wells, P. J. (1966). A study of the changes in hydrogen transport in an isolated rat heart preparation. *J. R. Micros. Soc.*, **86**, 151

15. Chayen, J., Bitensky, L., Butcher, R. and Poulter, L. (1969). *A Guide to Practical Histochemistry*, p. 88. (Edinburgh: Oliver and Boyd)

16. Niles, N. R., Chayen, J., Cunningham, G. J. and Bitensky, L. (1964). The histological demonstration of adenosine triphosphatase activity in myocardium. *J. Histochem. Cytochem.*, **12**, 740

17. Chayen, J. (1968). The histochemistry of phospholipids and its significance in the interpretation of the structure of cells. In S. M. McGee-Russell and K. F. A. Ross (eds.). *Cell Structure and its Interpretation*, p. 149 (London: Edward Arnold)

18. Braimbridge, M. V., Darracott, S., Clement, A. J., Bitensky, L. and Chayen, J. (1973). Myocardial deterioration during aortic valve replacement assessed by cellular biological tests. *J. Thoracic Cardiovasc. Surg.*, **66**, 241

19. Jennings, R. B., Sommers, H. M., Herdson, P. B., and Kaltenbach, J. P. (1969). Ischemic injury of the myocardium. *Ann. N.Y. Acad. Sci.*, **156**, 61

20. Hoelschen, B. (1965). Studies by electron microscopy on the effects of magnesium chloride–procaine amide or potassium citrate on the myocardium in induced cardiac arrest. *J. Cardiovasc. Surg.*, **12**, 163

21. Todd, G. J. and Tyers, F. O. (1975). Amelioration of the effects of ischaemic cardiac arrest by the intracoronary administration of cardioplegic solutions. *Circulation*, **52**, 111

22. Gay, W. A. Jr. (1975). Potassium-induced cardioplegia. *Ann. Thoracic Surg.*, **20**, 95

23. Zimmermann, A. N. E., Daems, W., Hülsmann, W. C., Snijder, J., Wisse, E. and Durrer, D. (1967). Morphological changes of heart muscle caused by successive perfusion with calcium-free and calcium-containing solutions (calcium paradox). *Cardiovasc. Res.*, **1**, 201

24. Ruigrok, T. J. C., Burgersdijk, J. A. and Zimmermann, A. N. E. (1975). The calcium paradox: a reaffirmation. *Eur. J. Cardiol.*, **3/1**, 59

25. Buckberg, G. (1972). Subendocardial ischemia after cardiopulmonary bypass. *J. Thoracic Cardiovasc. Surg.*, **64**, 669

26. Schaper, W., Schaper, J., Palmowski, J., Thiedemann, U. and Hehrlein, F. (1975). Ischemia-tolerance following cardioplegic arrest in human patients and in experimental animals. *J. Cardiovasc. Surg.*, **16**, 268

27. Søndergaard, T., Berg, E., Staffeldt, I. and Szczepanski, K. (1975). Cardioplegic arrest in aortic surgery. *J. Cardiovasc. Surg.*, **16**, 288

41

Low sodium-induced arrest in patients

I. H. RYGG AND G. PETERSEN

In 1964 Bretschneider[1] published his experiences with a cardioplegia solution which did not contain any sodium or calcium. It had, however, a local anaesthetic drug, novocaine, in a concentration of 0.3%, and a potassium content near normal for extracellular fluids. It was made more or less iso-tonic by means of mannitol and had a glucose content near the physiological range. Table 1 shows the composition of the solution used in our clinic.

Table 1   Bretschneider's solution (1000 ml)

Procaine hydrochloride	11.00 mmol	=	3.0 g
Potassium chloride	5.37 mmol	=	0.4 g
Glucose	5.05 mmol	=	1.0 g
Mannitol	274.50 mmol	=	50.0 g
Sterilized water – ad 1000 ml			
Chloride content	16.40 mmol		
pH 4.3			
Filtration through 0.45 μm filter			
Heat treated 120 °C – 20 min			

Because of the extracellular sodium depletion the action potential over the cell membrane cannot be created, and consequently the membrane will remain in its polarized resting condition. Calcium depletion has the effect of stopping the contractions, and procaine or novocaine is said to stabilize the membrane further by inhibition of sodium permeability and enzymatic activities of the ATPases.

Bretschneider ascribes the effect of his solution to a stabilization of the myocardial cells in a polarized diastolic condition, which is the least energy-requiring situation of the myocardial functional cycle. He proved this solution to be superior to any other known method of cardiac preservation during ischaemia and that easily reversed ischaemic periods of 2 h duration could be obtained at a myocardial temperature of 15 °C.

This method was soon taken into clinical use, and the first publication about clinical series came from Søndergaard and Senn[2] and from Reidemeister and his group[3].

Søndergaard and his group in Århus has used this method ever since then. He has until recently, however, used a precooling of the heart by perfusion with a cold mixture of arterial blood and saline followed by infusion of 500 ml Bretschneider's solution. All the fluid was sucked up from the right side of the heart.

Reidemeister has perfused with a pump at the rate of 700 ml/min of Bretschneider's solution for 5 min into the aortic root with aspiration of the resulting 3–4 l of fluid from the right side of the heart.

Rodewald and his group in Hamburg also use pumps for perfusion of the coronary arteries. He uses a mixture of low sodium and high magnesium-induced arrest (Kirsch's solution) followed by pressurized pump perfusion of a cold, oxygen-saturated solution with low sodium content for 8–10 min. Because of the magnesium content a thorough aspiration is necessary.

We have found some of these procedures and the use of this considerable amount of fluid to be rather cumbersome.

We have accordingly tried to simplify the procedure as much as possible by reducing the amount of Bretschneider's solution to such an extent that it is not necessary to suck up the fluid from the right atrium.

The only disadvantage mentioned by Bretschneider in allowing the solution to be mixed with the circulating blood volume was a drop in blood pressure, which could be counteracted by administration of calcium.

In our present procedure, then, the Bretschneider's solution serves three main purposes: to paralyse the heart by polarized myocardial membrane stabilization, to obtain some cooling of the heart and finally to serve as haemodilution of the circulating blood.

INFUSION PROCEDURE

The infusion is made from two bottles, each containing 1 l of the solution. As seen from Figure 1, the fluid leaves the bottles through two large needles with internal diameter of $2\frac{1}{4}$ mm. The two bottles are connected by means of silicone tubings and a Y-connector to a single silicone tube which goes to the operating table.

One important technical detail is a long stainless steel needle going right through the bottle with its tip well above the surface of the fluid. This needle is necessary for ensuring a free air passage into the bottle.

Infusion is made into the root of the aorta. Figure 2 shows another large-bore needle, used for puncture of the aortic root. For adult patients it has an internal diameter of 3–4 mm and is provided with a disc-like ring which stops against the aortic wall after puncture. The resistance to flow through this infusion set-up must be low. We have assessed that 400–500 ml/min of fluid should be able to pass from a level above the aorta of about 50 cm (35–40 mmHg).

Figure 2 also shows a 50 cc syringe used for infusion of the solution in newborns and young children. The needle is here provided with a stopper taken from a piece of rubber tube.

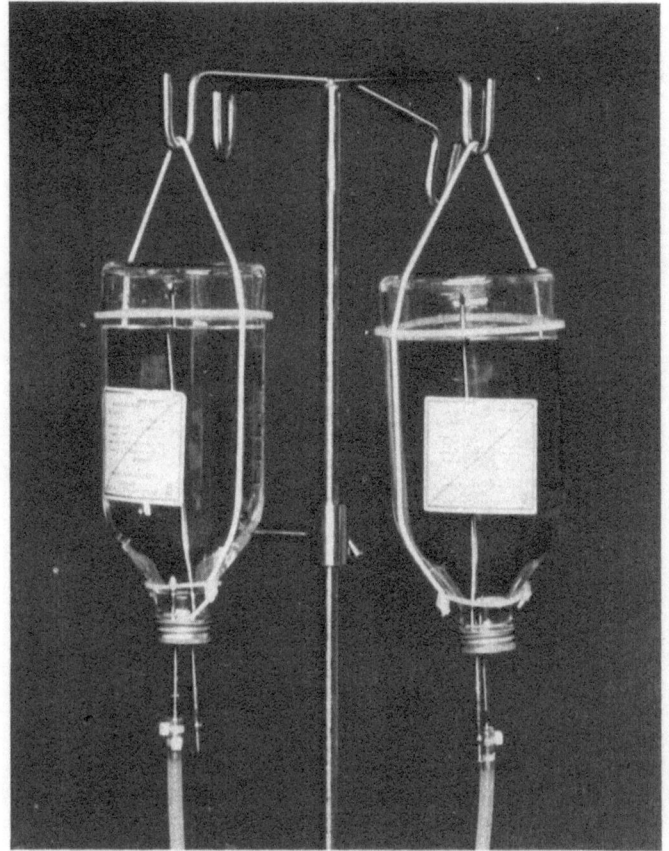

Figure 1 Infusion procedure (see text for explanation)

The steps shown in Table 2 are followed during infusion. The biggest amount of cardioplegic solution is used for cases with aortic valve insufficiency or combined insufficiency of the aortic and mitral valves. The time used for the infusion in such cases is 3–4 min, in other cases usually less than 2 min. The pressure in the aortic root drops to 20–30 mmHg during infusion.

The procedure followed in cases with aortic valve insufficiency is seen from Table 3. The large vent in the left ventricle is opened very shortly after the start of infusion, then closed again; and the left ventricle is allowed to distend in relation to the pressure in the aortic root. A distension to more than normal size has never been observed, and manual compression or massage of the heart has never been used.

Figure 3 shows crushed ice put around the heart after it has been cooled with the Bretschneider solution. We have not observed frostbite lesions of the myocardium nor phrenic nerve paralyses following this procedure.

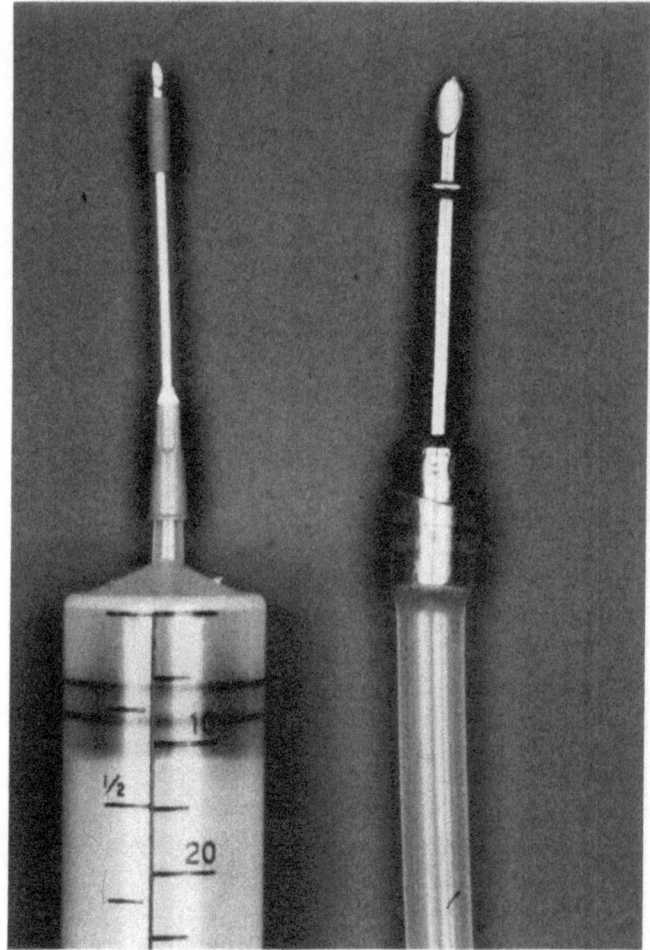

Figure 2   Large-bore needle used for aortic root puncture

Table 2   Procedure

1. The cannula is placed before aortic cross-clamping
2. Infusion of Bretschneider's solution, 3–5 °C
3. Infusion pressure: 50–70 mmHg
4. Infusion volume: 400–1200 ml in adults
   20–100 ml in children
5. Pieces of frozen isotonic glucose are placed in the pericardial sac

302

Table 3 Aortic insufficiency

1. The left ventricular vent is closed
2. The cannula is placed in the aortic root
3. The aorta is cross-clamped
4. The left ventricular vent is opened for a short time

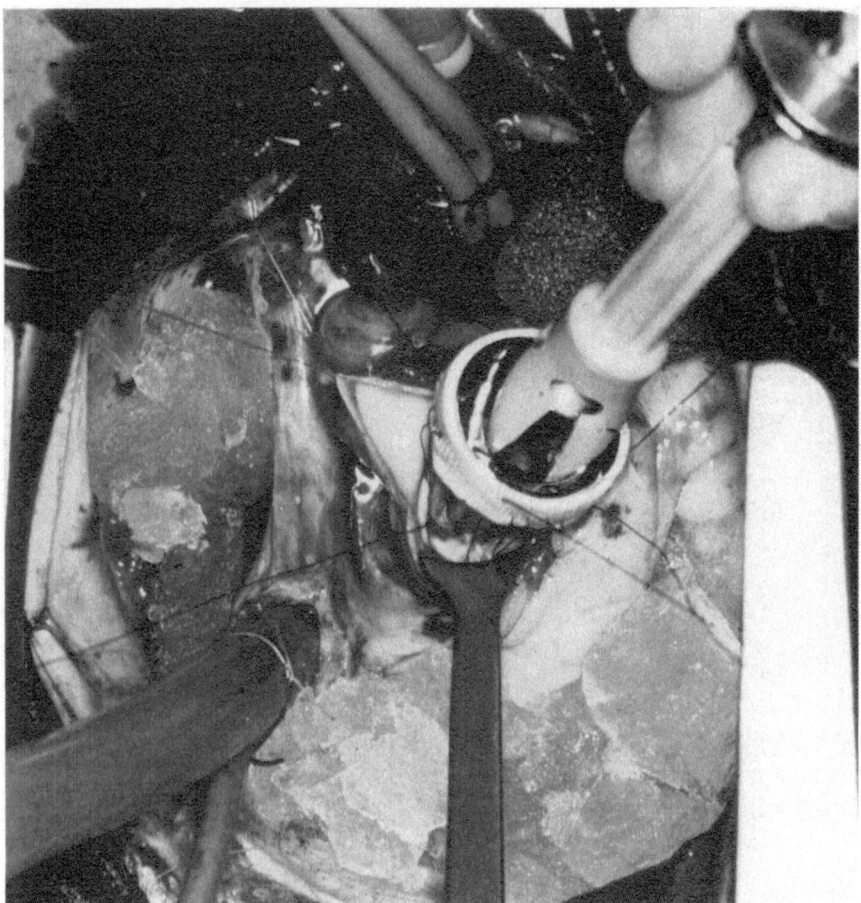

Figure 3 Crushed ice around the heart, after heart was cooled with the Bretschneider solution

COMPLICATIONS

We had at the beginning some minor complications, such as bleeding around the needle in cases with fragile aortic wall, puncture through the posterior wall of the aorta in small children, and blood loss because of insufficient occlusion around a caval cannula during aspiration from the right atrium, in one case early in the series when this procedure was still in use.

PATIENTS

It has been difficult to compare series from the time of coronary perfusion with the present series. Only for a group with isolated aortic valve disease has it been possible to find comparable parameters for perfusion, degree of haemodilution and hypothermia.

At the beginning we used Bretschneider cardioplegia only during aortic valve replacements. Accordingly, in multiple valve replacements the aortic valve was replaced first, and the other valve or valves after closure of the aorta and re-establishment of coronary perfusion at a temperature of 28–30 °C, usually with the heart in fibrillation.

This method has now been abandoned so that most of the cardiac operations have been completed during one uninterrupted period of cardioplegia.

The material consists of 145 patients with a postoperative observation time of 1–5 years, and the patients operated on in 1976, when low sodium arrest was used for all kinds of valve replacement.

The first group of 145 patients all had aortic valve replacement, 28 had aortic and mitral and four had triple valve replacement; 99 of the patients had isolated aortic valve disease, and four died within 30 days after the operation. Figure 4 shows the operative mortality (30 days) of 12 patients

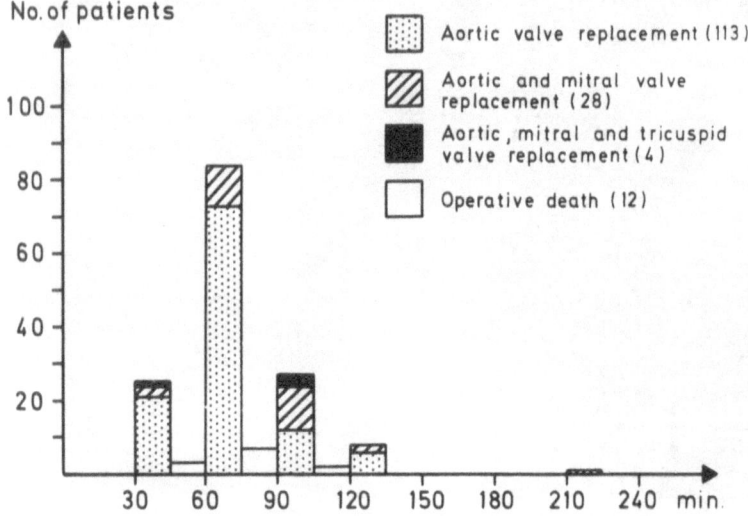

Figure 4 Operative mortality (30 days) of 12 patients related to cross-clamping time

related to the aortic cross-clamping time. No correlation is found. One patient with a cross-clamping time of 216 min had reperfusion of the coronaries with Bretschneider's solution after 126 min.

The cause of death is shown in Table 4. Seven of the patients had rheumatic heart disease, of whom four died of low cardiac output syndrome (LCOS). Only one died from acute myocardial infarction (AMI), and one patient had subendocardial infarction. This patient had the aortic valve replaced during

Table 4   Operative mortality (30 days)

Causes of death	Valves replaced	No. of patients
Low cardiac output syndrome	2 double ⎱ 2 triple ⎰	4
Acute myocardial infarction	double	1
Subendocardial infarction	double	1
Hepatitis	double	1
Atrioventricular dissociation	aortic	1
Stone heart	aortic	1
Hypovolaemic shock	aortic	1
Toxaemia	aortic	1
Tachycardia	aortic	1
TOTAL		12

low sodium arrest and the mitral valve replaced after re-established 'normal' coronary artery perfusion with the heart in fibrillation. One patient died from 'stone heart'.

The late mortality (1–5 years) of 11 patients in this group is shown in Table 5. Four of them were operated on for severe aortic incompetence and

Table 5   Late mortality (1–5 years)

Causes of death	Valves replaced	No. of patients	Time postoperative
Acute myocardial infarction	Aortic (1 homograft)	2	1½ years / 2 years
Cardiac failure	Aortic Double	2	1½ years
Endocarditis			2 months
	Aortic	3	4 months
			8 months
Sudden death	Aortic Double	2	1¼ years / 8 months
Pulmonary cancer	Aortic	1	1 year
Intracranial aneurysm	Aortic	1	2 years
TOTAL		11	

had severe myocardial fibroses of whom two had signs of acute myocardial infarction (AMI).

The other group of patients operated on in 1976 are listed in Table 6. Four

Table 6   Cardiac valve replacement in 1976

Valves replaced	No. of patients	Operative mortality (30 days)
Aortic	42	0
Aortic and mitral	13	2
Mitral	35	2
Aortic, mitral and tricuspid	1	0
Aortic and resection of aortic aneurysm	2	1
Aortic and resection of subvalvular aortic stenosis and mitral incompetence	1	1
TOTAL	94	6

patients with rheumatic heart disease, one patient with central aortic aneurysm and one patient with aortic incompetence and severe subvalvular stenoses and mitral incompetence died in connection with the operation. There was no operative mortality in cases with isolated aortic valve disease.

DISCUSSION

The operative mortality has in general decreased in recent years in patients receiving cardiac valve replacement, independent of the kind of myocardial preservation used during aortic cross-clamping. Accordingly it may be stressed that the operative mortality from different periods can hardly be used for evaluation of the benefit of one method of myocardial preservation over the other. The reason why we still think that the present method of cardioplegia bears some relation to the operative mortality in our series is the sudden fall in mortality observed from the very day we gave up isolated continuous coronary perfusion and started on the present method.

Even though the operative mortality had gradually decreased in our previous series from the initial 25%, it was still 14–15% in the last series before introduction of cardioplegia. In this series the incidence of stone heart condition preoperatively and the postoperative incidence of LCOS and early and late AMI was about 7%, 25% and 12% respectively. The occurrence of stone heart has now practically disappeared after a correctly performed cardioplegic procedure, and the significant drop in the incidence of LCOS and AMI including subendocardial infarction postoperatively is in our opinion in favour of the present method of cardioplegia.

A corresponding drop in the operative mortality after mitral valve replacement was observed when this kind of cardioplegia replaced our previous procedures of intermittent anoxic arrest and/or electrical fibrillation.

We strongly believe in our present practice of doing all the open heart surgery during one uninterrupted period of cardioplegia even if the aorta is cross-clamped for more than 2 h.

The simplification of the procedure as described here, with a simple gravity infusion of a comparatively small amount of cold Bretschneider's solution avoiding pumps and aspiration from the right atrium, has made this method easy and safe to use. The composition of the solution is the first one described by Bretschneider. We do not intend to alter this composition at the moment. The low pH in this solution is more than compensated for by the rapid and rather severe shift of the pH in the myocardium to the alkaline side during rapid cooling of the heart, a condition which we like to counteract.

Perhaps the most important factor in the procedure is the application of crushed ice around the heart immediately after the infusion. This lowers the temperature of the heart very effectively, and we have not observed any side effects of this direct application of ice on the heart, when it has been precooled with the Bretschneider solution.

Low sodium arrest as described is now used in almost all cases of open heart surgery including coronary surgery. For us it has proved to be better than any other method of myocardial preservation. A big advantage is the clean and dry field which makes surgery much easier to perform.

References

1. Bretschneider, H. J. (1964). Überlebenszeit und Wiederbelebungszeit des Herzens bei Normo- und Hypothermie. *Verh. Dtsch. Ges. Kreist.-Forsch.*, **30**, 11
2. Søndergaard, T. and Senn, A. (1967). Klinische Erfahrungen mit der Kardioplegi nach Bretschneider. *Langenbecks Arch. Klin. Chir.*, **319**, 661
3. Reidemeister, J. C., Heberer, G. and Bretschneider, H. J. (1967). Induced cardiac arrest by sodium and calcium depletion and application of Procaine. *Int. Surg.*, **47**, 535

42

Myocardial preservation during extended periods of ischaemia

Experimental results with a new cardioplegic solution ('Sbokos 3') solution

C. G. SBOKOS

This new cardioplegic solution is a modified potassium arrest solution, and has been developed at Harvard Medical School and the Massachusetts General Hospital, Boston, USA. It contains (See Table 1): potassium (24 mEq/l);

Table 1 Myocardial preservation: Sbokos 3 (S3) solution to induce cardiac arrest during cardiopulmonary bypass

Glucose	2.0 g/l
Sodium bicarbonate	1.0 g/l
Potassium chloride	1.87 g/l
Procaine HCl	2.0 g/l
Mannitol	30 g/l
Sterile distilled water	to final volume of 1000 cc

The analysed values of this solution are as follows:

Sodium	21 mEq/l
Potassium	24 mEq/l
Procaine	0.2%
Glucose	200 mg%
pH	7.7
Osmolality	285 mOsm/kg

Temperature of the solution before use: 3–4 °C

procaine (0.2%); sodium (21 mEq/l); glucose (200 mg%); mannitol (30 g/l) pH 7.7; and osmolality 285 mOsm/kg.

It is injected into the aortic root by a single bolus of 100–120 ml, immediately after cross-clamping the aorta. Its temperature before use is 3–4 °C.

This method fulfils most of the criteria for a safe, effective cardioplegic agent:

1. rapid onset of mechanical and electrical arrest;
2. dependable and rapid restoration of normal rhythm;

3. adequate cardiac function postischaemia;
4. absence of toxicity, secondary to the cardioplegic agent;
5. minimal or no biochemical aberrations during and after cardioplegia;
6. easy to use.

In order to evaluate the efficacy of this solution as compared to hypo-thermic and potassium arrest, an experimental protocol employing 90 and 120 min of ischaemia, with or without local cooling of the canine heart, was developed.

Adult mongrel dogs were studied with the use of a right heart–total bypass preparation (Figure 1), for determination of left ventricular function (LVF) curves—by relating left ventricular stroke work (LVSW) to mean left atrial pressure, at varying cardiac outputs, maintaining a fixed heart rate and mean aortic pressure—myocardial contractility (LVdp/dt), myocardial water

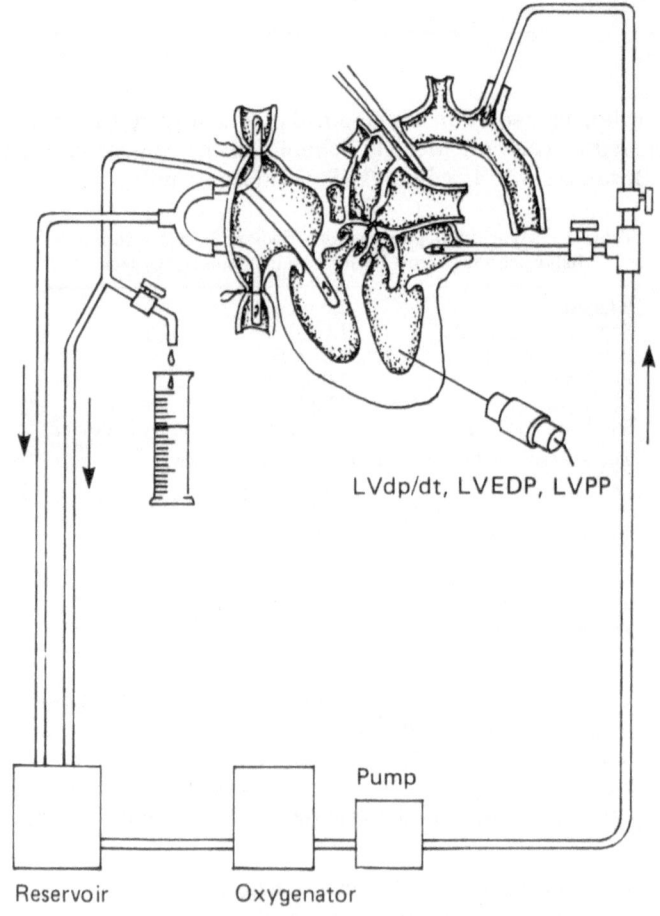

Figure 1 Right heart-total bypass arrangement

content, myocardial glycogen, coronary sinus lactate and pyruvate, and oxygen extraction of the heart.

Full-thickness biopsies of the left ventricle, for electronmicroscopic studies, were performed at varying intervals postischaemia, and the reactive hyperaemia, following reperfusion of the ischaemic heart, was carefully measured. Routine and subendocardial electrocardiograms were recorded.

Six groups of dogs were used in this part of our study, as detailed below:

1. 90 min ischaemia at 28 °C, with local cooling of the heart (core temperature 10–14 °C);

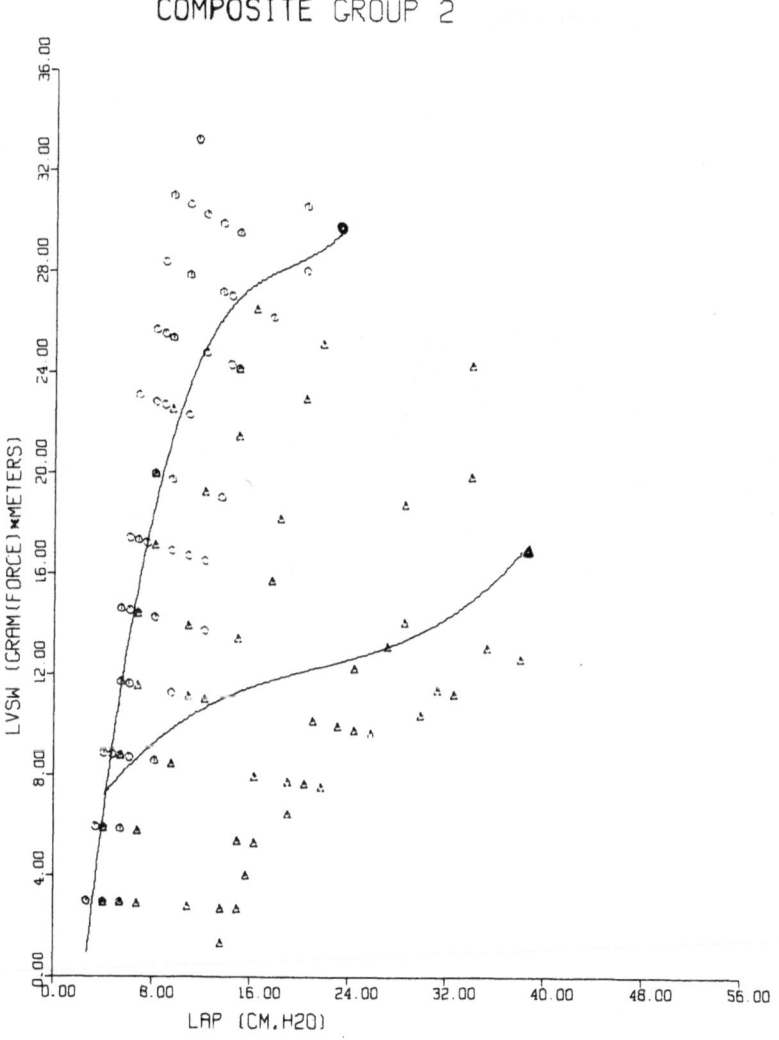

Figure 2 Composite group 2. 90 min ischaemia at 28 °C + local cooling (hypothermic arrest) (n = 6; O = control (preischaemia); △ = 35 min postischaemia)

311

2. 90 min K$^+$ arrest at 28 °C, with local cooling of the heart (core temperature 10–14 °C;
3. 90 min K$^+$ arrest at 28 °C; no local cooling;
4. 90 min 'Sbokos 3' solution arrest at 28 °C; no local cooling;
5. 120 min K$^+$ arrest at 28 °C, with local cooling (core temperature 10–14 °C);
6. 120 min 'Sbokos 3' solution arrest at 28 °C, with local cooling.

LVF decreased significantly following 90 min of hypothermic arrest, but did not change much after 90 min of hypothermic K$^+$ arrest (Figures 2 and 3).

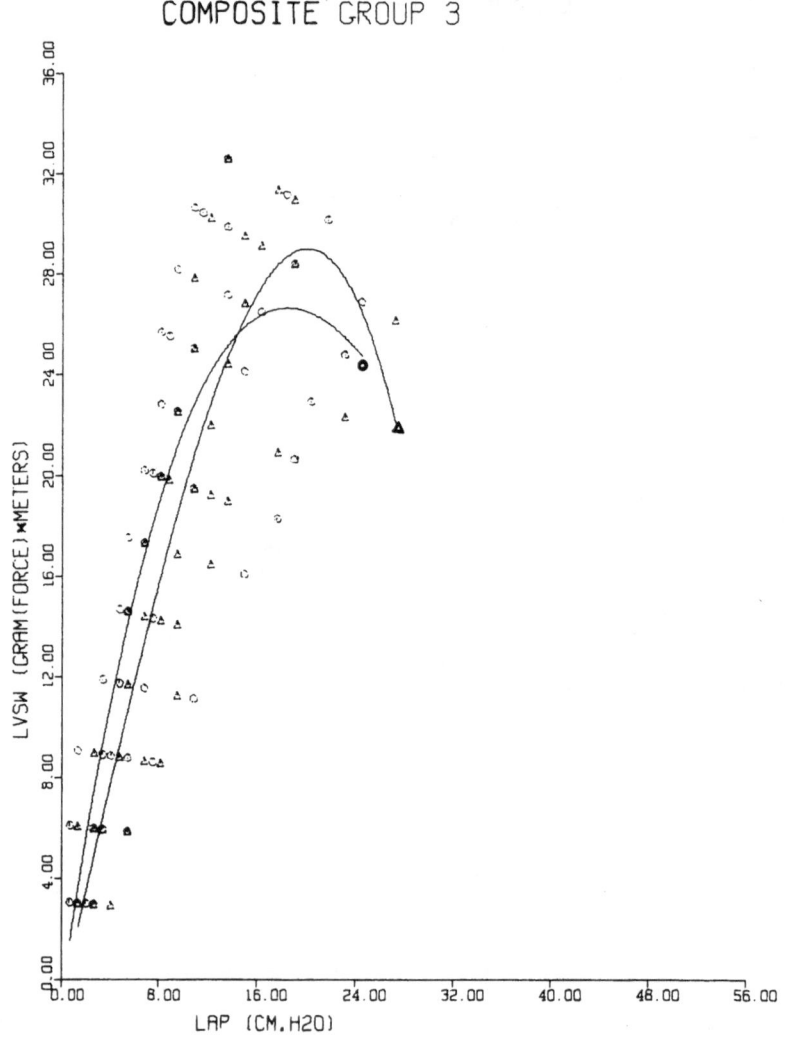

Figure 3 Composite group 3. 90 min ischaemia + local cooling: K$^+$ arrest (n = 6; ○ = control (preischaemia); △ = 35 min postischaemia)

There was, however, progressively severe depression in LVF, proportional to the cardiac output and to the postischaemia time, in the 90 mini schaemia with K^+ arrest without local cooling while not changing significantly in a similar group with 'Sbokos 3' (S3) solution arrest (Figures 4 and 5). It was interesting that the LVF was improving as the postischaemia recovery time was increased, in the S3 solution arrest group.

The difference in LVF between the K^+ arrest and the S3 solution arrest was much more obvious, and the superiority of S3 solution more striking,

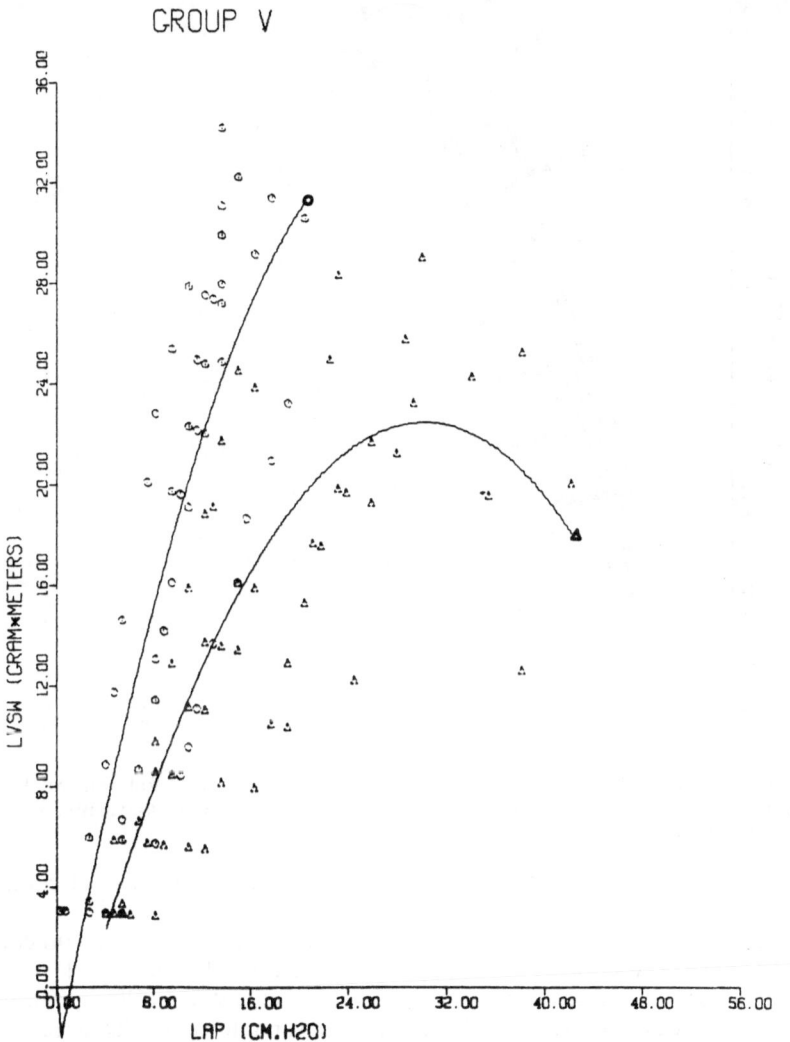

Figure 4 Group V. 90 min. ischaemia at 28 °C. No local cooling following K^+ arrest ($n = 6$; $\bigcirc$ = control (preischaemia). $\triangle$ = 35 min postischaemia) *Note:* In three experiments a third function study could not be completed, 60 min postischaemia

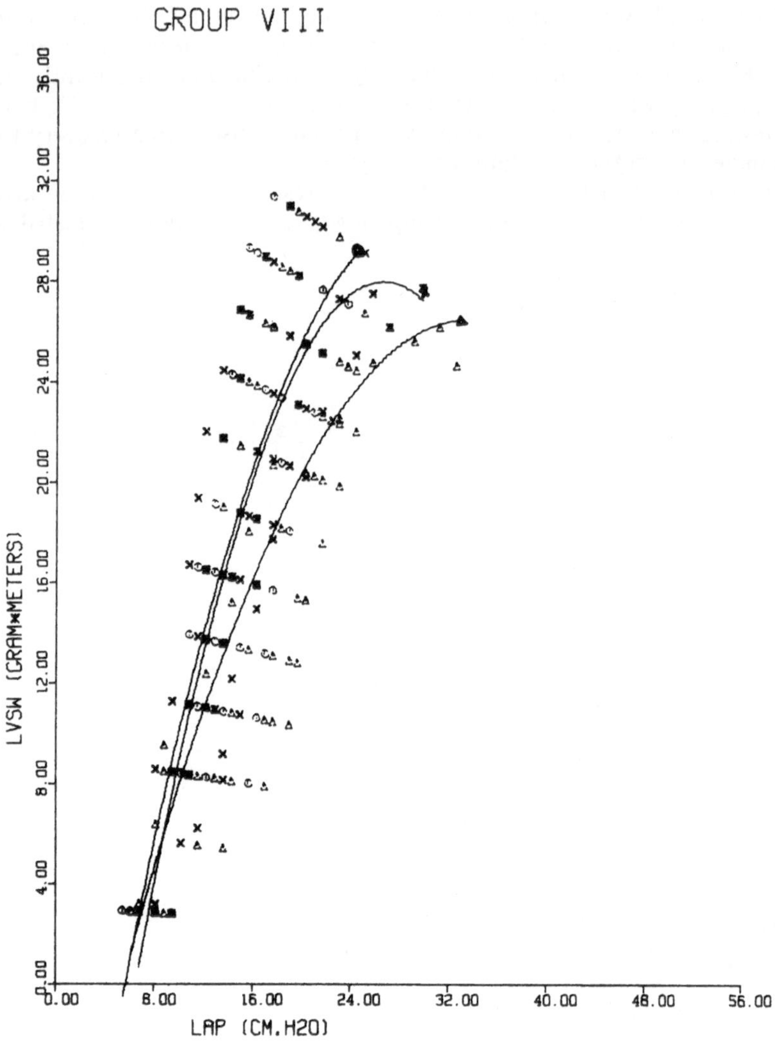

GROUP VIII

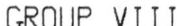

Figure 5 Group VIII. 90 min ischaemia at 28 °C. No local cooling following Sbokos 3 solution arrest (n = 6; ○ = control preischaemia; △ = 35 min postischaemia; × = 60 min postischaemia)

in the other two groups of 120 min arrest accompanied with local cooling (Figures 6 and 7).

The statistical analysis and comparison of these ventricular function curves, have been done by the 'analyses of variance techniques', at Harvard Medical School, and the superiority of S3 solution is statistically significant.

Left ventricular contractility (LVdp/dt), was variable but tended to parallel left ventricle function curves, although the statistical analysis of these curves is a more complex procedure, and is still in progress.

The same happened with subendocardial ECG recording, which is a more

GROUP VII.

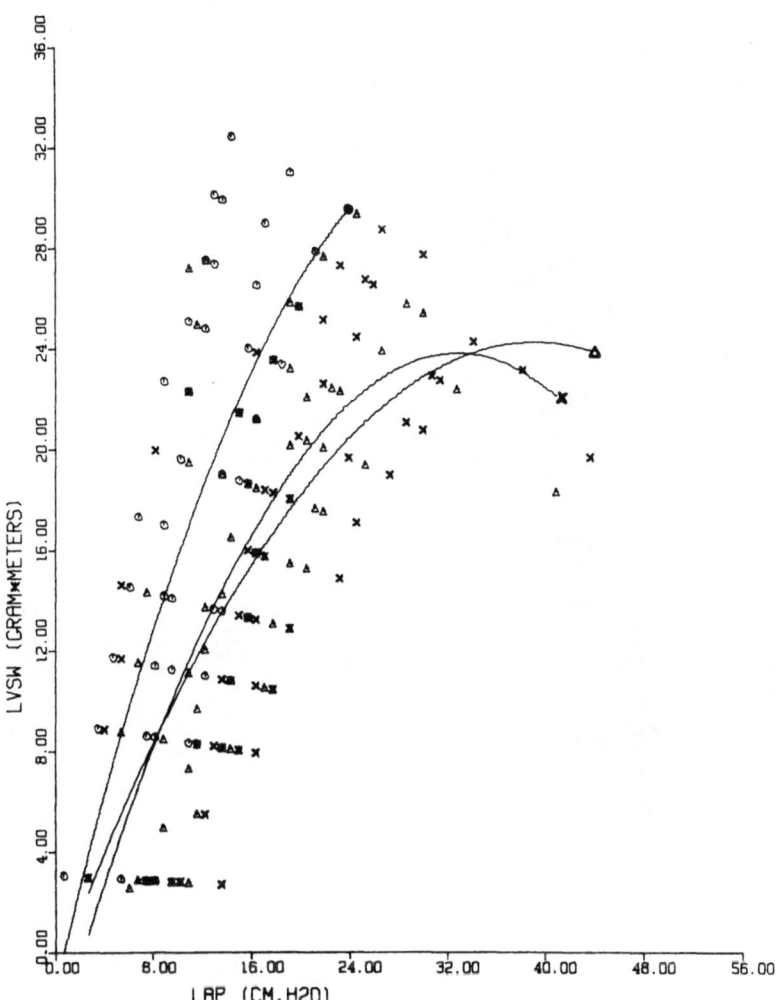

Figure 6 Group VII. 120 min ischaemia at 28 °C + local cooling following K⁺ arrest ($\bigcirc$ = control (preischaemia); $\triangle$ = 35 min postischaemia; $\times$ = 60 min postischaemia) *Note:* In two experiments postischaemia function studies at high flows could not be completed because of very high LA pressure

sensitive index of ischaemia in the open chest, than epicardial or routine ECG recordings. The subendocardial S–T segment changes, soon after cross-clamp was released, were less marked in the S3 group, in comparison with the hypothermic and K⁺ arrest experiments, and restored to preischaemia levels more quickly.

The electronmicroscopy examination of the left ventricle biopsies showed:

1. Ischaemic arrest with local cooling alone (the heart in ventricular fibrillation during ischaemia): after 90 min of cross-clamp, there is prominent

315

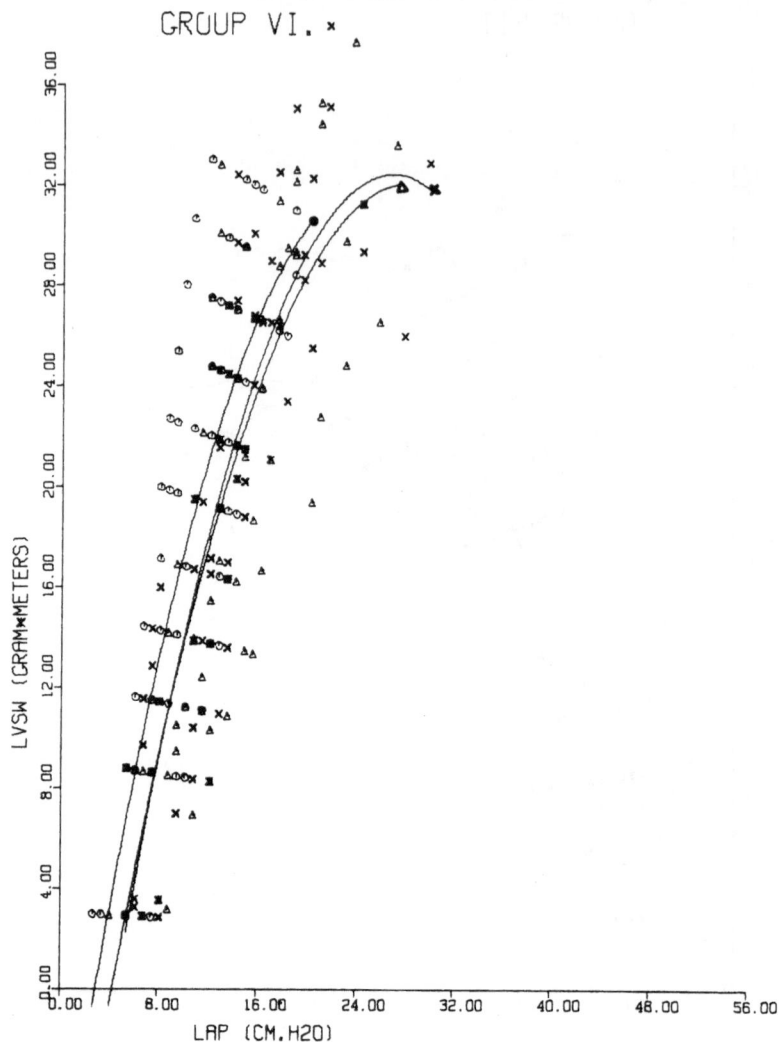

Figure 7 Group VI. 120 min ischaemia at 28 °C + local cooling following Sbokos 3 solution arrest (*n* = 7; ○ = control preischaemia; △ = 35 min postischaemia; × = 60 min postischaemia)

interstitial and intracellular oedema. There is dehiscence of intercalated discs and clearing of myofibrils in the I-band region.

2. K⁺ arrest: after 90 and 120 min of cross-clamp, there is minimal interstitial and intracellular oedema. Infrequent dehiscence of intercalated discs is present but there are no I-band changes.

3. S3 solution arrest: After 90 and 120 min of cross-clamp, oedema is not present. There are no myofibrillar changes and the intercalated discs are intact.

In summary, ultrastructural evaluation of these three types of myocardial arresting procedure demonstrates that the S3 solution produces less damage at the cellular and subcellular levels.

The water content of drill biopsies of the left ventricular (LV) free wall was expressed as a wet weight/dry weight (w/d) ratio. The increase in the w/d ratio, relative to its control value, is indicative of the oedema incurred during the period of ischaemia.

All groups exhibited this increase in myocardial water control (Table 2);

Table 2 Myocardial preservation: postischaemia oedema–oxygen extraction–reactive hyperaemia

Experimental group	w/d Ratio (% control)	Oxygen extraction (% control)	Reactive hyperaemia (% control)
90 min ischaemia at 28 °C (local cooling)	114.32 ± 3.30	9.37 ± 5.01	842.3 ± 98.7
90 min ischaemia + K⁺ arrest (local cooling)	109.25 ± 3.20	60.13 ± 34.87	754.7 ± 66.5
t test	p < 0.05	p < 0.01	p < 0.01
90 min ischaemia + K⁺ arrest (no local cooling)	105.96 ± 3.36	31.15 ± 22.02	805.7 ± 286.1
90 min ischaemia + Sbokos 3 arrest (no local cooling)	106.30 ± 3.26	61.88 ± 25.10	347.5 ± 81.5
t test	ns	p < 0.05	p < 0.001
120 min ischaemia + K⁺ arrest (local cooling)	107.10 ± 2.11	39.83 ± 17.07	567.7 ± 227.2
120 min ischaemia + Sbokos 3 arrest (local cooling)	106.69 ± 2.56	48.38 ± 22.83	347.5 ± 81.5
t test	ns	p < 0.01	p < 0.1

w/d = Wet/dry weight ratio = oedema
ns = not significant
p = probability obtained using Student one-tailed t test for unpaired data
Reactive hyperaemia: 2 min postischaemia

K^+ and S3 solution arrest seem equally adequate in maintaining low oedema, while local cooling increases oedema significantly ($p < 0.05$). Local cooling increases oedema in all cases, possibly because the heart is being bathed by the cooling solution.

The % O_2 extraction of control, 5 min postischaemia, is indicative of the myocardium's ability to extract O_2 from the coronary flow, after ischaemia; K^+ and S3 solution arrest were significantly better at increasing the % O_2 extraction of control than hypothermia alone. S3 solution arrest, however, with or without local cooling, was superior to K^+ arrest at a significant level of $p < 0.05$.

An increase in coronary blood flow, soon after release of the cross-clamp, relative to that value prior to the ischaemia intervention, was observed in all experiments (reactive hyperaemia). A value of 100% is indicative of a return to the pre-cross-clamp value.

Once again, S3 solution arrest is superior to K^+ arrest at a level of $p < 0.001$.

Looking at the biochemistry results of the coronary sinus blood samples, and particularly at the lactate/pyruvate ratio and extraction, it seems that they match with function curves in all groups, although we found it difficult to do any statistical analysis of these results.

Myocardial glycogen levels, at the end of the ischaemic insult are a good biochemical index of myocardial protection, and again, in our series, S3 solution preserves it better, although the number of experiments is not enough yet to make a final comment.

Finally, there were a few other observations worth mentioning:

(a) all hearts in both groups with Sbokos 3 solution arrest—90 min ischaemia at 28 °C without local cooling, and 120 min with local cooling—defibrillated spontaneously, immediately after reperfusion, while this did not happen in the other groups of experiments.

(b) In the experiments with the new solution, left ventricular function improved after reperfusion, while the opposite happened in the other groups.

(c) It was possible to come off bypass easily and quickly with minimum or no pulmonary oedema with S3 solution arrest in all experiments while in the hypothermic arrest group two out of six dogs could not come off bypass at the end of the experiment.

We conclude that this new solution produces immediate cardioplegia— K^+ and procaine-induced 'membranoplegia'—washes out the capillary bed during arrest, cools the heart internally, and might be effective as either a substitute or an adjunct to hypothermia.

43

Intraoperative protection of the heart: topical myocardial hypothermia

E. B. STINSON

It is apparent from the cyclical recrudescence of the subject of intraoperative myocardial preservation over the entire history of modern cardiac surgery that no perfect and universally accepted method has yet evolved. I would like, in this chapter, simply to describe our experience at Stanford with topical hypothermia for myocardial protection. At the outset, it probably should be pointed out that the term 'myocardial protection' represents at the present state of development of cardiac surgery a euphemism for minimizing myocardial injury during cardiac operations that involve interruption of coronary flow and arrest of ventricular contractions. Under experimental conditions nearly complete preservation of myocardial structure and function during cardiopulmonary bypass can be achieved by continuous normo-thermic or mildly hypothermic perfusion of a beating, vented heart that is performing minimal external work under conditions of physiological perfusion pressures and arterial oxygen content. Most cardiac operations, however, are facilitated greatly by a quiet and relatively bloodless field provided by both mechanical cardiac arrest and interruption of coronary perfusion. During periods of coronary non-perfusion ischaemic damage to the myocardium occurs in a time-dependent fashion as a function of the disproportion between metabolic demand and substrate supply, and negative imbalance in this relationship is expressed in depletion of intracellular myocardial levels of high energy phosphate compounds, obligatory anaerobic metabolism, and evidence of membrane injury and contractile dysfunction after restoration of coronary blood flow. This has been summarized elegantly in the presentation of Dr Hearse (Chapter 33 in this book). The magnitude of ischaemic damage during aortic cross-clamping can be decreased significantly by reduction of myocardial temperature and by sustained membrane depolarization with a hyperkalaemic extracellular fluid. In this chapter, however, I would like to describe our clinical experience with myocardial hypothermia induced by simple topical, or epicardial, cooling during periods of coronary perfusion.

Our technique for inducing topical myocardial hypothermia was first described in 1960 and since then various refinements have been added. Nevertheless, the technique is extremely simple, perhaps deceptively so, but its advantages can be fully exploited only by meticulous attention to detail.

First, in order to respond to various misconceptions regarding our technique of topical hypothermia, I would mention features that do not represent the technique as utilized at our centre. Electrolyte solution containing slush or ice crystals is not used, but rather 0.9 % sodium chloride solution stored in a refrigerator kept at 3–4 °C. This is available in 2 litre irrigation containers and is needed in this quantity in order to provide the volumes that we employ. The technique does not consist of initially irrigating the pericardial cavity with cold solution and then subsequently intermittently moistening the cardiac surface. It is important to cool the heart as thoroughly as possible at the beginning of the aortic cross-clamp interval and to maintain protective levels of myocardial hypothermia by continuous circulation of cold saline within the pericardial sac at 100–150 ml/min. It is important not to remove the solution from the refrigerator or ice container in which it is stored until immediately before use in order to avoid warming the solution to ambient termperature.

The following comments regarding details of our technique for topical hypothermia apply both to valve replacement and coronary artery bypass grafting. After establishment of cardiopulmonary bypass with haemodilution prime, ventricular fibrillation is induced by brief DC stimulation and the aorta is cross-clamped. Immediately before and after cross-clamping, cooling is initiated by lavage of the pericardial sac with 2 litre of 0.9 % saline stored at 3–4 °C. Topical cooling is then continued with an infusion of cold saline into the pericardial reservoir at 100–150 ml/min. The saline is simultaneously aspirated near the lower end of the sternotomy incision and the level of saline in the pericardium is maintained as high as possible; that is, immediately below the cardiotomy or aortotomy incision or the coronary artery site being operated upon. Maximal immersion of both ventricles in the cold saline pool is enhanced by orienting the operating table in a head-up position with tilting toward the left. Systemic cooling in the range of 30–33 °C is used and active warming is begun approximately 10 min before anticipated release of the aortic cross-clamp. Topical cooling is continued until restoration of coronary blood flow and defibrillation is accomplished 5–6 min later. All distal coronary artery anastomoses are performed sequentially during a single cross-clamp interval, and proximal anastomoses are constructed after release of the cross-clamp. During aortic or mitral valve replacement, additional myocardial cooling is achieved by lavage of the interior of the opened ventricular chamber with additional litre amounts of cold saline. This also accomplishes removal of residual particulate débris. In cases of concomitant valve replacement and coronary bypass grafting, valve excision and left ventricular lavage are first performed and then a second cold saline infusion line is placed into the interior of the left ventricle to combine endocardial with epicardial cooling during performance of the distal coronary artery anastomoses. Lastly, the valve substitute is inserted and the cardiotomy incision closed. All of these steps are carried out during a single cross-clamp interval.

There are several technical aspects of intraoperative management that may affect the quality of myocardial hypothermia achieved. Pericardial adhesions are always dissected in order to completely expose the entire cardiac surface to the cooling solution. Low flow cardiopulmonary bypass in the range of 40–50 ml/kg/min is used, generally resulting in perfusion pressures in the range of 40–60 mmHg. The warming effect of collateral circulation through bronchial or mediastinal vessels is therefore minimized. Also, we routinely utilize cannulation of both the superior and inferior vena cava in order to ensure complete emptying of the right side of the heart.

Measured left ventricular intramyocardial temperatures decrease gradually over a 5–10-min period after the initiation of cooling, but vary according to region and intramural depth. In the anterolateral left ventricular midwall, temperatures in the range of 15–18 °C can be obtained consistently, although a transmural gradient of 5–6 °C from subepicardium to subendocardium is usually present. Midwall temperatures in the dependent portion of the left ventricle are usually 2–3 °C lower than those reached anteriorly, or in the interventricular septum. Combined endocardial and epicardial cooling, when

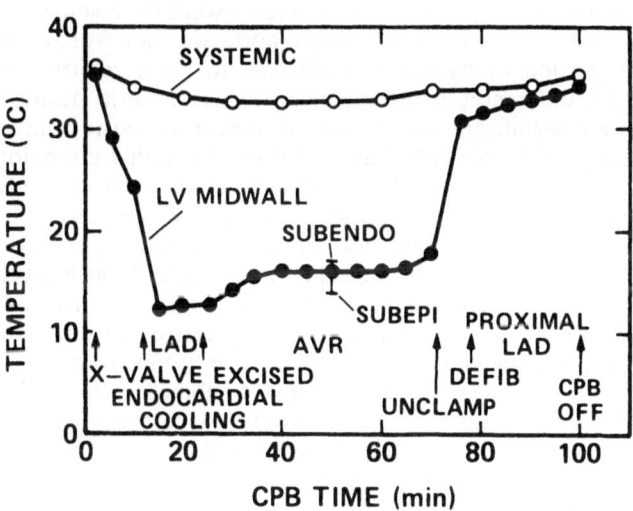

AVR + CABG

Figure 1 Systemic and left ventricular midwall temperatures during aortic valve replacement combined with coronary artery bypass grafting. The following features may be noted: the gradual fall in left ventricular midwall (anterolateral region) temperature during the first 10 min after aortic cross-clamping and valve excision, the lowest temperature achieved during combined endocardial and epicardial cooling (time of distal left anterior descending coronary artery anastomosis), general stability of the midwall temperature curve, and the temperature gradient from subepicardium to subendocardium

possible, results in a 3–4 °C decrease in midwall temperatures, as compared to external cooling alone.

Figure 1 illustrates typical systemic and left ventricular midwall temperatures during combined aortic valve replacement and bypass grafting of the left anterior descending coronary artery. This myocardial temperature curve is representative of those that we have measured in many cases, but it differs from those reported by many other investigators who have found less stable cooling of the myocardium utilizing topical hypothermia alone. The primary reason for this discrepancy probably relates to the detailed attention that we devote toward continuous and complete exposure of the heart to cold saline, as well as possibly to the technical features of our cardiopulmonary bypass system, as mentioned earlier.

It is difficult to provide convincing evidence for comparative superiority of the topical hypothermia technique versus other methods of preserving myocardial viability, mainly because of the lack of control data in our own experience. We did, however, compare topical hypothermia with continuous coronary perfusion for coronary bypass grafting in a study several years ago. In the continuous coronary perfusion group the aorta remained unclamped during the entire procedure, ventricular fibrillation was induced by brief DC stimulation, and the left ventricle was vented until immediately before defibrillation. In the clamped group topical hypothermia was provided during the entire period of aortic cross-clamping, no left ventricular vent was utilized, and the heart was defibrillated as soon as possible after release of the cross-clamp. These patient groups did not differ significantly in regard to preoperative risk factors or perfusion parameters except for a somewhat higher bypass flow rate in patients in whom the aorta was not cross-clamped, reflecting that portion of bypass flow directed to the coronary circulation. There were no differences in haemodynamic performance postoperatively, but there were significant differences in regard to postoperative serum enzyme levels (SGOT and LDH) and rates of myocardial infarction. In the clamped group serum enzyme levels were lower on each of the first four postoperative days than in the perfused group and the myocardial infarction rate was one half that encountered in the continuous perfusion group. Currently, the perioperative myocardial infarction rate at our institution with the topical myocardial hypothermia technique is 4.5 %. In this study of 304 patients there was no significant difference in operative mortality rates, being 0.6 % and 1.3 % for the clamped and unclamped groups respectively. These data indicate that myocardial hypothermia combined with a single aortic cross-clamp interval is preferable to continuous coronary perfusion with ventricular fibrillation for coronary bypass grafting, but obviously they do not support a claim for topical hypothermia as a uniquely preferable approach among all of those currently available.

We have further tried to quantify the usefulness of topical hypothermia for other cardiac operations by searching for correlations of cross-clamp time with postoperative outcome. In patients undergoing aortic valve replacement or mitral valve replacement since 1963 (stratified according to preoperative risk groups in terms of overall functional classification, left ventricular function, and the presence or absence of coronary artery disease) no correlation of cross-clamp time with outcome has been found. This is true for early survival rates, need for inotropic drugs, length of hospital stay, and survival rates at 1 year after operation for patients discharged from hospital.

These data indicate to us that myocardial hypothermia induced by topical cooling, as I have described, does afford satisfactory myocardial protection during periods of coronary non-perfusion. The advantages of this technique relate primarily to its simplicity and the superb operating conditions that it provides in terms of a quiet and relatively bloodless field and the ability to suture and retract a flaccid myocardium. Attention to detail ensures consistently protective levels of left ventricular hypothermia. A vent is unnecessary and the potential hazards associated with cannulation of the coronary artery orifices are averted. Clearly, there are disadvantages, and these relate primarily to gradual rather than abrupt cessation of cardiac electrical and mechanical activity and to temperature gradients in the left ventricular wall, both transmurally and regionally. In practice, we have found these gradients to be minimal. In this regard, however, I believe that the technique of perfusion-induced hypothermia with hyperkalaemic cardioplegic solutions introduced via the aortic root, in conjunction with topical cooling, may well enhance the quality of hypothermic myocardial preservation. I therefore look forward to the results of well-designed studies that will address not only the quality of early postoperative outcome, but also late postoperative cardiac morphology and function.

Section VIII
Transposition of the Great Arteries

44

The Mustard operation

J. P. BYRNE

Current results with the Mustard operation

Since the first Mustard operation was done at our institution in 1965, numerous changes in the overall management of patients with transposition of the great arteries (TGA) have been introduced. To assess our results with current techniques, a review of all Mustard operations done during 1974 and 1975 was undertaken.

During the 2-year period 98 patients underwent operation; 34 were less than 1 year old, and of these seven were 3 months or less. The exact diagnoses are recorded in Table 1. 129 previous procedures had been performed in these patients (Table 2). The most common was a balloon atrial septostomy (BAS) (83 patients), and 26 patients had the Blalock–Hanlon operation. Most of these patients were from abroad, as we no longer routinely perform the Blalock–Hanlon operation.

There were 63 patients with simple TGA, including eight patients with a

Table 1   Mustard operations (1974–75)—hospital deaths

	Number	Died	(%)
Simple TGA	63	4	6
TGA + PDA	8	4	50
TGA + VSD	7	3	42
TGA + VSD + PDA	1	1	—
TGA + VSD + LVOTO	9	0	—
TGA + VSD + LVOTO + TS	1	1	—
TGA + VSD + Coarctation + PDA	1	1	—
TGA + Coarc + PDA	3	0	—
TGA + LVOTO	4	0	—
TGA + TI	1	0	—
TOTAL	98	14	14%

Abbreviations are as explained in the text of this chapter

Table 2 Mustard operations (1974–75)
previous operations

Balloon atrial septostomy	83
Blalock–Hanlon	26
Blalock–Taussig	9
Pulmonary artery banding	5
Resection of coarctation	3
Ligation of patent ductus	2
Glenn shunt	1
Total	129

small ventricular septal defect (VSD). Four patients (aged 10 days, 3, 3 and 8 months) underwent emergency operation. Two underwent urgent operation at 3 and 5 months of age because of deterioration in their clinical status. The Brom trouser-shaped pericardial patch was used for the intra-atrial baffle. In general, the baffle was placed 'behind' the coronary sinus, in order to avoid damage to the atrioventricular node. In some cases, the coronary sinus was incised deep into the left atrium in order to provide a wider inferior vena caval pathway. In addition to these manoeuvres, care was taken to avoid damage to the atrioventricular node from retractors and intracardiac suckers. The pulmonary venous atrium was enlarged routinely in those patients with juxtaposition of the atrial appendages and in those in whom it was judged too small for primary closure.

In the simple TGA group, five patients underwent operation using profound hypothermia and circulatory arrest. The pulmonary venous atrium was enlarged in nine patients and in eight the coronary sinus was incised. The VSD was closed with interrupted sutures in five patients and left open in three patients.

Complex TGA

There were 35 patients in this group (Table 1), of which 14 had left ventricular outflow tract obstruction (LVOTO). Nine of these had a VSD, four had intact ventricular septum; another had VSD and tricuspid stenosis as well as LVOTO. At operation, an attempt was made to relieve the LVOTO directly. These patients were felt to be unsuitable for the Rastelli operation. However, one patient did poorly and underwent a successful Rastelli operation 2 weeks after the first. Another had a valveless left ventricle to pulmonary artery conduit placed to relieve the LVOTO.

Eight patients underwent ligation of a patent ductus arteriosus (PDA) at the time of the Mustard operation. Seven had patch closure of a large VSD, and four of these had undergone previous pulmonary artery banding. Three patients had undergone previous coarctation resection. Another had attempted complete repair of TGA, VSD, PDA and coarctation at the age of 2 months. Three patients in this group underwent emergency operation at 3 days, 7 days and 2 months of age. Seven were operated upon using hypothermia and circulatory arrest. The pulmonary venous atrium was enlarged in eight patients and the coronary sinus was incised in 13.

Follow-up ranged from 1 to 3 years (average 24.4 months). Cardiac rhythm has been assessed by serial standard electrocardiographic determination.

RESULTS

Simple TGA

There were four hospital deaths in this group (6.4%)—Table 2; two of these had undergone emergency operation. The mortality for elective operations is therefore 3.3%. Another patient operated upon urgently at 3 months of age left the hospital after operation, but died 1 month later.

Of the 59 patients who survived operation and left the hospital, six had junctional rhythm during the early postoperative period. This was transient in three and persists in three.

There have been no late deaths in this group. Two patients with caval obstruction and one with pulmonary vein obstruction required reoperation and all three survived.

Complex TGA

There were ten hospital deaths in this group (Table 1). Four patients with TGA and PDA died. Three patients with large VSD died. One patient with TGA, LVOTO and tricuspid and right ventricular hypoplasia died. Another died after attempted complete repair of TGA, VSD, PDA and coarctation at the age of 2 months. The last death in this group was due to unrecognized subaortic obstruction. Three of these patients had rhythm disturbances postoperatively.

Of the 25 survivors, three had transient rhythm disturbances postoperatively. One patient required peritoneal dialysis for 48 h and six were ventilated for longer than 48 h. There have been no late deaths, pulmonary vein or caval obstructions in this group. All patients have been in sinus rhythm at follow-up electrocardiographic examination.

DISCUSSION

Refinements in operative technique and postoperative care have improved our results over those of previous years. The mortality for elective operations in simple TGA is low. However, the risk for emergency or urgent operation remains high. The risk for repair of complex TGA remains high. Pulmonary vascular obstructive disease (PVOD) may develop early in patients with PDA, and two with VSD who died had signs of PVOD at postmortem examination. Patients with large VSDs should undergo closure at 4–6 months of age prior to development of PVOD. Small VSDs do not appear to increase risk and we have included them in the simple TGA group.

Rhythm disturbances, particularly supraventricular tachyarrhythmias, have been less frequent in this series of patients. However, arrhythmias were more frequent in the patients who did not survive the postoperative period, suggesting that they still contribute to mortality.

In summary, 82 of 97 patients (85%) are survivors 1–3 years postoperatively. (The patient who underwent Rastelli operation is excluded.) This figure for the group with simple TGA is 58 out of 63 (92%). Associated lesions, PVOD and emergency operations are factors which increase mortality. Other operations for repair of TGA, whether of the 'switch' type or alternate procedures for redirection of venous inflow are subject to these same risk factors. These procedures should be considered in the light of currently attainable results with the Mustard operation—particularly with regard to operative mortality.

Current results with the Mustard operation

Early Mustard operation has been accepted as the treatment of choice for most forms of transposition of the great arteries (TGA). The rationale is to relieve hypoxaemia and prevent the development of pulmonary vascular obstructive disease (PVOD) which is accelerated in the presence of a ventricular septal defect (VSD) or patent ductus arteriosus[1,2] (PDA). The prognosis of patients with transposition and PVOD has been considered very unfavourable. Those with markedly elevated pulmonary arterial resistance (PAR) were refused operation. In those with moderately elevated PAR the operative mortality as well as the late mortality are high. The results of surgery in patients with transposition, VSD, and PVOD were improved by Lindesmith's concept of the 'palliative' Mustard operation in which redirection of venous inflow is performed, but the VSD is left open[3].

At the Hospital for Sick Children, Great Ormond Street, 23 patients have undergone the 'palliative' Mustard operation between 1973 and 1976. Their ages were between $2\frac{1}{2}$ and 17 years; 19 patients had TGA with VSD, three had TGA with intact ventricular septum and one had double outlet right ventricle, VSD and malposition of the great arteries.

All patients were severely cyanosed and had markedly limited exercise tolerance. Arterial oxygen saturation ranged between 45 and 79% (mean 65). The mean haemoglobin value was 19 g/%, and was less than 16 g/% in only one patient. Mean calculated pulmonary arterial resistance was 17 units/m^2. It was less than 8 units in one patient; between 8 and 10 units in three and over 10 units in the remaining patients.

In 20 patients who underwent the Mustard operation the VSD was left open. The three patients with intact ventricular septum underwent the Mustard operation and in addition a VSD was created. This was done via an apical left ventriculotomy[4].

All patients survived the operation and have improved. Follow-up varies from 4 to 40 months (mean 14 months). There have been no late deaths, venous obstructions or arrhythmias in this group. Postoperative arterial oxygen saturation ranges from 75 to 96% (mean 89%). Serum haemoglobin is significantly reduced from preoperative values, the postoperative mean value is 13 g/%. Five patients have been restudied approximately 1 year after operation. No significant change in PAR has been noted.

We have found this to be a gratifying approach to the patient with TGA and PVOD. Those patients with PAR greater than 8 units/m^2 undergo the palliative Mustard operation while in those with less than 6 units/m², we close the VSD. Those with a resistance between 6 and 8 units should be considered on an individual basis. Although the palliative Mustard operation achieves satisfactory early symptomatic improvement, the long-term results are unknown. The increased awareness of the early development of pulmonary vascular obstructive disease in patients with TGA should lead to earlier diagnosis and treatment prior to the development of PVOD.

References

1. Newfeld, E. A., Paul, W. H., Muster, A. J. and Idriss, F. S. (1974). Pulmonary vascular disease in transposition of the great arteries. *Am. J. Cardiol.*, **34**, 75
2. Lindesmith, G. G., Stanton, R. E., Lurie, P. R., Takahishi, M., Tucker, B. L., Stiles, Q. R. and Meyer, B. W. (1975). An assessment of Mustard's operation as a palliative procedure for transposition of the great vessels. *Ann. Thoracic Surg.*, **19**, 514
3. Viles, P. H., Ongley, P. A. and Titus, J. (1969). The spectrum of pulmonary vascular disease in transposition of the great arteries. *Circulation*, **40**, 31
4. Stark, J., de Leval, M. R. and Taylor, J. F. N. (1976). Mustard operation and creation of ventricular septal defect in two patients with transposition of the great arteries, intact ventricular septum and pulmonary vascular disease. *Am. J. Cardiol.*, **38**, 524

45

A current technique for the Mustard operation

J. STARK

Anaesthesia and monitoring do not differ from other open heart procedures for congenital heart defects. The heart is approached through a midline sternotomy and care is taken not to open either of the pleural spaces. Pericardium is removed for a patch, as illustrated in Figure 1. On the right side, the incision is parallel with the right phrenic nerve and about 15–20 mm anterior to it. The size of the patch is as described by Brom. The flat diameter of the superior vena cava (SVC) and inferior vena cava (IVC) is measured. The patch is then cut according to these measurements (Figure 2): A–B is the distance between the left upper and lower pulmonary veins (estimated); E–D is twice the diameter of the SVC, D–F is twice the diameter of the IVC a is about 30°, R is 90°; distance C–D is a mean of E–D and D–F. These measurements are helpful, but adjustments are often necessary because the anatomy of each atrium differs. If adhesions after previous intrapericardial operations are very dense, a weaveknit patch (Thackeray's No. MT 44) can be used. The ascending aorta is then cannulated for arterial return: IVC through the right atrium/IVC junction, SVC directly. A left atrial line is placed through the right upper pulmonary vein (Figure 3).

Care is taken not to let any air into the right atrium during cannulation because the tricuspid valve is a systemic atrioventricular valve. A vent is inserted into the right ventricle. On cardiopulmonary bypass, the perfusate is cooled to 25 °C and at this temperature the aorta is cross-clamped. The right atrium is opened, stay-stitches placed and the remnant of the atrial septum excised (Figure 4). The raw area is then covered with single stitches and the patch is sutured in place using double-armed 4–0 prolene. The suture line starts between the left atrial appendage and the left pulmonary veins. It is important not to bring the suture lines too close together on the lateral atrial wall, to avoid future obstruction of the pulmonary veins (Figure 5).

Point D on the baffle is sutured, with a second double-armed stitch, to

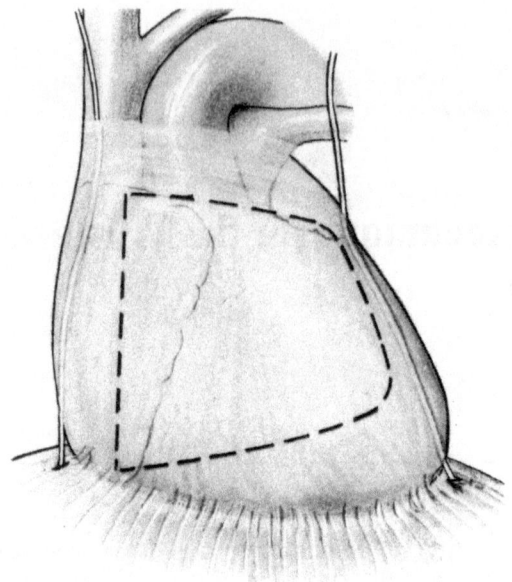

Figure 1   Pericardium removed for a patch

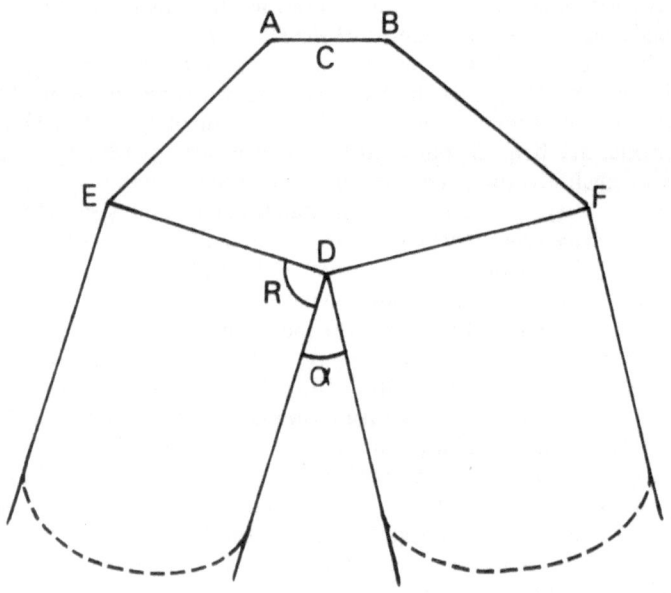

Figure 2   Calculation of the size of the patch (see text)

334

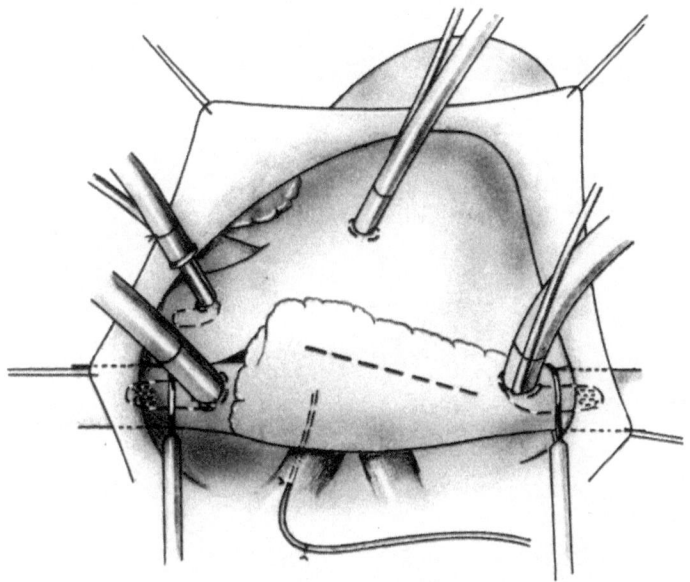

Figure 3 Preparation of the heart

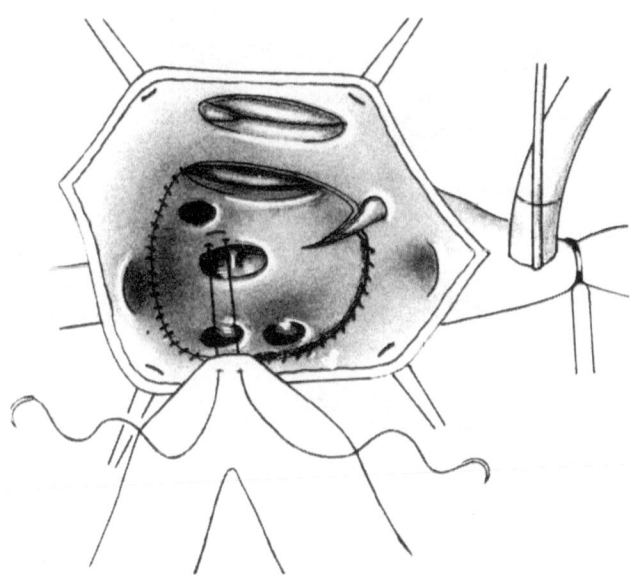

Figure 4 Positioning of the patch

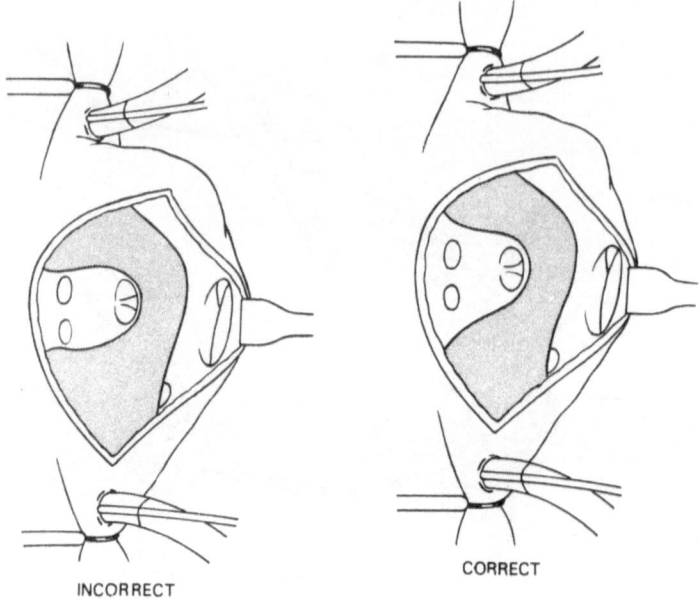

Figure 5 Correct and incorrect suture lines on the atrial wall

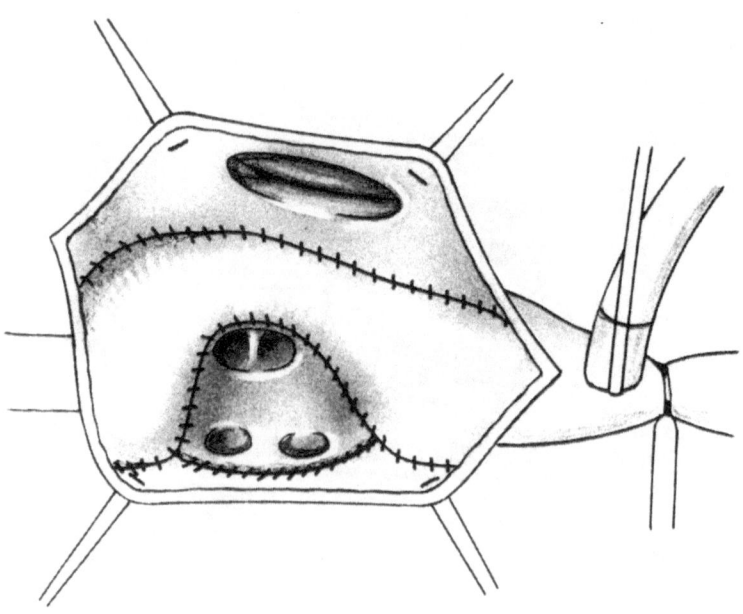

Figure 6 Completed patch

the remnant of the atrial septum. The lower part of the baffle is sutured either behind the coronary sinus, thus leaving the coronary sinus to drain with the pulmonary veins, to the tricuspid valve. Alternatively, the coronary sinus can be cut deep into the left atrium and then the lower suture line run through the floor of the coronary sinus, diverting its blood with the IVC blood to the mitral valve. In both techniques, the area of the atrioventricular node and bundle of His is not crossed with stitches. The completed patch is shown on Figure 6.

When the distance between the SVC and IVC is too short or when, after insertion of the baffle, uncertainty persists whether the new pulmonary venous atrium is too small, we prefer to enlarge it with an outside patch. An incision is extended across the crista terminalis, down between the right upper and right lower pulmonary veins. An oval patch of dacron is then stitched in place with prolene sutures. This separates the upper and lower pulmonary veins and enlarges the pulmonary venous atrium.

The patient is then re-warmed and the atriotomy closed. Prior to completion of this suture line, the heart is electrically fibrillated and an aortic needle vent inserted through a pursestring suture. Caval snares are released and all air is evacuated. When the filbrillator is removed, the heart usually resumes sinus mechanism spontaneously. Bypass is gradually discontinued, keeping the left atrial (pulmonary venous atrial) pressure at about 10–12 mmHg.

All patients are intubated with a nasotracheal tube and ventilated on a volume-cycled respirator usually for 12–24 h. Infants may be weaned off the respirator using a constant positive airway pressure system. Atrial lines are usually removed the following morning and mediastinal and pericardial drains taken out 1–2 h later.

COMPLICATIONS AFTER MUSTARD'S OPERATION

Several complications can occur after Mustard's operation. Obstruction of the SVC, IVC, or pulmonary veins has been encountered more often in patients in whom a dacron, rather than pericardial, patch was used[4]. In a series of 317 survivors of Mustard's operation in the period 1965–75, obstruction was noted in 16 patients in whom a pericardial patch had been used (7%) and in 29 (33%) in whom a dacron patch had been used. Refinements in operative technique decreased this high incidence. In 1974 and 1975, there were 97 survivors of the Mustard operation and only three developed obstruction (3%).

Dysrhythmias have been noted in all large series of Mustard operation. Amongst 14 patients who died after Mustard's operation at the Mayo Clinic[5] none was in sinus rhythm. El-Said et al.[6] observed 60 survivors of Mustard operation and only three remained in sinus rhythm at the last follow-up visit. We believe that atrial dysrhythmias are related to the operative technique, in particular to the preservation of the area of the subatrial node during cannulation, the atrial incision and suturing in the area of the atrioventricular node[7]. Atrial flutter and atrioventricular dissociation were more common in the beginning of our series. Amongst the first 49 survivors, only

40% showed sinus rhythm at the last follow-up. This increased to 73% in the next group of 63 survivors, while since 1971, 80% of 166 survivors remained in sinus rhythm on the clinic ECG.

It should be noted that only the 24-h ECG monitoring can give us a true picture of postoperative rhythm disturbances (see Tynan, Chapter 53 in this book).

Tricuspid valve incompetence is another complication which may occur[8]. Occasionally, a patient with transposition of the great arteries presents with tricuspid incompetence (TI) before the operation. In only one of our patients was the TI severe enough to require tricuspid valve replacement at the time of Mustard operation. A Hancock heterograft was used, and the child remains well 2 years and 4 months after the operation.

Doubts still exist about the right ventricular function in patients with transposition of the great arteries over a long period of time. At present, no adequate data are available for evaluation.

Acknowledgment

Figures 1, 2, 3, 4, 5, 6 are reproduced by kind permission from Churchill Livingstone, *Operative Surgery* (1977).

Bibliography

Mustard, W. T., (1964). Successful two-stage correction of transposition of the great vessels. *Surgery*, **55**, 469

Stark, J., de Leval, M. R., Waterston, D. J., Graham, G. R. and Bonham-Carter, R. E. (1974). Corrective surgery of transposition of the great arteries in the first year of life. Results in 63 infants. *J. Thoracic Cardiovasc. Surg.*, **67**, 673

Stark, J. (1973). Primary definitive intracardiac operations in infants. Transposition of the great arteries. In J. W. Kirklin (ed.) *Advances in Cardiovascular Surgery*, p. 101. (New York: Grune and Stratton)

Stark, J. (1976). Operation results for transposition of the great arteries. In: *Clinical Application of Current Technique and Treatment in Cardiology. Advances in Cardiology* Vol. 17, p. 20

Isaacson, R., Titus, J., Meredith, J., Feldt, R. H. and McGoon, D. C. (1972). Apparent interruption of atrial conduction pathways after surgical repair of transposition of the great arteries. *Am. J. Cardiol.*, **30**, 533

El-Said, G., Rosenberg, H. S., Mullins, C. E., Hallman, G. L., Cooley, D. A. and McNamara, D. G. (1972). Dyshyrhmias after Mustard's operation for transposition of the great arteries. *Am. J. Cardiol.*, **30**, 526

Stark, J. (1977). Surgical treatment of patients with transposition of the great arteries. *Johns Hopkins J.* (Special Issue)

Tynan, M., Aberdeen, E. and Stark, J. (1972). Tricuspid incompetence after the Mustard operation for transposition of the great arteries. *Circulation*, **45** (Suppl. I), 111

46

Long-term results of the Mustard operation

J. F. N. TAYLOR AND J. STARK

One hundred and sixty-four survivors of the Mustard operation were assessed in 1975. Attention was focused on the lifestyle and physical achievements of the survivors. The original operation was performed between 1965 and 1971. The follow-up period was, therefore, 4–10 years.

There were 36 late deaths, occurring 2 months to 6 years postoperatively. The main or contributory causes of the deaths were arrhythmias, obstructions of pulmonary and/or systemic venous inflow and tricuspid incompetence. Right ventricular function was not found to be a factor limiting a good functional result.

Fifty-six of the survivors attend normal schools and participate in sporting activities. A further 46 lead unrestricted lives, but with some complication (e.g., arrhythmia or tricuspid regurgitation). Twenty-one patients were restricted by a severe arrhythmia. Severe neurological deficits were present in seven survivors. It was not possible to assess the nine patients living abroad, although they are known to be alive.

47

Reoperation for complications of the Mustard operation: technical considerations

R. J. SZARNICKI

With further understanding of the pathophysiology and anatomy of transposition of the great arteries, and continued improvements in surgical techniques, the incidence of complications following the Mustard operation continues to decline.

Any institution dealing with this problem in significant numbers will continue to encounter occasional complications which require reoperation for correction. Obstructions to the caval and pulmonary venous pathways, as well as tricuspid insufficiency, have been reported by many groups. Approach through a median sternotomy incision is used by many surgeons, and the hazards with this approach are well known. Because of previous excision of the anterior pericardium, the surface of the right ventricle is densely adherent to the posterior aspect of the sternum and the risk of entering this chamber, thus damaging the coronary vessels, is high. Frequently, because of obstruction, large collateral vessels are encountered in the anterior mediastinum and this increases the risk of excessive blood loss during dissection.

Direct cannulation of the inferior vena cava and superior vena cava are necessary when reoperating on a patient with a previous Mustard operation. This dissection is frequently very tedious and difficult, and injury to the phrenic nerve is a common result. At our institution, we operated upon all patients with complications of the Mustard operation through a right thoracotomy incision. The patient is positioned with the thorax elevated 40–45° from the horizontal while the hips remain flat on the operating table. The incision is made in the 5th or 6th intercostal space, transecting the sternum if necessary.

The adhesions between the right lung and atrium are carefully separated,

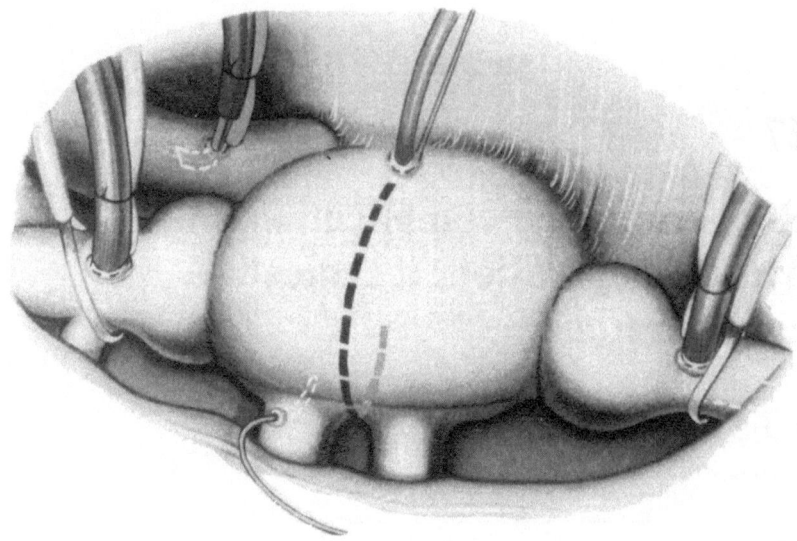

Figure 1   Transverse atriotomy

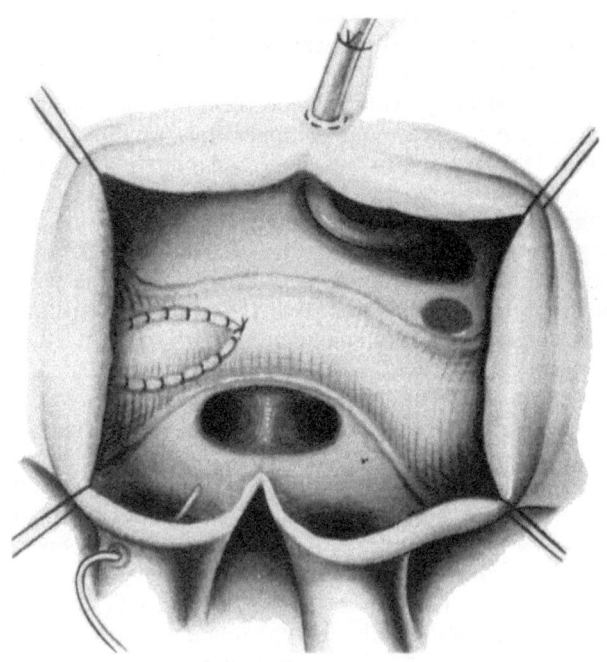

Figure 2   Exposure of previous Mustard patch

342

avoiding the phrenic nerve. Adhesions between the right ventricle and sternum are left untouched. The superior and inferior venae cavae are cannulated directly, as is the ascending aorta. A vent is inserted to the right atrial appendage and the atriotomy is made transversely and extends posteriorly between the right upper and lower pulmonary veins. A left atrial line is inserted through the upper pulmonary vein (Figure 1).

When the perfusion temperature is reduced to 25 °C, the aorta is cross-clamped and the pulmonary venous atrium is opened. The vent is then advanced across the tricuspid valve into the right ventricle. Traction sutures are placed anteriorly and posteriorly, eliminating the need for intracardiac retractors. Exposure of the previous Mustard patch is excellent (Figure 2).

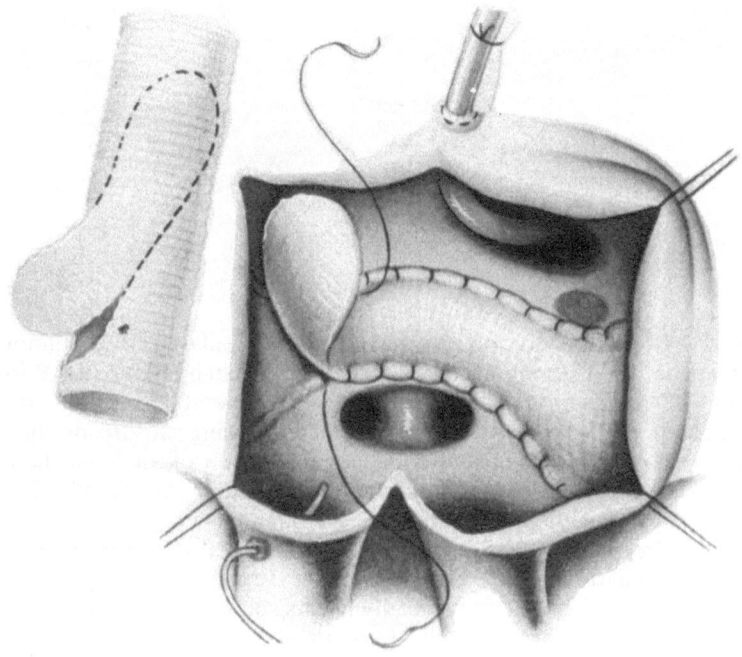

Figure 3   Insertion of elliptical dacron patch

In cases of isolated superior vena caval obstruction, the old patch is incised longitudinally in the region of the obstruction, and an elliptical dacron patch is then inserted to allow ample room for the passage of systemic venous blood (Figure 3). In cases of obstruction to both the superior and inferior venae cavae, the old patch is excised, leaving a small rim along the previous suture line to allow firm placement of sutures during placement of the new baffile. The new patch is constructed from a large woven dacron tube cut obliquely. This enables easier placement of the patch without kinking

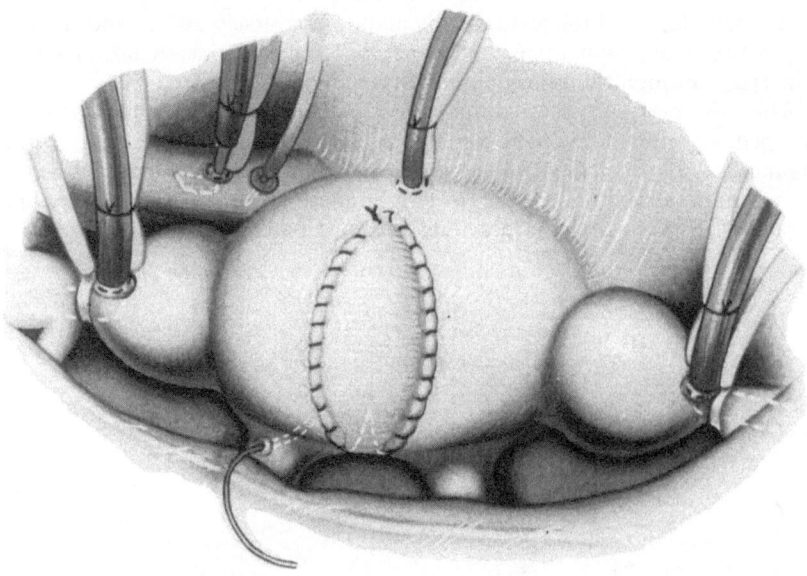

Figure 4   Enlargement of pulmonary atrium with oval dacron patch

(Figure 3). In all reoperations we have routinely enlarged the pulmonary venous atrium by inserting an oval-shape dacron patch (Figure 4). Prior to releasing the aortic cross-clamp, an aortic needle vent is inserted for the evacuation of air. The heart is then fibrillated during closure of the pulmonary venous atrium to ensure complete evacuation of air from the right ventricle. The vent is then withdrawn and the heart fibrillated. Cardiopulmonary bypass is discontinued in the usual manner.

Repair or replacement of the tricuspid valve is also simplified by this approach. Evacuation of air is carried out by the needle vent and the right ventricular vent. Cardiac activity usually begins spontaneously but defibrillation, if necessary, is not difficult. Exposure of intracardiac pathways is excellent without the need for intracardiac retractors. Postoperative bleeding has not been a major problem because of the minimal dissection used with this approach.

48

Management of transposition of the great arteries with left ventricular outflow tract obstruction

R. J. SZARNICKI

A systolic pressure gradient across the left ventricular outflow tract in transposition of the great arteries (TGA) is a common finding. In the majority of cases, this can be explained on the basis of high flow across this region.

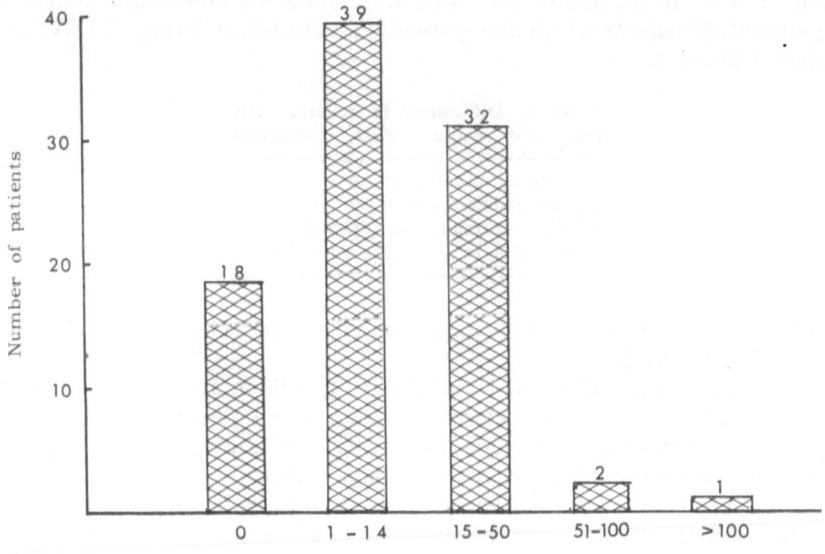

Systolic left ventricular to pulmonary artery gradient (mmHg)

Figure 1 Left ventricular to pulmonary artery gradient in 92 cases of simple TGA transposition of the great arteries

With interatrial redirection of venous return (the Mustard operation) this gradient is usually abolished.

Figure 1 shows the range of left ventricular outflow tract obstruction (LVOTO) gradients encountered in 92 patients with simple TGA. Over 96% of these patients had gradients less than 50 mmHg.

There are, however, well-recognized anatomic abnormalities which produce obstruction to the left ventricular ejection. These occurred in 18 out of 368 patients (or 5% of the total) who had the Mustard operation for TGA between 1965 and 1975. Six distinct types of anatomic obstruction have been described (Table 1). In these patients, pressure gradients ranged from 30 to 220 mmHg.

Table 1 Anatomic causes of left ventricular outflow tract obstruction in simple transposition of the great arteries

1. Subpulmonary fibrous ring or membrane
2. Anomalous attachment of mitral apparatus
3. Diffuse narrowing of subpulmonary conus
4. Bulging of muscular left ventricular septum
5. Aneurysm of the membranous ventricular septum
6. Pulmonary valvular or supravalvular stenosis

Relief of anatomical obstruction to LVOTO by a direct approach either through the pulmonary artery or mitral valve can be difficult, if not impossible. Risk of injury to the mitral valve apparatus, and/or the conduction system is significant. Situations which may present difficulties in relieving LVOTO are listed in Table 2.

Table 2 Difficulties in relieving left ventricular outflow tract obstruction

1. Diffuse muscular stenosis
2. Inaccessible due to posterior position
3. Major coronary artery branches
4. Mitral valve apparatus is involved

Our current policy in the management of simple TGA with LVOTO is outlined in Figure 2.

All children with TGA and LVOTO have a balloon atrial septostomy at the time of initial cardiac catheterization. At 8–12 months of age a Mustard operation is performed, and relief of the LVOTO is attempted. Those with a residual gradient are managed in one of three ways.

Those who have a left ventricular pressure which is less than or equal to systemic pressure with a near normal pulmonary artery pressure generally do well and are followed up. Those who have equal ventricular pressures at the completion of the Mustard operation with normal pulmonary artery pressure are followed up as well. If in the follow-up period there is evidence of clinical deterioration, progression of the LVOTO, a left ventricle to pulmonary artery conduit would be considered.

In the last group who have either systemic or suprasystemic pressures in the left ventricle with a low pulmonary artery pressure at the time of completion of the Mustard operation, a left ventricle to pulmonary artery conduit is inserted at that time.

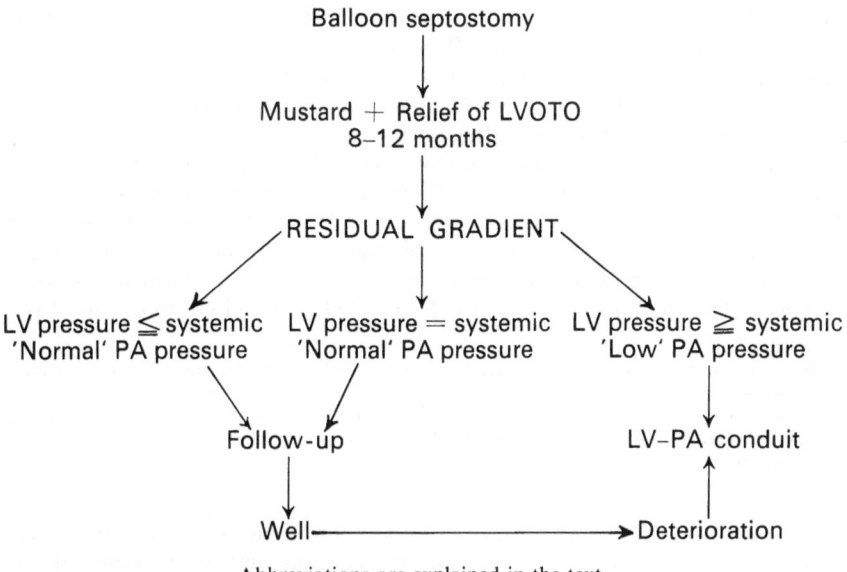

Abbreviations are explained in the text

Figure 2 Transposition of the great arteries and left ventricular outflow tract obstruction—management policy

Although progression of the left ventricle to pulmonary artery gradient has been observed in patients who were recatheterized prior to the Mustard operation, this has not been observed in patients after redirection of venous return, except in one patient who had an emergency Mustard operation at 3 days of age. At recatheterization, suprasystemic pressures were noted in the left ventricle, and two muscular ventricular septal defects were noted. In spite of this the patient remains well. Another operation to relieve this gradient may prove necessary in the future.

In our experience, we have encountered three patients in whom the left ventricular pressure was suprasystemic with a low pulmonary artery pressure at completion of the the Mustard operation. Resection of the obstructing lesions was impossible. In this group a left ventricle to pulmonary artery conduit was used. Our first experience with this problem occurred in a child with TGA, a small restrictive ventricular septal defect and acquired pulmonary atresia following a previous pulmonary artery band. A Blalock–Taussig shunt was necessary to maintain pulmonary blood flow. The left ventricle to pulmonary artery pressure gradient was 220 mmHg. At operation a valveless conduit was inserted from the left ventricle to pulmonary artery because the Hancock prosthesis was not available at that time. The small ventricular septal defect was left open because of concern regarding persistent elevation of left ventricular pressures.

The distal anastomosis of the conduit was created to the right of the aorta with the right pulmonary artery because of previous adhesions in the region of the Blalock anastomosis. In this position the conduit of necessity traverses the mediastinum beneath the sternum increasing the risk of compression. We would currently make every effort to avoid this position. This child's postoperative course was complicated by a low cardiac output which required prolonged inotropic support. He ultimately recovered completely and remains well 2 years 9 months after operation[1].

A few critical technical points deserve mention regarding insertion of such a conduit. While making the left ventriculotomy extreme care must be taken to avoid injury to major coronary arteries and the papillary muscles of the mitral valve. The pericardium and pleura are routinely opened widely posterior to the phrenic nerve to allow posterior displacement of the conduit (Table 3). The thymus is now routinely resected to avoid compression of the

Table 3 Technical points during insertion of left ventricular to pulmonary artery conduit

1. Avoid coronary arteries and papillary muscles of mitral valve during ventriculotomy
2. Open pericardium and pleura widely posterior to phrenic nerve
3. Thymectomy

distal anastomosis. A postoperative angiogram done 4 months postoperatively in our patient who had a valveless conduit inserted demonstrates a gradual increase in pressure throughout the body of the conduit with no abrupt pressure gradients. In spite of this excellent result we recommend the use of a valved conduit in this position to avoid the potential postoperative problems related to the pulmonary insufficiency.

To date we have used the left ventricle to pulmonary artery conduit in three patients, with one death.

Reference

1. Singh, A. K., Stark, J. and Taylor, J. F. N., (1976). Left ventricle to pulmonary artery conduit in treatment of transposition of the great arteries, restrictive ventricular septal defect and acquired pulmonary atresia. *Br. Heart J.*, **38**, 1213

49
Rastelli operation

M. R. DE LEVAL

The operation proposed by Rastelli in 1969[1] for patients with transposition of the great arteries (TGA), ventricular septal defect (VSD) and left ventricular outflow tract obstruction (LVOTO) has tremendously improved the prognosis for those patients. The poor results obtained in the past were mainly related to the difficulties in relieving the LVOTO. The principle of the operation consists of redirecting the blood at ventricular level, through the VSD, in such a way that the left ventricle empties into the aorta and the right ventricle empties into the pulmonary artery through an extracardiac valved conduit. In this way, there is a physiological and anatomical correction, since the ventricular arterial discordance is also dealt with.

INDICATIONS FOR OPERATION

If an infant with TGA + VSD + LVOTO presents with serious cyanosis or cyanotic spells, our present policy is still to perform a systemic to pulmonary artery shunt and delay the Rastelli operation until the patient is 3–4 years of age. This policy is based on the fact that palliative surgery is very helpful in that condition for small children, on the fact that the results of Rastelli operation in the young age group have been less satisfactory than in older patients and also on the fact that an adult-sized conduit can be inserted when the patient is 3–4 years of age.

SURGICAL TECHNIQUE

We perform the Rastelli operation with conventional cardiopulmonary bypass, moderate hypothermia and intermittent cross-clamping of the aorta. In many patients, the first step in the operation consists of dealing with a previous systemic to pulmonary anastomosis. Most patients have an atrial septal defect (natural or created) which needs closure. Next, a longitudinal ventriculotomy is performed on the right ventricle. The direction of the incision points towards the main pulmonary artery which usually lies to the left of the aorta (d-TGA). The VSD is then inspected. If its diameter is smaller than the diameter of the aortic annulus, it is enlarged to prevent any obstruction from the left ventricle to the aorta. A large patch of dacron velour is then used to build the intraventricular tunnel, redirecting the blood from the left ventricle to the aorta. Before this, we usually try to approximate the cusps of the pulmonary valve through the VSD if they are accessible. The main pulmonary artery is then doubly ligated and the distal anastomosis of a valved conduit (homograft or heterograft) to the pulmonary artery is performed. Finally, the valved conduit is anastomosed to the right ventricle.

RESULTS

Between July 1971 and July 1976, we operated upon 25 patients. Their ages ranged from 2 to 14 years (mean 9.3 years). There were four hospital deaths (16%), and four late deaths. One patient died at reoperation for residual VSD, another died in biventricular failure 11 weeks after reoperation for a residual VSD. Two sudden deaths remained unexplained 5 and 13 months respectively postoperatively. The overall mortality was, therefore, 32%–which is fairly similar to the recently reported mortality for 59 patients operated upon at the Mayo Clinic between 1968 and 1975[2]. In that group, there were 11 early deaths and five late deaths, which accounts for an overall mortality of 28%.

References

1. Rastelli, G. C. (1969). A new approach to 'anatomic' repair of transposition of the great arteries. *Mayo Clin. Proc.*, **44**, 1
2. Marcelletti, C., Mair, D. D., McGoon, D. C., Wallace, R. B. and Danielson, G. K. (1976). The Rastelli operation for transposition of the great arteries. Early and late results. *J. Thoracic Cardiovasc. Surg.*, **72**, 427

50
Atrial inversion for transposition of the great arteries using an intra-atrial dacron baffle: surgical technique and results

H. OELERT

From 1974 until March 1977 atrial inversion for transposition of the great arteries (TGA) was performed 103 times; 40% of the children were under 1 year of age, the youngest being 6 days old. In this child TGA was complicated by an intact atrial septum and a large patent ductus arteriosus (PDA) draining into the left pulmonary artery. Because of azygos continuation with absence of the inferior vena cava, atrial septostomy could not be performed. This child, and 13 similar infants under 6 months of age therefore underwent emergency total correction.

Out of the 103 patients, 60 had simple transposition with an intact ventricular septum (see Table 1). In eight patients a PDA was also present and in another eight there was left ventricular outflow tract obstruction (LVOTO); 13 patients had large but otherwise uncomplicated VSDs, while in eight cases VSDs were associated with severe pulmonary vascular disease, and atrial inversion was the only procedure done. A VSD was associated with LVOTO in six patients: two had a banded pulmonary artery, one had valvular and three subvalvular pulmonary stenosis. Subvalvular obstruction of the left ventricular outflow tract was considered a contra-indication to atrial inversion alone when the systolic pressure gradient exceeded 60 mmHg.

Our surgical technique followed Mustard's principles. Instead of pericardium a weave-knit dacron vascular prosthesis was used in all cases and was considered superior to other prosthetic material because of its pliability, its natural bend and absence of fuzzing on the edges. The material makes intra-operative handling easy and does not tend to fold.

The graft is tailored like an eye-mask (Figure 1). As a point of technical detail we consider it important to anchor the apex of the convexity of the patch not exactly opposite the deepest point of its concavity but rather

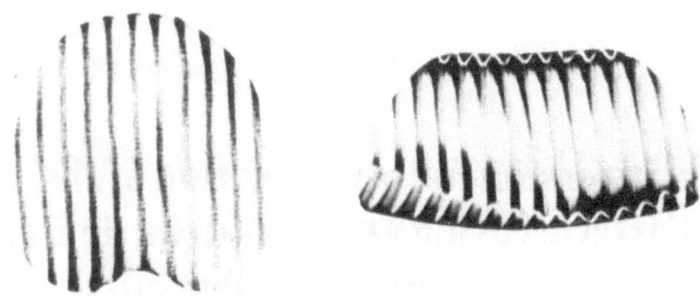

Figure 1 Shape of the dacron prosthesis used for atrial inversion in transposition of the great arteries (TGA). Posterior (left pulmonary venous) border. Anterior (interatrial septal) border

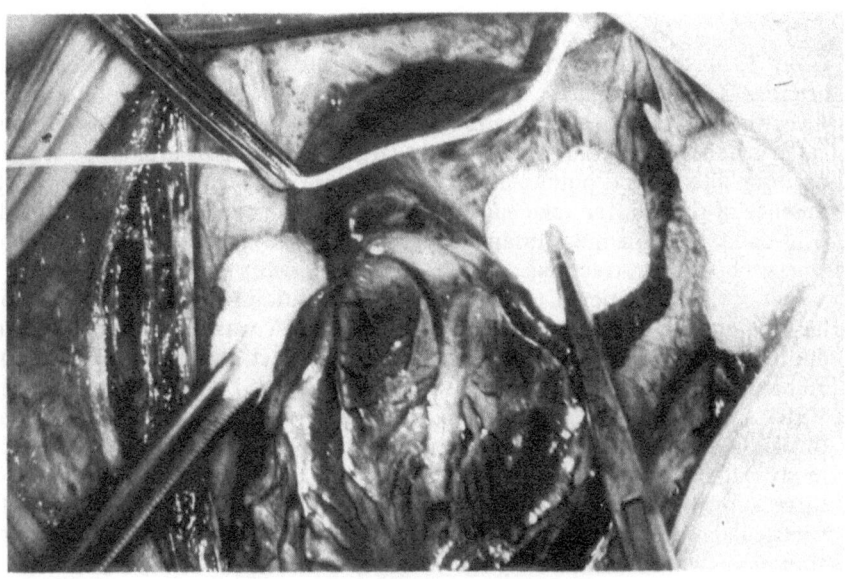

Figure 2 Line of the atrial incision going across the interatrial groove down into the right upper pulmonary vein

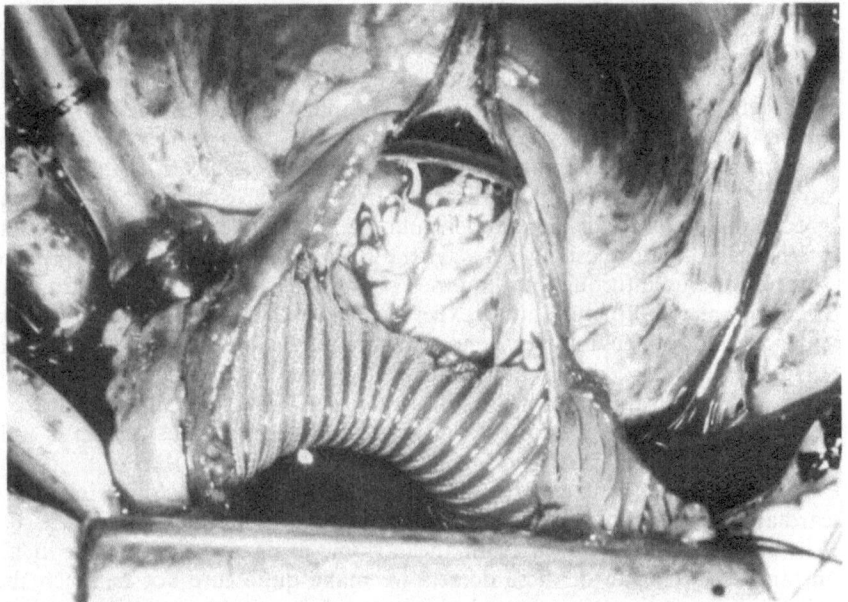

Figure 3 The intra-atrial dacron baffle after its complete insertion

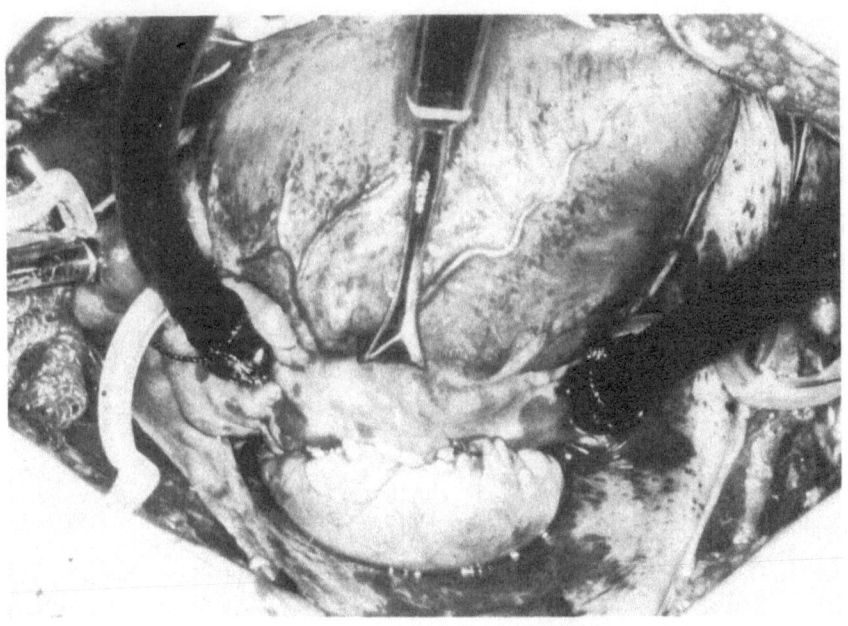

Figure 4 Operative view of the pulmonary venous atrium which has been enlarged with a pericardial patch. Notice the intact atrial wall close to the atrioventricular sulcus

some-what cephaled in agreement with the more superior position of the pulmonary venous inflow route. The coronary sinus usually was not slit and therefore remained on the pulmonary venous side. Only in two cases with persistent left superior vena cava the coronary sinus was incised and its blood directed into the systemic venous channel.

With respect to enlargement of the pulmonary venous atrium an oblique atriotomy is done from a point near the tricuspid valve across the interatrial groove directly into the right upper pulmonary vein (Figure 2). For insertion of the dacron prosthesis in between the two atria, continuous 5-O prolene sutures were used throughout. Figure 3 shows the baffle after its insertion has been completed. In our initial experience we never used pericardium for enlargement of the pulmonary venous atrium but have done so routinely since 1976—in the last 51 patients. An operative view of the pericardial patch anchored within the biatrial incision is given in Figure 4. On the postoperative chest X-ray (Figure 5) the enlarged pulmonary venous atrium is well outlined on the right heart side.

When an open ductus arteriosus was present, it was closed intrapericardially by ligature or more simply by a large haemoclip (Figure 6). All VSDs could be closed from the atrium, using a dacron patch in all instances. In closure of these defects we make quite sure not to touch the tricuspid annulus, rather taking the limbus underneath the ring in order not to produce tricuspid insufficiency. There has been neither complete heart block

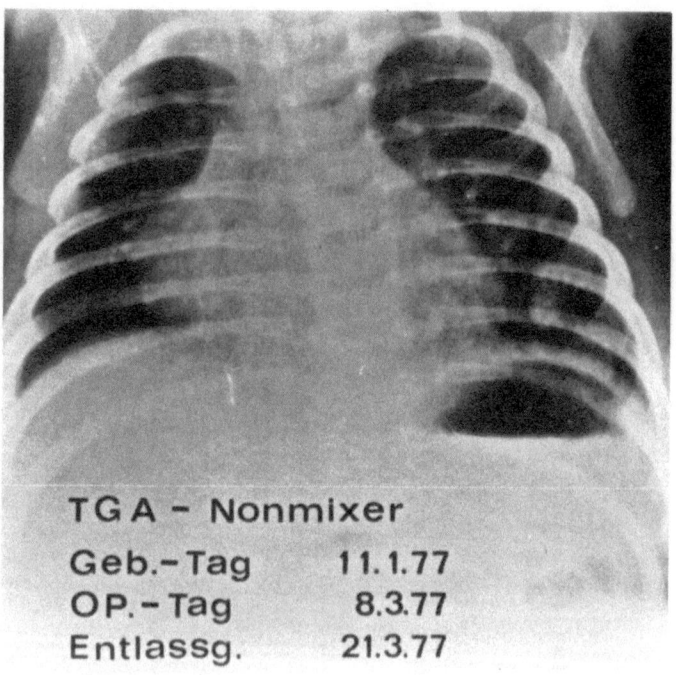

Figure 5   Postoperative chest X-ray after the Mustard operation for TGA with enlargement of the pulmonary venous atrium. Notice the atrial bulge on the right heart side

nor recurrence of VSD or tricuspid incompetence in the early or late post-operative period. LVOTO of significant degree was treated by pulmonary valvotomy in one case or by excision of the subvalvular stenosis through the pulmonary artery or, more recently, through the left atrium and the retracted mitral valve in the others.

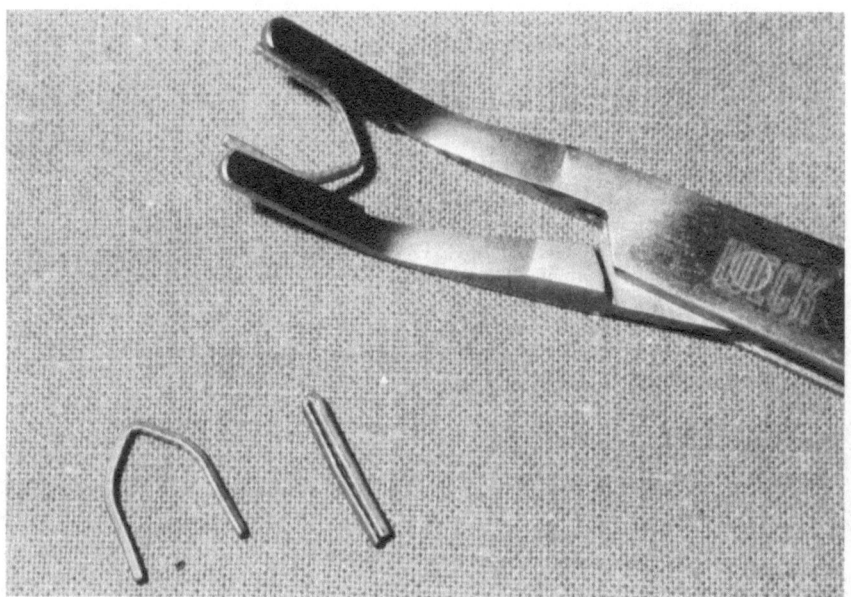

Figure 6   Haemoclips for duct closure via a median sternotomy incision[1]

All operations were performed using extracorporeal circulation and moderate hypothermia of 28 °C. Flow of 2.4 l/m² was reduced occasionally when indicated. Circulatory arrest under deep hypothermia was not considered advantageous or necessary. The aorta was cross-clamped in two periods for performing the posterior and superior suture line of the intracardiac baffle. The heart lung machine was filled with albumin in glucose solution with 0.5 litre of blood added in patients under 8 kg.

Among the 68 children with TGA and intact ventricular septum, and in the 13 cases with a large but otherwise uncomplicated VSD there were no hospital deaths (Table 1). One of eight patients died after palliative atrial inversion in progressive cyanosis and acute right heart failure.

On the other hand, among the 14 patients with LVOTO three died because of incomplete release of the narrowing at the time of operation. In one the ventricular septum was intact, in the other two a large VSD or multiple VSDs were present. All of these patients were over 1 year of age. The overall mortality was 4% in all 103 patients.

In the more recent series, from the beginning of 1976, when primary enlargement of the pulmonary venous atrium was included in every patient undergoing the Mustard procedure, only one of 51 patients did not survive

Table 1 Solitus concordant TGA with and without associated anomalies: diagnoses and early results in 103 patients operated on between 1974 and March 1977

	Infants	Children	Total	Early deaths
TGA, intact VS	26	34	60	—
TGA, intact VS, PDA	5	3	8	—
TGA, intact VS, SPS	2	6	8	1
TGA, VSD	7	6	13	—
TGA, VSD, SPS (intracardiac repair)	—	6	6	2
TGA, VSD, PVD (palliative Mustard)	—	8	8	1
TOTAL	40	63	103	4

TGA = transposition of the great arteries; VS = ventricular septum; VSD = ventricular septal defect; PDA = patent ductus arteriosus; SPS = subvalvular pulmonary stenosis; PVD = pulmonary vascular disease

Table 2 Solitus concordant TGA with and without associated anomalies: diagnoses and early results in 51 patients operated on between 1976 and March 1977

	Infants	Children	Total	Early deaths
TGA, intact VS	7	17	24	—
TGA, intact VS, PDA	4	2	6	—
TGA, intact VS, SPS	2	5	7	—
TGA, VSD	6	2	8	—
TGA, VSD, SPS (intracardiac repair)	—	3	3	1
TGA, VSD, PVD (palliative Mustard)	—	3	3	—
TOTAL	19	32	51	1

Abbreviations as in Table 1

operation (Table 2). In this child, who has had TGA, VSD and LVOTO, the mitral valve was injured during subpulmonary muscular resection through the pulmonary artery and had to be replaced.

During the follow-up period, three infants died of pulmonary venous channel obstruction not recognized in outside hospitals, six patients were reoperated upon successfully, four because of pulmonary venous obstruction, two because of pulmonary venous and superior vena cava (SVC) obstruction. The reoperation consisted of inserting a large woven dacron patch (Figure 7, a–c) into the pulmonary venous channel and in two cases a piece of weave-knit dacron into the baffle. Significantly, all these children had their Mustard operation in the first 6 months of life, and in none had an atrioplasty been performed during primary repair. For facilitating reoperation a right anterior approach was used and in cases of pulmonary venous obstruction alone only the SVC was intubated with a single right-angled catheter, draining the entire

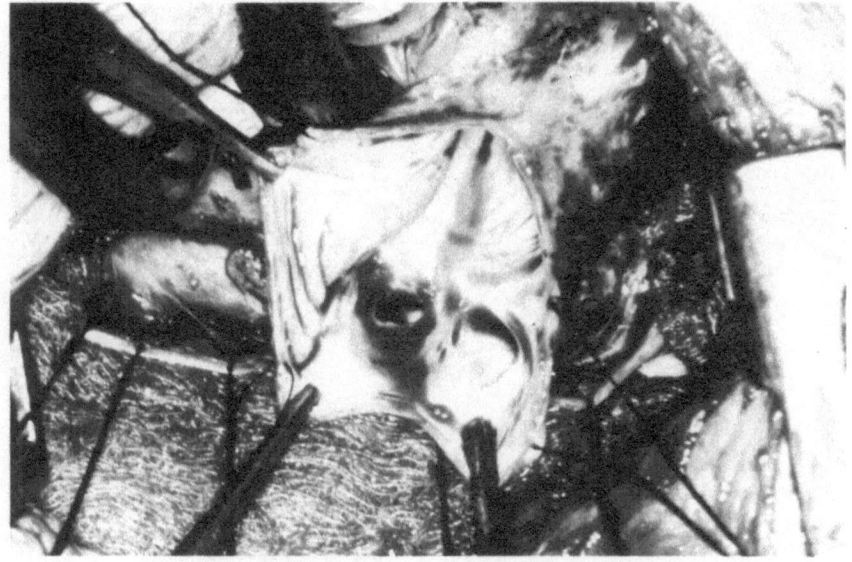

(a)

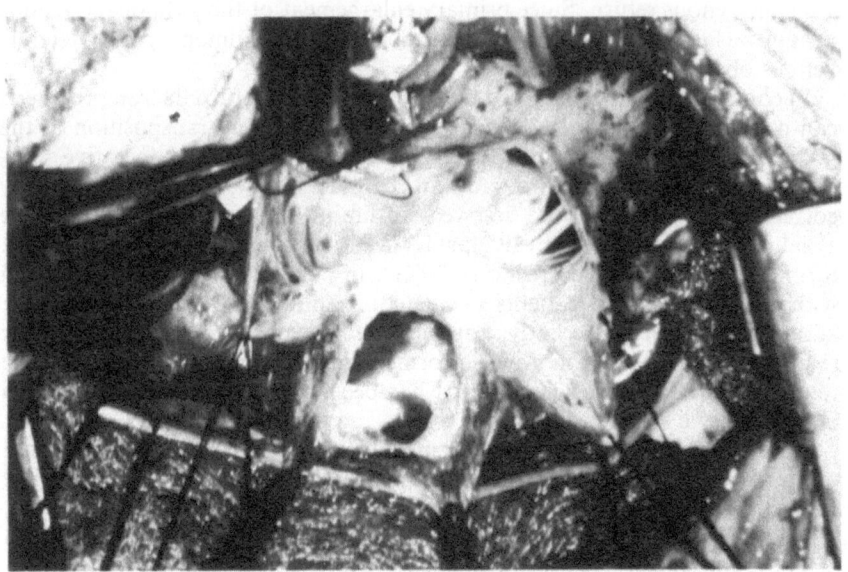

(b)

Figure 7 Late pulmonary venous obstruction after the Mustard operation for TGA without primary pulmonary venous atrioplasty; (a) operative view of the stenosis between both pulmonary venous atria; (b) enlarged opening between the proximal and distal pulmonary venous atrial chamber; (c) reconstruction of the pulmonary venous atrium by insertion of a large dacron prosthesis

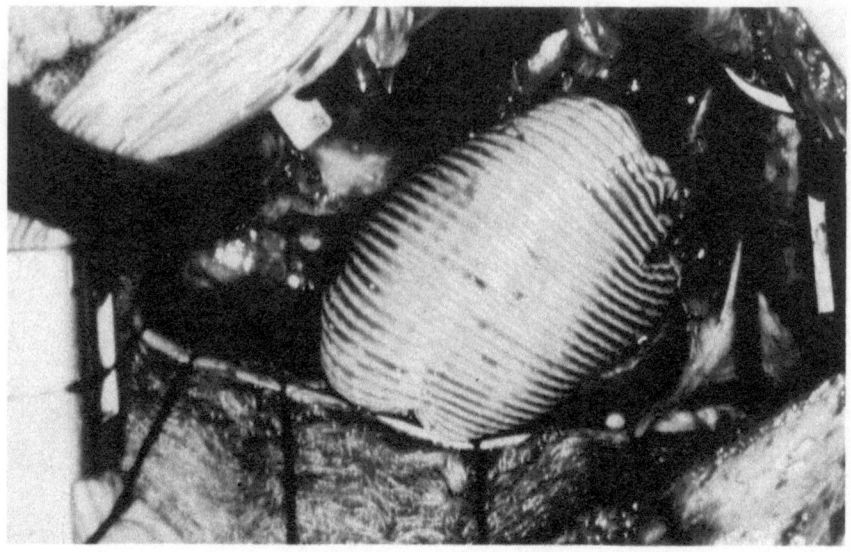

Figure 7   (c)

systemic venous return. Since primary enlargement of the pulmonary venous atrium was employed in the last 51 patients neither pulmonary nor systemic venous obstruction had occurred.

In conclusion, it may be stated that atrial inversion with a dacron prosthesis can now be done with a negligible hospital mortality in transposition of the great arteries with or without VSD. For reasons of simpler operative technique and possible narrowing of the cardiac inflow, we prefer to delay correction to the end of the first year of life in the presence of an effective atrial communication. Subvalvular LVOTO of significant degree poses a formidable obstacle to correction of TGA in our hands, and was associated with three deaths in 14 patients so treated, in spite of the fact that they were all older than 1 year. Recently, however, we have changed our technique for relief of LVOTO. This is now performed through the left atrium and the retracted mitral valve after the heart has been completely relaxed by means of cardioplegic solution[2].

Since late obstruction of one or more of the venous channels occurred primarily in babies operated upon as emergencies and only in those not receiving an atrioplasty which extends into the right upper pulmonary vein, this simple additional manoeuvre is considered mandatory in early correction of TGA, and since 1976 is now being used in all cases.

References

1. Oelert, H. and Frank, G. (1976). *Thoraxchir.*, **24**, 131
2. Oelert, H., Laprell, H., Piepenbrock, S., Luhmer, I., Kallfelz, H. C. and Borst, H. G. (1977). Emergency and non-emergency intra-atrial correction for transposition of the great arteries in 43 infants *Thoraxchir.*, **25**, 305

51
Transposition of the great arteries

J. F. N. TAYLOR

Transposition is the single most common cyanotic congenital heart lesion to present in early infancy. Here only the uncomplicated forms of transposition will be considered. Cyanosis is evident from the first day of life, if not from birth. At this time, this may be the only recognizable abnormality. During the neonatal period, murmurs may not be present or may be trivial. The second heart sound is always single, but this can be a difficult physical sign at this age. The chest X-ray and electrocardiogram in early life remain within normal limits. It will be several weeks before the expected cardiac enlargement and plethora are evident radiographically and-right ventricular hypertrophy electrocardiographically. The young infant becomes ill as hypoxaemia increases and acidaemia becomes progressively more severe. These are the physiological consequences of the deranged circulation whereby insufficient saturated blood from the pulmonary veins enters the systemic arterial circulation.

Treatment at this stage primarily consists of creating an adequate inter-atrial communication by balloon atrial septostomy[1]. This allows equal volumes of saturated pulmonary venous blood to reach the systemic arteries, and of desaturated blood from the venae cavae to enter the pulmonary circulation. A systemic arterial oxygen saturation of 60–65% is commonly achieved.

As these young infants are ill at the time of presentation and diagnosis, the degree of invasive investigation mandatory in the immediate evaluation of the cyanotic neonate or infant is kept to a minimum. It is the practice of this unit to perform a balloon atrial septostomy immediately the diagnosis of transposition is established without necessarily undertaking angiocardio-graphy. It is not necessary at this stage to define absolutely the presence or otherwise of a persistent ductus arteriosus or ventricular septal defect. Their presence at this time will not alter the immediate management, and of more importance is their continuing presence. Management in this unit necessitates complete investigation at 4–5 months of age, including detailed angiocardiography. At this time, knowledge of the pulmonary flow and pressure within the pulmonary artery will give an indication of the pulmonary vascular response to the disordered circulation and indicate how significant are the additional lesions, if present.

If there is no indication of a rising pulmonary vascular resistance, and the systemic arterial oxygen saturation remains satisfactory (not less than 60%), the Mustard operation is undertaken at 8–12 months of age. The age at which the operation is performed is reduced if cyanosis becomes progressively more severe. (Indeed if cyanosis is persistently severe after balloon atrial septostomy, then immediate reinvestigation proceeding to Mustard operation is indicated whatever the age or weight of the infant). If the pulmonary resistance is elevated, the Mustard operation is also performed with closure of the ventricular septal defect and persistent ductus arteriosus as indicated. These additional lesions may be left for correction at the time of the Mustard operation at 8–12 months of age, only if their presence does not cause an additional significant change in the haemodynamic status.

It is important to remember that the left ventricular pressure does not always reflect the pulmonary artery pressure. There is frequently a gradient from the left ventricle to pulmonary artery appearing at subvalvular level in an otherwise uncomplicated transposition. In most, the magnitude of the gradient is related to the magnitude of the pulmonary blood flow, and does not exceed 50 mmHg. Gradients greater than this, and some gradients less than 50 mmHg, are associated with recognizable angiocardiographic abnormalities of the left ventricular outflow. These include apposition of the anterior leaflet of the mitral valve with the interventricular septum in systole[2], excessive hypertrophy of the upper part of the interventricular septum, and fibrosis occurring as a ring or tunnel below the pulmonary valve (pulmonary valvular stenosis has not been observed in the absence of a ventricular septal defect). It is considered important to recognize the causes of a gradient between the left ventricle and pulmonary artery before undertaking the Mustard operation. Not all represent obstruction, or indeed restriction, of pulmonary flow. Any attempt at surgical intervention could damage the mitral valve apparatus or the conducting mechanism (particularly the left bundle). When true obstruction is present and remains severe (that is, there is at least systemic pressure in the left ventricle after the Mustard operation), consideration should be given to bypassing the obstruction with a valved conduit from the left ventricle to pulmonary artery[3].

References

1. Rashkind, W. J. and Miller, W. W. (1966). Creation of an atrial septal defect without thoracotomy: a palliative approach to complete transposition of the great arteries. *J. Am. Med. Assoc.*, **196**, 991
2. Silove, E. D. and Taylor, J. F. N. (1973). Angiographic and anatomical features of subvalvar left ventricular outflow obstruction in transposition of the great arteries. The possible role of the anterior mitral valve leaflet. *Ped. Radiol.*, **1**, 87
3. Singh, A. K., Stark, J. and Taylor, J. F. N. (1976). Left ventricle to pulmonary artery conduit in treatment of transposition of the great arteries, restrictive ventricular septal defect and acquired pulmonary atresia. *Br. Heart J.*, **38**, 1213

52

Diagnosis of double outlet right ventricle (DORV) by M-mode echocardiography

D. G. GIBSON

Double outlet right ventricle is one of a group of conditions in which relations between the great arteries, ventricles and atrioventricular valves may be abnormal. The way in which M-mode echocardiography can be used in the

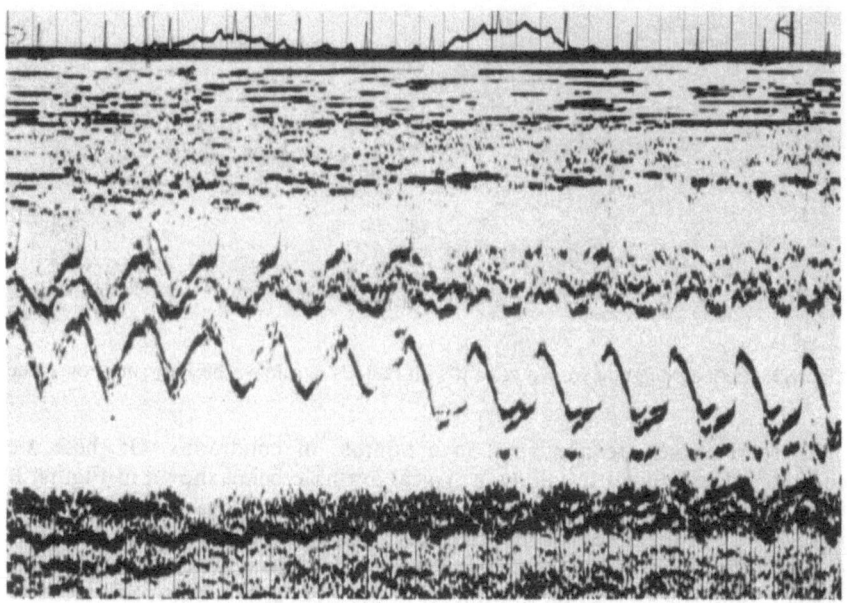

Figure 1 Slow sweep from aortic root to left ventricular cavity in a patient with classical d-transposition of the great arteries. Normal aortic–mitral and aortic–septal continuity is shown

diagnosis of such conditions is illustrated in Figure 1, a record taken from a patient with classical d-transposition. In this example, the transducer was initially directed at the aortic root, and during the course of the recording its angle was changed, so that the beam passed through the atrioventricular valves, and finally through the cavity of the posterior ventricle. In this way, it is possible to demonstrate that the anterior border of the posterior great artery is normally continuous with the interventricular septum, and the posterior border of the posterior great artery with the posterior atrioventricular valve. It is necessary to use the terms 'posterior great artery' and 'posterior atrioventricular valve' because it is not possible, on such a sweep, to distinguish between pulmonary artery and aorta or between mitral and tricuspid valves.

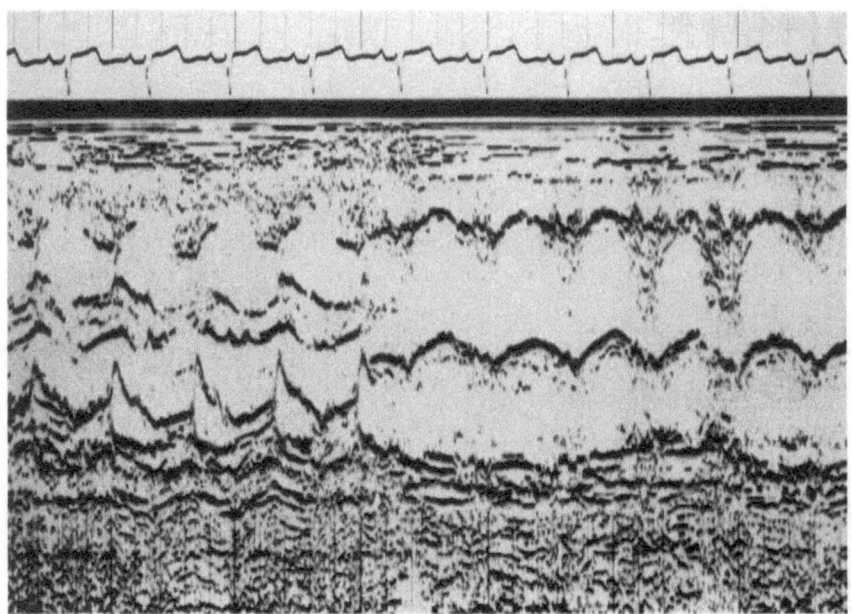

Figure 2   Echocardiogram from a patient with Fallot's tetralogy, showing aortic over-ride

These relations are abnormal in a number of conditions. Of these the commonest is Fallot's tetralogy, a typical example being shown in Figure 2. Here, the left-hand end of the record represents the ventricular cavity and the right-hand end the time that the transducer was directed towards the posterior great artery. It is apparent that in this patient the interventricular septum was not continuous with the anterior border of the great artery, but is considerably posterior to it, indicating the presence of over-ride. The mitral valve is continuous with the posterior border of the great artery, although it is unusual in being at a rather deeper level. The degree of over-ride could be quantified from such a record, but it is apparent that this differs at different times in the cardiac cycle, as during systole the aorta moves forwards and the interventricular septum backwards.

The echocardiogram of a patient with double outlet right ventricle and subaortic ventricular septal defect is shown in Figure 3. Here, there is clearcut discontinuity between the posterior atrioventricular (AV) valve and the posterior border of the great artery, which is, in fact, continuous with the anterior AV valve. Unfortunately, M-mode echocardiography is not a wholly reliable means of demonstrating the presence or absence of aortic–mitral

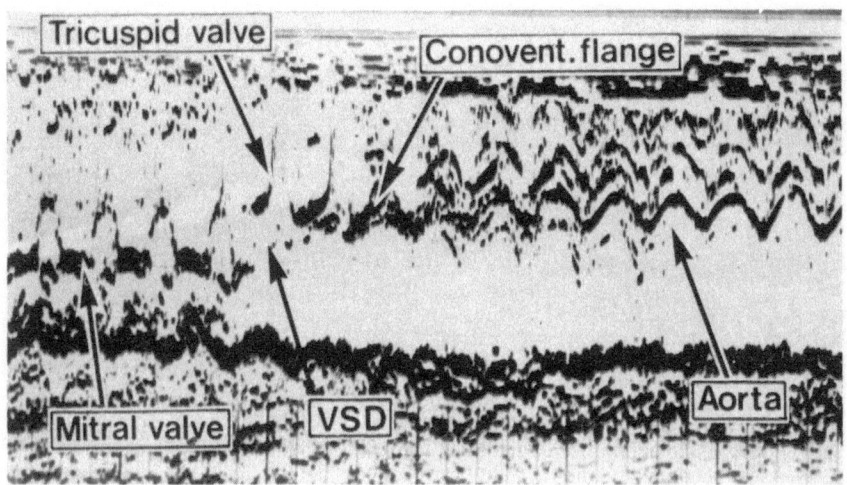

Figure 3 Echocardiogram from a patient with double outlet right ventricle, showing loss of continuity between posterior AV valve and posterior great artery, which is displaced forwards

discontinuity, and misleading results may appear, an example being given in Figure 4. This patient had a truncus arteriosus, whose relation to the septum is clearly apparent. In addition, there appears to be aortic–mitral discontinuity of a degree comparable to that in the patient illustrated in Figure 3. Similar appearances were present at angiography, and also at surgery. However, careful dissection at autopsy revealed that there was, in fact, fibrous continuity between the two.

Echocardiography can also be used to diagnose the origin of both great arteries from the posterior ventricle, an example being shown in Figure 5. Here, the mitral valve and posterior septum are seen on the left; and to the right, a larger anterior and a smaller posterior great artery arise directly from the posterior ventricle. In this particular patient, the posterior great artery was shown to be a pulmonary artery and the posterior ventricle was morphologically left.

It appears, therefore, that M-mode echocardiography may have value in such patients as a technique complementary to angiography in defining relations between the great arteries, interventricular septum and atrioventricular valves. However, like angiography, it is subject to limitations, some of which have been indicated.

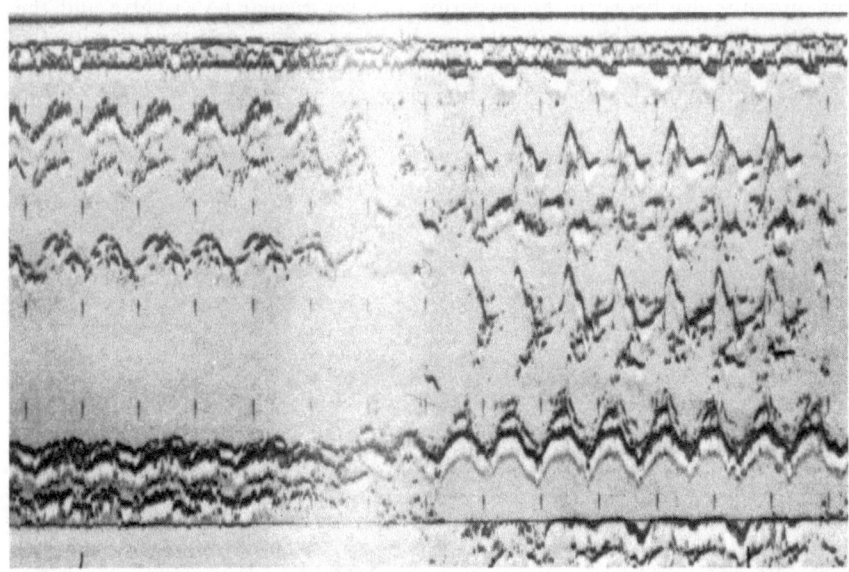

Figure 4 Echocardiogram from a patient with truncus arteriosus showing over-ride with apparent loss of continuity with the mitral valve

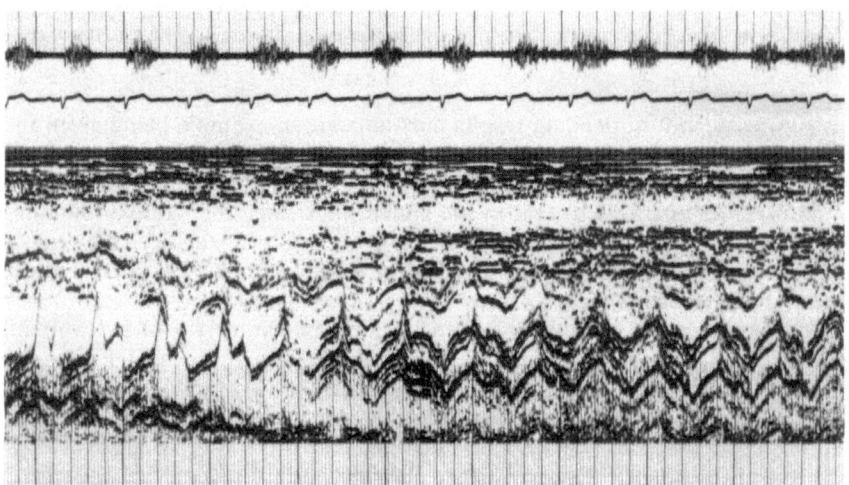

Figure 5 Echocardiogram from a patient with douole outlet left ventricle, showing both great arteries arising posterior to the interventricular septum

53
Arrythmias after the Mustard operation: a study of 24-h tape monitoring

M. TYNAN, D. S. REID AND A. GOODWIN

The frequency with which arrhythmias occur as a consequence of the Mustard operation for transposition of the great arteries (atrioventricular concordance with ventriculoarterial discordance) has given considerable cause for concern. The incidence varies widely from series to series[1-3] and appears to increase with increasing time after the operation[3]. All previous studies have relied on random standard ECGs and thus may not reflect the true incidence of arrhythmias. We therefore studied all the survivors of the Mustard operation, who were available to us, using 24-h tape monitoring of the ECG.

CASE MATERIAL AND METHODS

Twenty-four-hour tape recordings of the ECG were performed, on an outpatient basis in 21 survivors of the Mustard operation for transposition. The time which had elapsed after the operation was from 1 month to 9 years 11 months (mean 2 years 10 months). The operations had been performed in a variety of centres by a variety of surgeons so no attempt has been made to relate the results to surgical techniques. Prior to the Mustard operation, standard ECGs showed all patients to be in sinus rhythm, 24-h tapes confirmed this in eight patients but one showed atrioventricular Wenckebach which was related to digitalis toxicity and responded to cessation of digoxin treatment.

RESULTS

In six patients the standard ECG showed an arrhythmia (Table 1); in all cases this was confirmed on the 24-h tape. In three patients, however, the tape-recording revealed further abnormalities suggesting that the arrhythmia was of greater severity than had been suspected. Thus, patient 4 had evidence of sinus node disease with asystolic episodes of up to 3½ s, patient 5 had evidence of atrioventricular conduction abnormalities in addition to his junctional rhythm, and in patient 6 the sinus node disease was found to be associated with heart rates of 40 at times. The findings in patients 4 and 5 explained episodes of syncope which both had reported. In both patients permanent pacemakers were implanted as a result of these investigations.

Table 1   Patients with known arrhythmias

Patient	Standard ECG	24-h Tape
1	Atrial flutter with episodes of junctional rhythm	As for the standard ECG
2	Wandering pacemaker	As for the standard ECG
3	Complete heart block	As for the standard ECG
4	Paroxysmal supraventricular tachycardia	Paroxysmal supraventricular tachycardia, sinus bradycardia with asystole of up to 3½ s duration
5	Junctional rhythm	Junctional rhythm with idioventricular escape. Lowest heart rate recorded—34 beats/min
6	Sinus bradycardia	Sinus bradycardia, 2:1 sinoatrial block, slowest heart rate recorded 40 beats/min

In four patients, whose standard ECGs showed sinus rhythm, the 24-h tape revealed an unsuspected arrhythmia. These are listed in Table 2. At the present time these arrhythmias have not required treatment but in cases 8, 9 and 10 the recording of heart rates of less than 45 beats/min occurring at times identifies these patients as being at risk.

Table 2   Arrhythmias found on the 24-h tape in patients with sinus rhythm on the standard ECG

Patient	
7	Atrioventricular Wenckebach
8	Sinus bradycardia. Lowest recorded heart rate—34 beats/min
9	SA block with episodes of atrioventricular dissociation. Lowest recorded heart rate—43 beats/min
10	Sinus bradycardia, 2:1 Sinoatrial block. Lowest recorded heart rate 37 beats/min

Finally, in two further patients, apparently in sinus rhythm, the 24-h tape showed one to have frequent ventricular premature contractions and the other to have a minor degree of sinus slowing with junctional escapes.

CONCLUSION

In a series of 21 patients who had had the Mustard operation for transposition, 24-h tape monitoring of the ECG revealed definite arrhythmias in four out of 15 patients thought to be in sinus rhythm, and a further two were found to have minor rhythm disturbances which could presage serious arrhythmias but may well be within the limits of normality[4,5]. When considering the incidence of arrhythmias occurring as a consequence of the Mustard operation, 24-h tape monitoring of the ECG provides information which is not available on random standard ECGs alone. No statement can be made regarding the incidence of arrhythmias without the use of this technique. However the method is of probably greater clinical importance in assessing the severity of both unsuspected and known arrhythmias.

References

1. Aberdeen, E. (1971). Correction of uncomplicated cases of transposition of the great arteries. *Brit. Heart J.*, **33**, Supplement 66–68
2. Ebert, P. A., Gay, W. A. and Engle, M. A. (1974). Correction of transposition of the great arteries: Relationship of the coronary sinus and post-operative arrythmias. *Ann. Surg.*, **180**, 433
3. El-Said, G., Rosenberg, H. S., Mullins, C. E., Hallman, G. L., Cooley, D. A. and McNamara, D. G. (1972). Dysrhythmias after Mustard's operation for transposition of the great arteries. *Am. J. Cardiol.*, **30**, 526
4. Clarke, J. M., Hamer, J., Skelton, J. R., Taylor, S. and Venning G. R. (1976). The rhythm of the normal heart. *Lancet*, **ii**, 508
5. Raftery, E. B. and Cashman, P. M. M. (1976) Longterm recording of the electrocardiogram in a normal population. *Postgrad. Med. J.*, **52**, Suppl. 7, 32

Section IX
Complicated atrioseptal defects

54
Complicated atrioseptal defects

Compiled by Sally P. Allwork

---

(1) THE ANATOMY OF THE ATRIA *S. P. Allwork*

The atria are readily recognized by their auricles, which are an almost infallible guide to the morphology of the chamber (Figure 1). The right auricle is somewhat triangular or 'tongue'-shaped with a large os which is continuous with the atrial cavity. It is thin-walled and has pectinate muscles when viewed from within. The left auricle, by contrast, is by its eponym, ear-shaped, but finger-like describes it rather more accurately. It has a small os which separates it from the body of the left atrium. It too has pectinate muscles, denoting its developmental origin, like the right auricle, from the primitive heart tube. The auricles are the sole, recognizable survivors, as it were, of the primitive atrium.

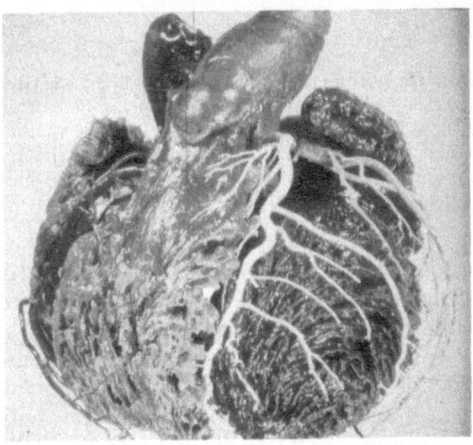

Figure 1   A cast of a normal adult heart (frontal view). The right auricle is triangular in shape, while the left is 'ear'- or 'finger'-shaped

The right atrium (Figure 2) is a thin-walled chamber whose anterior aspect is trabeculated. It receives the superior vena cava superiorly. A shallow depression, the sulcus terminalis, is usually distinguishable on the outside of the atrium between the superior vena cava and the right auricle. This sulcus is seen inside the cavity as the crista terminalis separating the trabeculated anterior part from the smooth-walled posterior part of the atrium derived from the sinus venosus and the endocardial cushions. The chamber receives numerous venae cordae minimae. The inferior vena cava enters the right atrium on its diaphragmatic surface. Its opening is guarded by a low rim of valve tissue, the Eustachian valve, which is continued upwards towards the

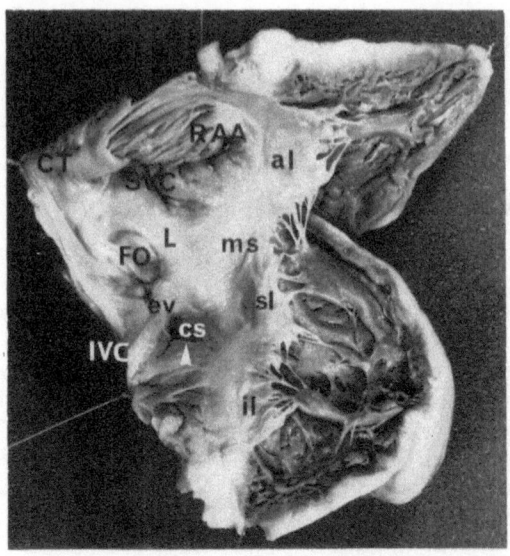

Figure 2   The anatomy of the normal right atrium. The right auricle (RAA) is trabeculated, and the crista terminalis (CT) separates it from the smooth-walled atrium. The fossa ovalis (FO) is bounded anteriorly by the limbus fossa ovalis (L). The inferior vena cava (IVC) enters the chamber on its diaphragmatic aspect and is guarded by the Eustachian valve (ev). The coronary sinus (cs) and its valve are arrowed in white; MS = membranous septum; al, sl, and il are the leaflets of the tricuspid valve

opening of the coronary sinus. This vein, too, has a little valve, the Thebesian valve. The atrioventricular node lies in the small triangle (of Koch) formed by the tendon of Todaro, the coronary sinus and the tricuspid annulus. The tendon is not very easy to see in living subjects. Immediately above the Eustachian valve lies the thin fossa ovalis, and between this fossa and the tricuspid annulus is a conspicuous bar of muscle, the limbus fossa ovalis. The tricuspid leaflets are more or less divided into three discrete parts: the inferior, medial and superior leaflets. The atrioventricular part of the membranous septum lies on the atrial septum above the commissure of the inferior and septal leaflets.

The left atrium (Figure 3) is, compared with the right, a relatively featureless structure. It receives four pulmonary veins but it is devoid of a crista terminalis, has no venous valves, no venae cordae minimae and is not trabeculated. In most adults, even the valve of the foramen ovale is rather hard to see. However, in about 25 % of normal adults, the foramen ovale is probe-patent. The posterior wall of the chamber is derived from the incorporation of the primitive pulmonary veins into the chamber, and the endocardial cushions.

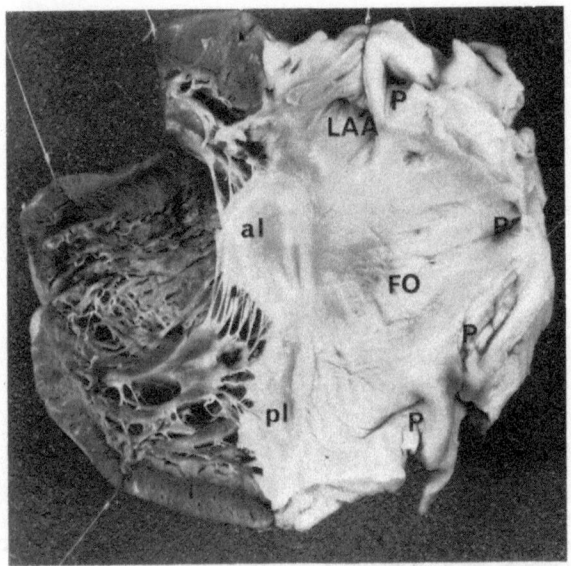

Figure 3 The left atrium is relatively featureless, compared with the right. It receives four pulmonary veins (P) posteriorly, the fossa ovalis (FO) is not always well seen. The left auricle (LAA) has a small os separating it from the left atrium; al, pl = anterior and posterior mitral leaflets

(2) THE DIAGNOSIS OF ATRIAL SEPTAL DEFECTS AND VENOUS ANOMALIES D. H. Fitchett

Accurate diagnosis of atrial septal defects and venous anomalies is necessary even today when hypothermia is so rarely utilized. The diagnosis may influence the surgeon's choice of incision and he should have available as much information as will aid him in planning the operation.

Preoperative investigations must distinguish the diagnoses of ostium secundum atrial septal defect (ASD), ostium primum ASD, single atrium, and anomalous pulmonary venous drainage, as well as associated intra-cardiac anomalies (for example, in ostium secundum ASD: moderate pulmonary stenosis 15 %, mitral stenosis 7 %, anomalous pulmonary veins 11 %[1]).

The physical signs of a left-to-right shunt at atrial level are similar in all defects; however the presence of cyanosis must suggest total venous mixing (i.e. single atrium or total anomalous pulmonary venous drainage), and a pansystolic murmur the atrioventricular canal defect. Extracardiac anomalies such as seen in the Ellis–van Creufeld syndrome (chondrodysplasia and polydactyly) may be associated with a single atrium.

The plain posteroanterior chest X-ray sometimes indicates the diagnosis of anomalous pulmonary venous connection, particularly in the supracardiac form of total anomalous pulmonary drainage and anomalous venous drainage of the right lower lobe (scimitar syndrome) (Figures 4, 5a and b).

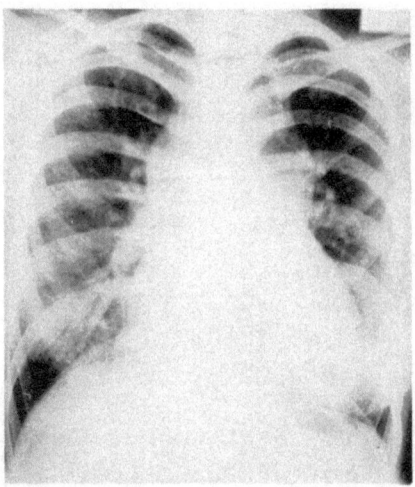

Figure 4 Anteroposterior chest X-ray of an adult woman with supracardiac totally anomalous pulmonary venous connection

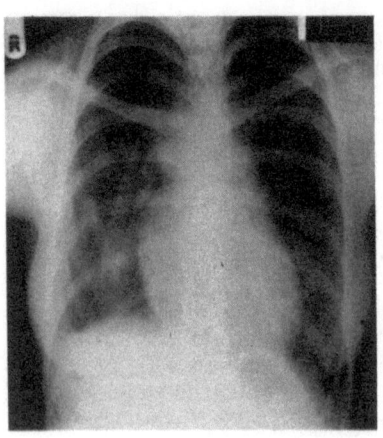 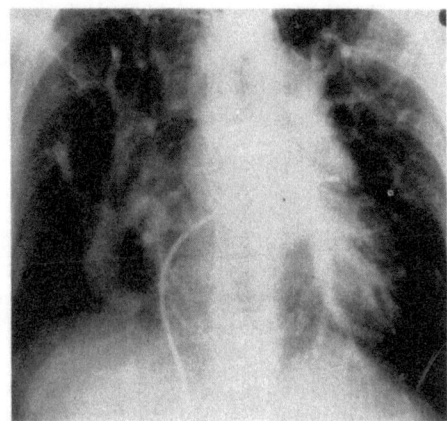

Figure 5a Anteroposterior chest X-ray of an adult with hemi-anomalous pulmonary venous connection to the inferior vena cava (scimitar syndrome); **5b** venous phase of a pulmonary arteriogram in the same patient demonstrates the right pulmonary vein entering the inferior vena cava above the diaphragm

An electrocardiogram is the most specific means of differentiating the uncomplicated ostium primum ASD from the ostium secundum defect. In 95% of ostium secundum defects the mean frontal QRS vector is between 0 and +180° (Figure 6) whereas about the same proportion of ostium primum defects have characteristic left axis deviation (Figure 7). Cardiac catheterization is probably only indicated when a diagnosis other than a 'simple' ostium secundum ASD is suspected on clinical, radiological, and electrocardiographic grounds. From the position of the catheter across the defect, and the site at which a step-up in oxygen saturation occurs, it may be

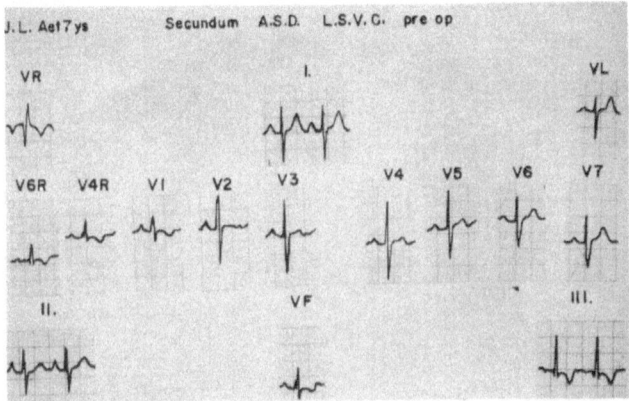

Figure 6 The characteristic electrocardiogram of a 7-year-old child with a secundum atrial septal defect. Note the right axis deviation and partial right bundle branch block

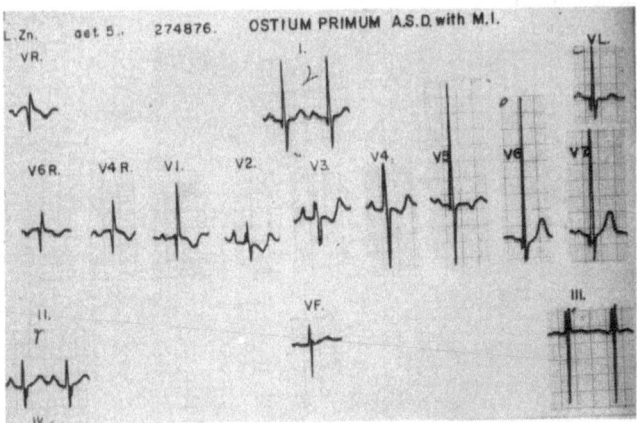

Figure 7 The electrocardiogram in a 5-year-old with an ostium primum atrial septal defect and associated mitral regurgitation. In contrast to Figure 6 note the left axis deviation and left ventricular hypertrophy

possible to determine the type of atrial septal defect (i.e. sinus venosus ostium secundum, ostium primum or inferior vena cava). The presence of a persistent left superior vena cava may be suspected and then sought should the catheter not enter the brachiocephalic vein.

A left ventricular angiogram in the 15° right anterior oblique projection may demonstrate an endocardial cushion defect with the characteristic deformity of the outflow tract seen during diastole (Figure 8) and mitral regurgitation and a cleft in the mitral valve in systole (Figure 9). A pulmonary arteriogram with visualization of the venous phase will opacify anomalous pulmonary veins (see, for example, Figure 5b) which can be precisely located by injecting contrast into them.

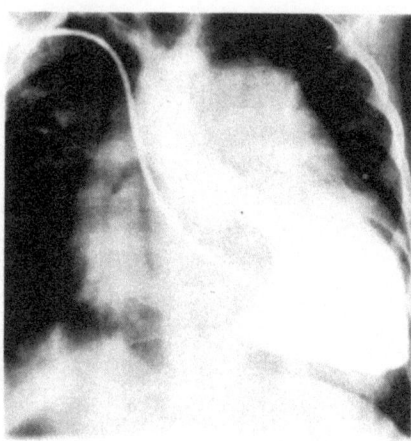

Figure 8 Anteroposterior left ventricular angiogram in atrioventricular canal defect (diastolic frame). Note the left ventricular outflow tract is elongated and displaced superiorly (gooseneck deformity)

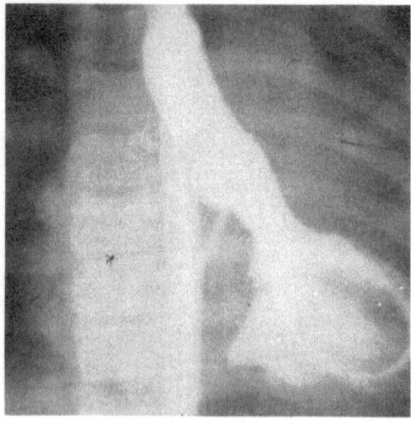

Figure 9 Anteroposterior left ventricular angiogram cardiogram in atrioventricular canal defect. Note that the cleft mitral valve is well seen during systole

Despite all these aids to diagnosis the most specific obstructions in re-
solving the differential diagnosis are arterial desaturation and the electrocardiogram (Table 1)[2]. However, a number of anomalies are overlooked and
misdiagnosed, as will be seen in subsequent sections.

Table 1 Diagnosis of atrioseptal defects

	Cyanosis	ECG QRS axis deviation
Ostium secundum	—	Right
Ostium primum	··	Left
Single atrium	⊦	Left
Total anomalous pulmonary venous drainage	⊣·	Right

Acknowledgements

Figures 4, 5, 8 and 9 are reprinted by permission of C. M. Oakley, and M. J.
Raphael, *Cardiac Radiology* (Blackwell, to be published).

(3) COMPLICATED CASES OF ATRIAL SEPTAL DEFECTS
R. K. Walesby

Table 2 shows the number of solitary atrial septal defects surgically closed at
Hammersmith Hospital between 1967 and 1976. Cases of patency of the foramen ovale and complex disorders in which an atrial septal defect was associated (for example, tetralogy of Fallot, complete atrioventricular canal and
totally anomalous pulmonary venous connection) are excluded. The three
deaths among the secundum defects were due to brain damage and acute
mitral regurgitation in two, while the third had had reclosure of the defect.

Table 2 Surgically corrected atrial septal defects (ASD) 1967–76

Total ASDs	185		
Primum ASDs	12	5 males	2 deaths
		7 females	
Secundum ASDs	173	48 males	3 deaths
		125 females (ratio—1:2.6)	

Anomalies associated with the 173 cases of secundum defect are given in
Table 3. Age at time of operation is shown in Table 4. The distribution of
venous anomalies in 31 cases appears in Table 5.

377

**Table 3   Associated additional abnormalities
with 173 secundum ASDs**

12 pulmonary stenosis
6 mitral valve disease (non-rheumatic)
4 VSDs
2 VSDs and pulmonary stenosis
2 primum ASDs and secundum
2 tricuspid valve disease
1 patent ductus arteriosus
1 aortic valve disease

8 left superior vena cava
1 left inferior vena cava

VSD = ventricular septal defect

Table 4   Age distribution at closure of ASDs

0–9	10–19	20–29	30–39	40–49	50 +
50	44	22	22	18	17

**Table 5   Secundum ASDs with anomalous
venous connections**

Secundum ASD and PAPVD	9
Inferior caval ASDs and PAPVD	3
Sinus venosus defects and PAPVD	9
Common atrium	2
Left SVC	8

PAPVD = partially anomalous pulmonary
venous drainage; SVC = superior vena cava

Anomalies of the Atrial septum - SINUS VENOSUS DEFECT

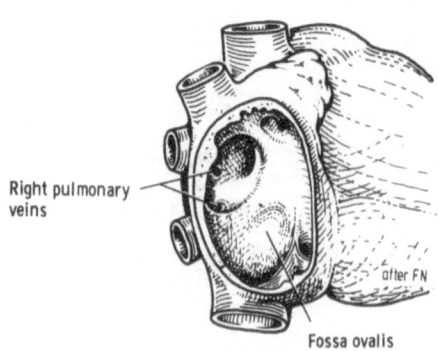

Right pulmonary veins

after FN

Fossa ovalis

Figure 10   Diagrammatic representation (redrawn from Netter, 1969) of a sinus venosus
type of atrial septal defect

In eight patients, one or more right pulmonary veins entered the right atrium directly. In five, the veins entered the chamber independently of the superior vena cava, and in three, the right upper lobe vein entered immediately below the superior cava, causing a bulge or dilatation in the atrial wall.

Figure 10 shows the typical anatomy of the sinus venosus type of defect. Anomalous connection of the right pulmonary veins occurred in four of our patients with sinus venosus defects. In two, the upper and lower veins entered the right atrium independently; in one, the upper lobe vein joined the superior vena cava at the cavoatrial junction; and in one, a common vein entered the superior cava at a distance from the atrium.

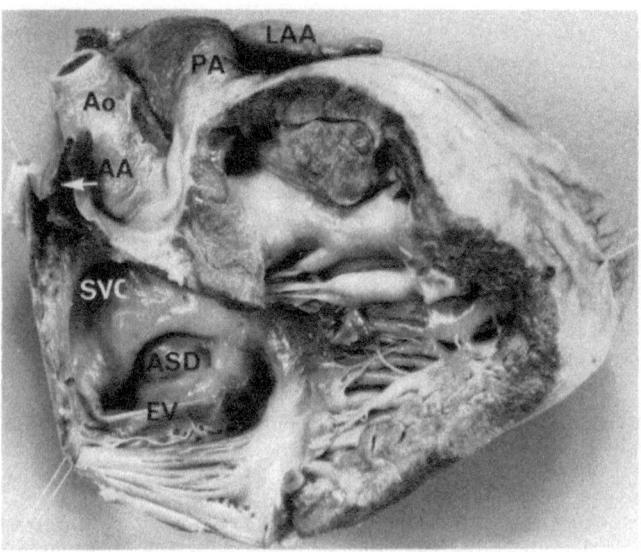

Figure 11 Photograph of the heart of a child with the tetralogy of Fallot (untreated), with an inferior vena cava type of atrial septal defect. Note that the Eustachian valve (EV) is very large, and directs most of the flow directly into the left atrium through the defect (ASD); RAA = right auricle, SVC = superior vena cava, Ao = aorta, PA = pulmonary artery, LAA = left auricle. (The compiler is indebted to Dr R. H. Anderson for allowing her to photograph this specimen)

Figure 11 shows an inferior atrial septal defect with the inferior cava straddling it. This defect was found at operation in five patients. In one of these the right lower lobe vein entered the atrium above the inferior vena cava, while in another the upper lobe vein entered below the superior vena cava, far distant from the defect. In the third case, a very large Eustachian valve acted as a baffle, directing the inferior caval blood through the defect into the left atrium. The fourth case had a hepatic vein confluent with the coronary sinus, while the fifth had a common right pulmonary vein entering the inferior vena cava (scimitar syndrome, see Figure 5a and b).

Figure 12 illustrates a common, or single, atrium encountered in three of our patients. In one of these, the common right pulmonary vein entered the right side of the chamber close to the superior vena cava while the two left veins entered on the left. In the second, the right lung was drained by a common vein entering the right side between the two cavae, while the left had a common vein opening into the left side rather anteriorly. The third case had a bizarre orientation of the atrium relative to the ventricles so that the pulmonary venous connections (two common veins as in the second case) entered the chamber anteriorly rather than posteriorly.

Anomalies of the Atrial septum - COMMON ATRIUM

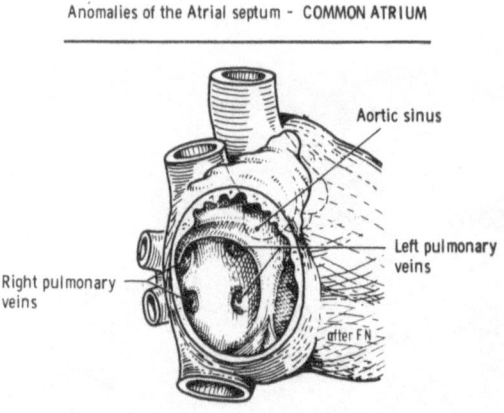

Figure 12 Diagram to show the anatomy of a common or single atrium. Note the relationship of the aortic valve (dotted lines) to the defect

Table 6 shows the diagnoses with which these patients came to operation, and Table 7 demonstrates that despite careful preoperative assessment of patients with apparently isolated secundum defects, a significant number of cases still come to operation with additional anomalies either undiagnosed or misdiagnosed. Atrial septal defects may still present a surgical challenge, even today.

Table 6   Preoperative diagnoses

Secundum ASD and PAPVD	
Correct	2
Not diagnosed	4
Misdiagnosed	3
Sinus venosus	
Correct	1
Uncommitted	4
Misdiagnosed as	
ASD and PAPVD	5

Abbreviations as Table 5

Table 7   Diagnosis of atrial septal defect

	Correct diagnosis	Not diagnosed	Misdiagnosed
1967		× ×	
1968			×
1969	×		
1970		× ×	×
1971		× × × ×	×
1972	× ×		
1973		× ×	
1974			
1975		×	×
1976		× × × ×	×
	3	15	5

(4) REROUTING OPERATIONS   *R. N. Sapsford*

The general principles of planning a rerouting operation for unexpectedly complicated atrial defects are much the same as for any other operation on bypass. Moderate hypothermia and aortic cross-clamping may be necessary, and a left ventricular vent may be desirable.

In particular, though, *all* the veins entering the heart should be carefully and accurately identified, both from without and within. Furthermore, the orifices of the coronary sinus and left atrial appendage (left auricle) must be identified, as must the Eustachian valve. The size and position of the defect must be assessed, as this operation is to reroute blood, rather than merely to close a defect. The specific details of this procedure are summarized in Table 8.

Table 8   Specific principles

1. Never close by direct suture
2. Ensure that the atrial septal defect is large enough. If not, enlarge it by excising the residual septum
3. Ensure that there is no shelf either anterior to, or posterior to, the abnormally situated vein orifices
4. Always patch (pericardium or two-way stretch Dacron)
5. Stay clear of pulmonary vein orifices
6. Use a voluminous patch

With respect to sinus venosus defects (Figure 10) it is desirable to explore the lesion digitally to determine the most suitable site for cannulating the superior vena cava for bypass. Either the vein itself or the right auricle may be suitable. Figure 13 illustrates diagrammatically what one is trying to achieve with this operation.

Concerning defects with partially anomalous pulmonary venous connection on the right side, digital exploration of the chamber will reveal:

(a) the size of the defect—(it may need enlargement);

(b) the existence of a right lateral margin to the defect;

(c) the relationship of the anomalous vein or veins to it.

Figure 13 shows the nature of the operation for this malformation.

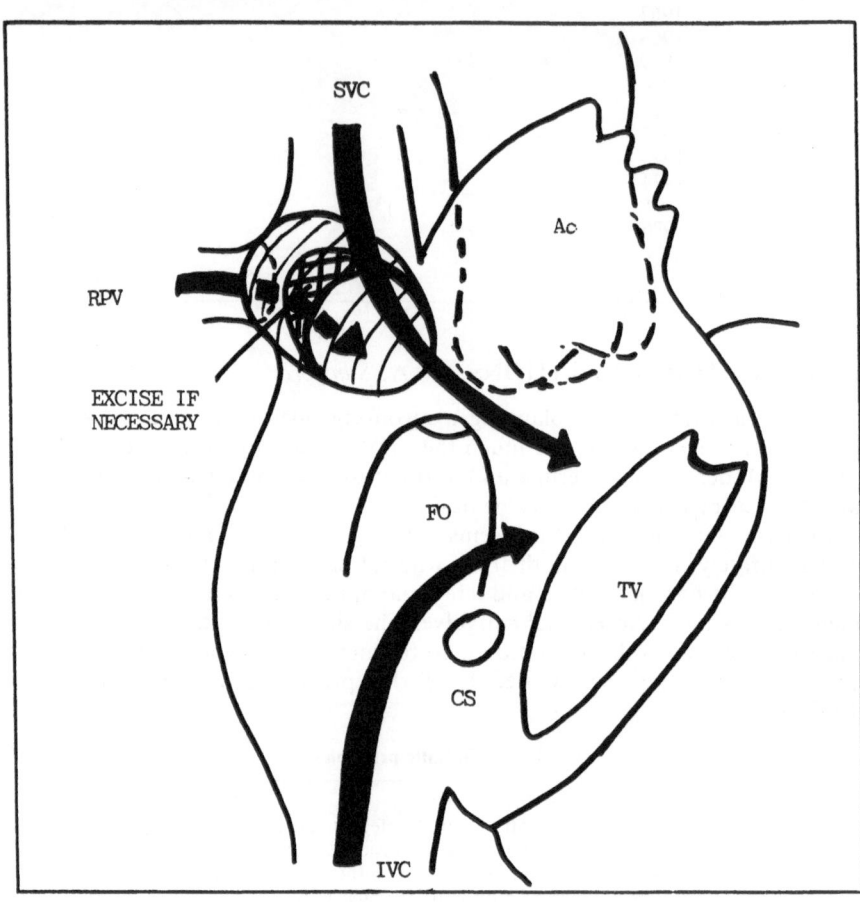

Figure 13 Diagrammatic representation of the technique to reconstruct the venous connections in (superior) sinus venosus atrial septal defect A = aorta, SVC = superior vena cava, RPV = right pulmonary vein, CS = coronary sinus, TV = tricuspid valve, IVC = inferior vena cava, FO = foramen ovale

The scimitar syndrome (Figures 5a and b) presents a particular set of circumstances to the surgeon. A right anterolateral thoracotomy is preferred to median sternotomy in this anomaly, so that the right pulmonary vein may more readily be exposed from the lung hilum to its confluence with the inferior vena cava above the diaphragm. This completed, divide the confluence between clamps, and close the resulting deficiency in the inferior vena cava. Next, establish cardiopulmonary bypass with hypothermia if necessary. If the cut end of the right pulmonary vein is long enough, it may be anastomosed to the right wall of the left atrium. If it is not, then it must be anastomosed to the right wall of the right atrium, just anterior to the septum. In either case, the atrial septal defect must of course be closed, and in the latter case, it may (probably will) need enlargement before patching both in a manner similar to that for right partial anomalous pulmonary venous connection (Figure 14).

Where the termination of the inferior vena cava is doubtful, or if it enters the left atrium either directly or when its flow is so determined by a large Eustachian valve, the following procedure should be utilized. First, the lower margin of the defect should be identified digitally; then if possible, separate the margins of the defect from the Eustachian valve. The snare on the inferior caval cannula must be placed as low as possible, the vein having been cannulated through the defect. The placing of the snare necessitates division of the posteroinferior pericardium and the peritoneal reflection around the inferior vena cava.

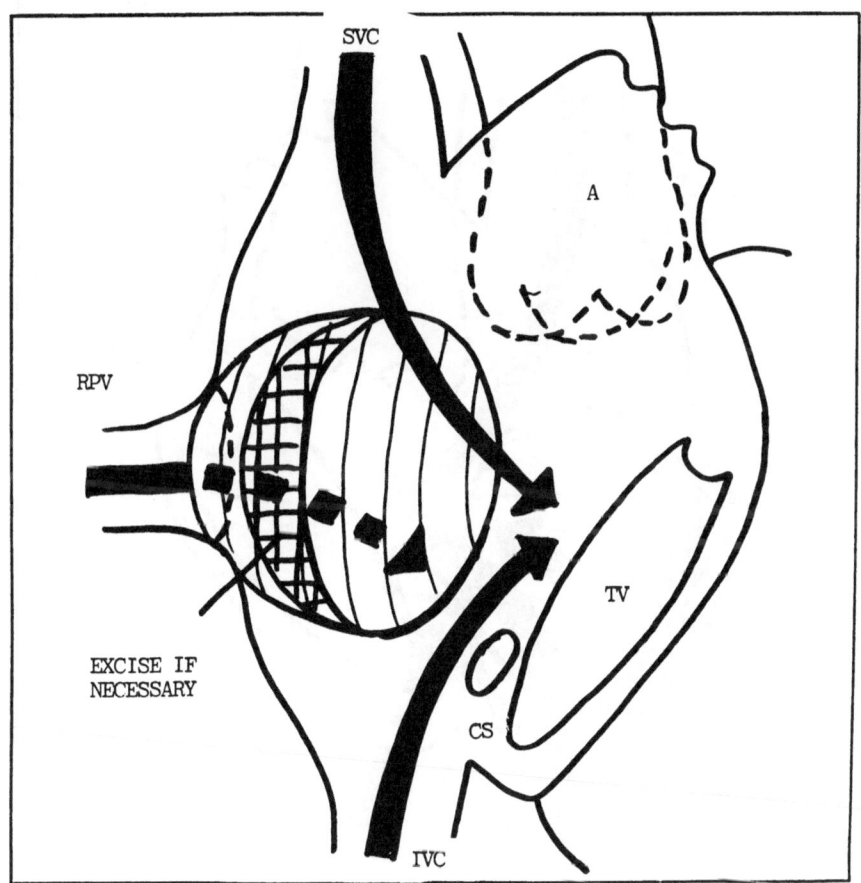

Figure 14 Diagrammatic view of the operation for right hemi-anomalous pulmonary venous connection. Abbreviations as in Figure 13

The presence of a left superior vena cava must always be determined, either from the preoperative investigation, or from the initial examination of the heart at the beginning of the operation. As we have seen, left superior cavae are not always known about in advance. When present, a left superior vena cava almost always enters the coronary sinus, which usually has a large orifice. Sometimes, but not often, the vein opens into the left atrium, and rarely it has a fenestration into the left atrium as it passes to the coronary sinus.

(5) JUXTAPOSITION OF THE AURICLES *S. P. Allwork*

Juxtaposition of the auricles is that rare condition in which they lie side by side either to the left or the right of the origins of the great arteries (Figure 15). The disorder was first described by Birmingham[3] in 1893 in a Dublin fishwife

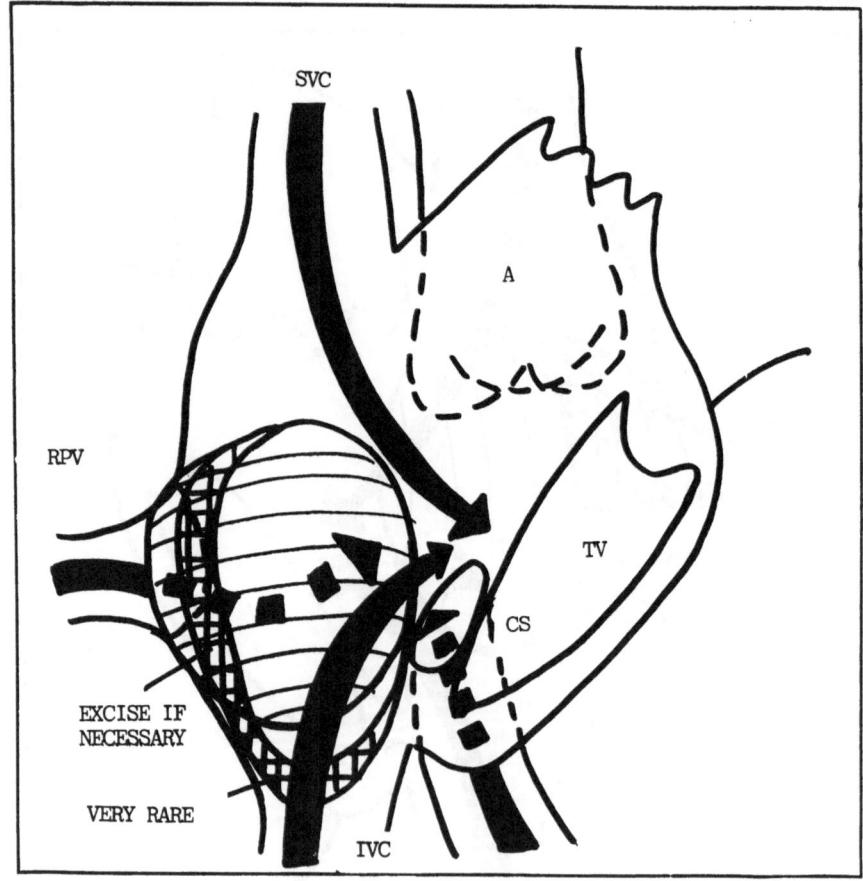

Figure 15 Diagram to show the operation to reroute venous flow in inferior vena cava atrial septal defect with an anomalous pulmonary vein (see text). Abbreviations as in Figure 13

with double outlet right ventricle, and since then quite a number of reports have appeared. Left juxtaposition is far more common than right, in a ratio of 14:1.

Although a wide range of ventriculoarterial anomalies are usually associated with juxtaposition of the auricles, we are concerned here with the atrial malformation. Figure 17 shows the typical anatomy of the atria, which is always abnormal, but relatively constant. The atrial septum, if present, is at right angles to that of the posterior ventricular septum. One can see very clearly what Mr Sapsford meant in section (4) of this chapter when he emphasized the need positively to identify both the topography of the defect and the os of the auricle. The right os looks like a large defect, but the inferior rim of the defect is identified by the shallow sill of septum primum. A large atrial septal defect is usually present, but in one case in our recent series[4] only a patency of the foramen ovale occurred. This opening, however, lay in the superior part of the septum, and this probably explains the difficulties reported[5] in entering the left atrium during catheterization of such patients.

The venous connections are normal in juxtaposition of the auricles, but a significant number of patients have a persistent left superior vena cava entering the coronary sinus (Figures 16 and 17).

The morphogenesis of the malformation is uncertain, but it is probably associated with failure of lateral expansion of the primitive atrioventricular

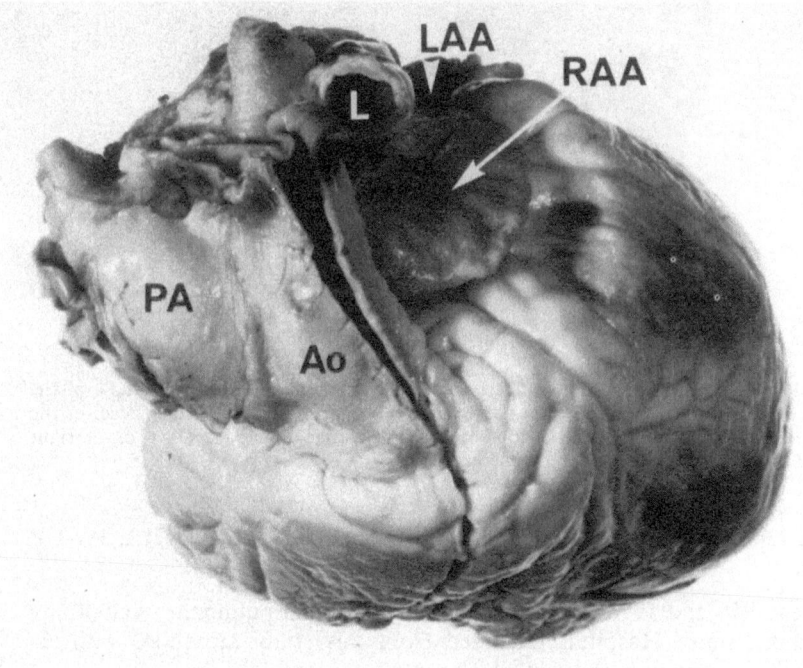

Figure 16 The heart in left juxtaposition of the auricles; LAA = left auricle, RAA = right auricle, PA = pulmonary artery

canal because hypoplasia of the contralateral side of the heart is commonly associated.

It has been said that juxtaposition of the auricles is readily diagnosed on the plain chest film, but in our series, even retrospectively, it was in fact unusual rather than usual to be able to predict this extreme atrial anomaly.

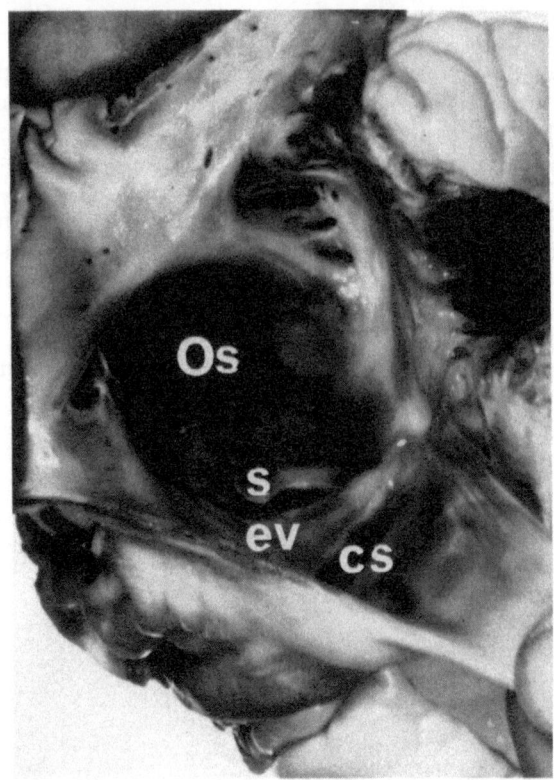

Figure 17 The right atrium of the heart illustrated in Figure 16. Note the plane of the remnant of the atrial septum (S) and the enlarged coronary sinus (CS) which receives the left superior vena cava. Note the numerous venae cordae minimae; Os = os of right auricle; ev = Eustachian valve

(6) PULMONARY VALVE STENOSIS—LONG-TERM FOLLOW-UP
U. Nair

Between 1958 and 1976, 54 patients underwent open pulmonary valvotomy at Hammersmith Hospital. Excluded from this study are those with infundibular obstruction, those in which ventricular septal defect was associated and those with transposition of the great arteries and pulmonary atresia. This follow-up therefore concerns only pure, valvular pulmonary stenosis.

The age and sex of the patients are given in Table 9. The age at which the diagnosis of pulmonary valve stenosis was made ranged from birth to 41 years but the mean age was 12 years. The interval between diagnosis and operation ranged from 1 to 35 years, with a mean of 10 years.

Table 9 Patients operated upon for pulmonary valve stenosis at Hammersmith Hospital from 1958 to 1976 (open pulmonary valvotomy on cardiopulmonary bypass)

Total number of patients studied:	54
Age	
Range	2–45 years
Mean	13 years
Sex	
Male	29
Female	25
Ratio: male:female	9:7

Patency of the foramen ovale was associated with pulmonary valve stenosis in 30 cases (55%) and one patient had a patent ductus arteriosus.

All but one of the patients underwent cardiac catheterization. Right ventricular pressure ranged from 62 to 207 mmHg, with a mean pressure of 117 mmHg, while the gradient across the pulmonary valve ranged from 40 to 180 mmHg with a mean gradient of 93 mmHg.

The range of pressures recorded in the operating room is expressed in Table 10.

Table 10   Pressures at the time of operation

Peak RV pressure before valvotomy:
Range: 60–300 mmHg
Mean: 119 mmHg

Peak RV pressure after valvotomy:
Range: 30–150 mmHg
Mean: 66 mmHg

Gradient across the pulmonary valve before valvotomy
Range: 25–275 mmHg
Mean: 91 mmHg

Gradient across the pulmonary valve after valvotomy
Range: 2–120 mmHg
Mean: 40 mmHg

RV = right ventricular

With respect to the morphology of the pulmonary valve, 45 (83%) of the patients had a tricuspid pulmonary valve, while it was bicuspid in only five cases (9%). Four patients (8%) had a diaphragm obstructing outflow from the infundibulum.

The size of the valves before operation was not always available, but in those with this datum the mean increase in valve diameter achieved by open pulmonary valvotomy was 11 mm. One patient suffered a femoral artery thrombosis following decannulation of the femoral artery.

Two patients died in the early postoperative period; both, regrettably, from overtransfusion. None of our own patients has come to reoperation, but a second valvotomy was performed at Hammersmith Hospital on a boy of 14 who had had his first operation in infancy. Details of his case history have been described in detail elsewhere[6].

During the follow-up period (longest–19 years) two patients have had episodes of gross right heart failure. Both of these were cyanosed before operation and had marked effort intolerance.

Six of our 52 surviving patients have been lost to follow-up, but most of those still attending have gained considerable relief of symptoms – 96% are asymptomatic compared with only 6% before operation; none is now cyanosed (20% before valvotomy); none has growth retardation (19% before); and none has chest pain, whereas 13% complained of chest pain before operation. Of the operated patients 4% still complain of exertional dyspnoea, compared with 89% with this symptom before operation.

References

1. Wood P. (1968). *Diseases of the Heart and Circulation.* (London: Eyre and Spottiswoode)
2. DuShane, J. W., Weidman, W. H., Brandenberg, R. O. and Kirklin, J. W. (1960). Differentiation of intra-atrial communications by clinical methods: ostium secundum, ostium primum, common atrium and total anomalous venous connection. *Circulation,* **21,** 363
3. Birmingham, A. (1893). Extreme anomaly of the heart and great vessels. *J. Anat. Physiol.,* **27,** 139
4. Allwork, S. P., Urban, A. E. and Anderson, R. H. (1977). Left juxtaposition of the auricles with 1-position of the aorta. Report of 6 cases. *Br. Heart J.,* **39,** 299
5. Ellis, K. and Jameson, A. G. (1963). Congenital levoposition of the right atrial appendage. *Am. J. Roentgenol.,* **89,** 984
6. Samarrai, A. A. R., McCloy, R. and Ablett, M. B. (1976). Biloculate false aneurysm of the right ventricle after cardiac surgery. *Br. Heart J.,* **38,** 297

Index